REAL-WORLD NURSING SURVIVAL GUIDE:
COMPLEMENTARY
& ALTERNATIVE THERAPIES

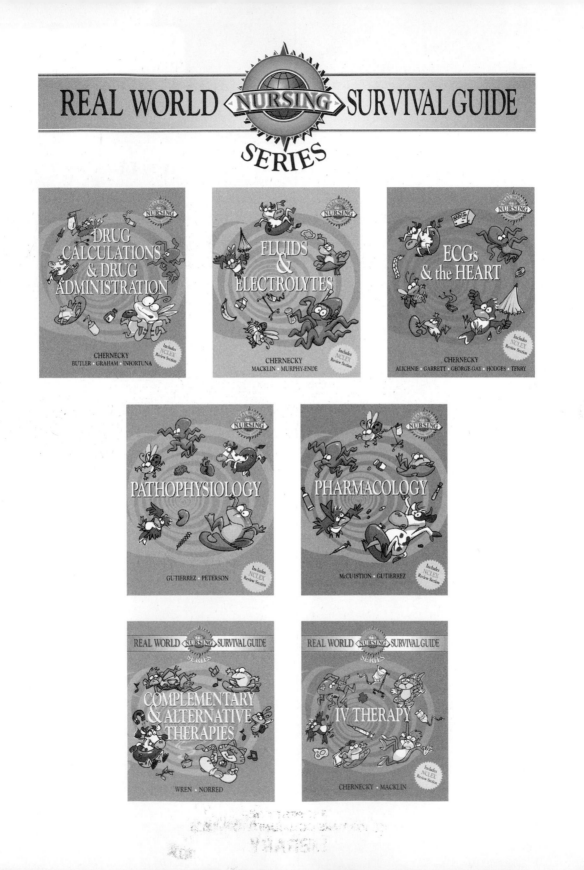

REAL-WORLD NURSING SURVIVAL GUIDE:

COMPLEMENTARY & ALTERNATIVE THERAPIES

KATHLEEN R. WREN, CRNA, PHD
Program Director, Nurse Anesthesia Program
School of Nursing
Louisiana State University Health Sciences Center
New Orleans, Louisiana

CAROL L. NORRED, CRNA, MHS
Clinical Instructor and Researcher, Department of Anesthesiology
University of Colorado Health Sciences Center
Denver, Colorado
Adjunct Clinical Professor, Nurse Anesthesia Program
College of Health Sciences, Old Dominion University
Norfolk, Virginia

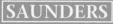

SAUNDERS
An Imprint of Elsevier Science

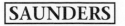

An Imprint of Elsevier Science

The Curtis Center
Independence Square West
Philadelphia, Pennsylvania 19106-3399

REAL-WORLD NURSING SURVIVAL GUIDE:
COMPLEMENTARY & ALTERNATIVE THERAPIES   ISBN 0-7216-0022-0

DEDICATION

This book is for the two most important men in my life. Dad (M. Robert Hicks), I still think of you every day and miss you a bit more. Tim, with you at my side, I have all I need.

Kathy Wren

This book is dedicated in eternal love for Caitlin, Stephen, and Sterling.

Carol Norred

NOTICE

Nursing is an ever-changing field. Standard safety precautions must be followed, but as new research and clinical experience broaden our knowledge, changes in treatment and drug therapy may become necessary or appropriate. Readers are advised to check the most current product information provided by the manufacturer of each drug to be administered to verify the recommended dose, the method and duration of administration, and contraindications. It is the responsibility of the licensed health care provider, relying on the experience and knowledge of the patient, to determine dosages and the best treatment for each individual patient. Neither the publisher nor the editor assumes any liability for any injury and/or damage to persons or property arising from this publication.

International Standard Book Number 0-7216-0022-0

Vice President and Publishing Director, Nursing: Sally Schrefer
Acquisitions Editor: Robin Carter
Developmental Editor: Kristin Geen
Project Manager: Catherine Jackson
Designer: Amy Buxton
Cover Designer and Illustrator: Chris Sharp, Ted Bolte, GraphCom Corporation

Printed in the United States of America

Last digit is the print number: 9 8 7 6 5 4 3 2 1

About the Authors

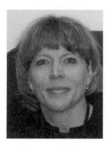

Kathleen R. Wren, CRNA, PhD, is a Certified Registered Nurse Anesthetist with degrees from Union College (BS in nursing), Rush University (MS in nursing), and University of Nebraska (PhD). Kathy has clinically practiced in several hospitals across the middle plains and as a partner in an anesthesia service business. She began a career in academic nursing at the Medical College of Georgia before moving to Louisiana State University Health Sciences Center where she is the program director of the Nurse Anesthesia Program. In addition to her administrative responsibilities, Kathy also maintains an active clinical practice at Charity Hospital in New Orleans. She is a speaker, researcher, and published author in the field of nurse anesthesia. She is also active in the Seventh-day Adventist Church and enjoys life with her husband of 21 years and 2 teenaged children.

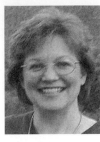

Carol L. Norred, CRNA, MHS,* is a Certified Registered Nurse Anesthetist with a Master's degree in Health Science from Texas Wesleyan University, Graduate School of Nurse Anesthesia. Currently, her institutional predoctoral training is provided through a National Research Service Award funded by the National Center for Complementary and Alternative Medicine and the National Heart Lung and Blood Institute (HL T32 07085). Carol is a clinical instructor in the Department of Anesthesiology and a doctoral student in the School of Nursing at the University of Colorado Health Science Center, Denver, Colorado. Carol has extensively studied the use of complementary and alternative medicines by patients who have undergone surgery, funded by grants from Sigma Theta Tau and the American Peri-Operative Registered Nurses Foundation. She is an internationally and nationally recognized speaker, researcher, and published scholar in the area of complementary and alternative medicine. Her research has also been reported on television's *PBS Healthweek*, and *ABC 20/20*, as well as local and national newspapers including the *Rocky Mountain News*, *New York Times*, and *The Washington Post*.

Carol's web site, "Healing Emergence: Alternative Medicine in Anesthesiology," can be found at http://www.carolnorred.mybravenet.com.

*Sources of support: The manuscripts for accupressure, aromatherapy, echinacea, ephedra, garlic, magnets, and St. John's wort were written by Ms. Norred. Ms. Norred collaborated in writing manuscripts for prayer and therapeutic touch. These manuscripts were developed with support from a grant award HLT3207085 at the University of Colorado Health Sciences Center, funded by the National Center for Complementary and Alternative Medicine and the National Heart, Lung and Blood Institute, National Institutes of Health.

Contributors

Chuck Biddle, CRNA, PhD
Professor of Nurse Anesthesia and Clinical Staff Anesthetist
Medical College of Virginia
Virginia Commonwealth University
Richmond, Virginia

Cheryl Bourguignon, PhD, RN*
Postdoctoral Fellow, CAM Research Training Program
Center for the Study of Complementary and Alternative
   Therapies
University of Virginia
Charlottesville, Virginia

Rosa Bustamante-Forest, RN, MPH, MN
Assistant Professor of Clinical Nursing
School of Nursing
Louisiana State University Health Sciences Center
New Orleans, Louisiana

Karen D'Huyvetter, MS, ND†
Postdoctoral Fellow, CAM Research Training Program
Center for the Study of Complementary and Alternative
   Therapies
University of Virginia
Charlottesville, Virginia

Audrey Elizabeth Emmett
Feng Shui Consultant and Founder
Life Harmony Dynamics
New Orleans, Louisiana

Ursula Frieman, BSN
Homeopathic Consultant
University of Colorado Hospital, Pain Practice Medicine
   Clinic
Denver, Colorado

Daniel I. Galper, PhD‡§
Postdoctoral Fellow, CAM Research Training Program
Center for the Study of Complementary and Alternative
   Therapies
University of Virginia
Charlottesville, Virginia

Deborah Delaney Garbee, APRN, MN, CNS, CNOR
Instructor of Clinical Nursing
School of Nursing
Louisiana State University Health Sciences Center
New Orleans, Louisiana

Mike Jacobs, MSN, RN, CEN, CCRN
Clinical Assistant Professor
College of Nursing
University of South Alabama
Mobile, Alabama

Elizabeth J. Monti, MSN, CRNA
Assistant Professor
Medical College of Georgia
Augusta, Georgia

*Sources of support: The manuscript for chondroitin and glucosamine was developed with support from grant award T32-AT-00052 CAM Research Training Program funded by the National Center for Complementary and Alternative Medicine, National Institutes of Health.

†Sources of support: The manuscript for fish oil and vitamin C was developed with support from grant award T32-AT-00052 CAM Research Training Program funded by the National Center for Complementary and Alternative Medicine, National Institutes of Health.

‡Sources of support: The manuscript for relaxation therapy was developed with support from grant award T32-AT-00052 CAM Research Training Program and K30-AT-00060 CAM Clinical Research Curriculum Program funded by the National Center for Complementary and Alternative Medicine, National Institutes of Health.

§Sources of support: The manuscript for hypnosis was developed with support from grant award T32-AT-00052 CAM Research Training Program funded by the National Center for Complementary and Alternative Medicine, National Institutes of Health.

Susan Orlando, RNC, MS, NNP
Doctoral Student
School of Nursing
Louisiana State University Health Sciences Center
New Orleans, Louisiana

Christine A. Pollock, RN, PhD
Associate Professor of Clinical Nursing
School of Nursing
Louisiana State University Health Sciences Center
New Orleans, Louisiana

Shannon M. Powell, MN, CRNA
Instructor
Medical College of Georgia
Augusta, Georgia

Francelyn M. Reeder, RN, CNM, PhD
Associate Professor
School of Nursing
University of Colorado Health Sciences Center
Denver, Colorado

Elizabeth B. Schomaker, CRNA
Brennan Healing Science Practitioner and Nurse
    Anesthetist
Shriner's Burn Institute
Cincinnati, Ohio

Annita Stansbury, RN, MSN, CNS
Adjunct Faculty, Nursing Program
Front Range Community College
Fort Collins, Colorado

Ann Gill Taylor, MS, EdD, RN, FAAN[*†‡§||]
Betty Norman Norris Professor of Nursing
Director, Center for the Study of Complementary
    and Alternative Therapies
University of Virginia
Charlottesville, Virginia

Jean Watson RN, PhD, HNC, FAAN
Distinguished Professor of Nursing
Endowed Chair in Caring Science
University of Colorado Health Sciences Center
Denver, Colorado

Allison E. Williams, RN, ND, MEd, CMT, BCIAC
Doctoral Student
University of Colorado Health Sciences Center
Denver, Colorado

Timothy Wren RN, MS
Assistant Professor, Adult Nursing
School of Nursing
Louisiana State University Health Sciences Center
New Orleans, Louisiana

*Sources of support: The manuscript for chondroitin and glucosamine was developed with support from grant award T32-AT-00052 CAM Research Training Program funded by the National Center for Complementary and Alternative Medicine, National Institutes of Health.

†Sources of support: The manuscript for fish oil and vitamin C was developed with support from grant award T32-AT-00052 CAM Research Training Program funded by the National Center for Complementary and Alternative Medicine, National Institutes of Health.

‡Sources of support: The manuscript for relaxation therapy was developed with support from grant award T32-AT-00052 CAM Research Training Program and K30-AT-00060 CAM Clinical Research Curriculum Program funded by the National Center for Complementary and Alternative Medicine, National Institutes of Health.

§Sources of support: The manuscript for hypnosis was developed with support from grant award T32-AT-00052 CAM Research Training Program funded by the National Center for Complementary and Alternative Medicine, National Institutes of Health.

||Sources of support: The manuscript for reflexology was developed with support from grant award K30-AT-00060 CAM Clinical Research Curriculum Program funded by the National Center for Complementary and Alternative Medicine, National Institutes of Health.

Faculty & Practitioner Reviewers

Alan P. Agins, PhD
Adjunct Associate Professor
Brown University Medical School
Providence, Rhode Island

Linda Hein, MSN, RN, CNS, HNC, CHTP, CST, RM
Owner, Healing Connections
Vancouver, Washington

Stephen P. Kilkus, RN, MSN
Associate Professor
College of Nursing and Health Sciences
Winona State University
Winona, Minnesota

Jane A. Madden, MSN, RN
Assistant Professor
Deaconess College of Nursing
St. Louis, Missouri

Student Reviewers

FEATURED STUDENT REVIEWER

Jeffrey M. Waddell is a nontraditional student in the BSN program at Pittsburg State University in southeast Kansas. He will graduate in May 2003 and plans to earn his master's degree and become a nurse practitioner with an emphasis in rheumatology while working either in a critical care setting or in an emergency department. He eventually plans to obtain a PhD and teach in nursing. In 1995 he started as an emergency medical technician and eventually became a nationally registered and certified medical assistant, working several years for a rheumatology practice in the Kansas City area. While in nursing school, he worked as a phlebotomist and as an emergency room technician at Olathe Medical Center in Olathe, Kansas. In addition, he served as vice president of his nursing class and president of the state executive board for the Kansas Association of Nursing Students. In April 2002 he was elected to the board of directors of the National Student Nurses' Association (NSNA) and was appointed chair of the Membership Committee in addition to serving on the "Breakthrough to Nursing" and "Image of Nursing" committees. Jeff makes his home in Pleasanton, Kansas, with his wife Maggie and stepdaughter Kyla and looks forward to remaining active in nursing leadership and politics.

STUDENTS

Shelly Bryant
Valencia Community College
Orlando, Florida

Janice J. Carter
Saint Louis University School
of Nursing
St. Louis, Missouri

Brandi E. Dingler
Medical College of Georgia
Athens, Georgia

Marni Dodd
Medical College of Georgia
Athens, Georgia

Debbie Eidam
Valencia Community College
Orlando, Florida

Jessica J. Fay
Saint Louis University School
of Nursing
St. Louis, Missouri

Cindy Green, RN, CCE
Georgia League for Nursing
Columbus, Georgia

Lora L. Gregory
Valencia Community College
Orlando, Florida

Sarah Hacker
Saint Louis University School of
    Nursing
St. Louis, Missouri

Bridget Hamed, RN
Oakland Community College
Waterford, Michigan

Tricia B. Harrison
Beth-El College of Nursing and Health
    Sciences
University of Colorado
Colorado Springs, Colorado

Elizabeth Hunnicutt
Macon State College
Macon, Georgia

Amy M. Johnson
Beth-El College of Nursing and Health
    Sciences
University of Colorado
Colorado Springs, Colorado

Kelly Knox
Medical College of Georgia
Athens, Georgia

James C. Reedy
Saint Louis University School of
    Nursing
St. Louis, Missouri

Constance Riopelle
Oakland Community College
Waterford, Michigan

Raelynn Schäfer, BS
Valencia Community College
Orlando, Florida

Kelly Swift
University of Iowa
Iowa City, Iowa

Sara Wyldwood
Saint Louis University School of
    Nursing
St. Louis, Missouri

Preface

Alternatives to conventional medicine and therapies have taken our country by storm. More and more frequently, nurses and other health care providers are encountering patients who are taking complementary medicines and using alternative therapies as they seek to improve their health status. As such, nurses need to be aware of the advantages and disadvantages of the uses of these medications and therapies by their patients. This text will help you understand complementary and alternative medications (CAMs) and complementary and alternative therapies (CATs). It will also help you integrate both into your traditional nursing course content.

Complementary & Alternative Therapies is the sixth book in the *Real World Nursing Survival Guide Series*, which has been created in response to input from nursing students. Focus groups held at the National Student Nurses' Association convention identified helpful methods to achieve mastery of new information. Their responses were used to design the basic structure and approach behind the *Real World Nursing Survival Guide Series*. In addition, throughout the development of this book, nursing students and faculty evaluated and critiqued its content.

The book is divided into four parts. **Part I: Pharmacologic Therapies** presents 30 of the most commonly used CAMs. The CAMs are further divided into separate sections for "Herbs" and "Vitamins and Dietary Supplements." For each CAM, consistent headings emphasize specific nursing actions. "What It IS" provides a general description of the CAM. "What You NEED TO KNOW" discusses actions, doses, side effects, indications and uses, and contraindications and precautions. "What You DO" is designed specifically for you, the nurse, and highlights what you should do for the patient under your care. This section highlights important information about patient history, potential drug interactions, and patient education. The "Do You UNDERSTAND" heading refers you to related learning activities in Part III that will help reinforce your knowledge.

As you learn about CAMs, it is important to remember a couple of important points. First, CAMs are only loosely regulated by the Food and Drug Administration (FDA) because of their status as diet supplements. The result is that many CAM preparations do not contain what they say they do. In fact, some preparations may not contain *anything* they say they do; rather, filler ingredients or—at times—even harmful substances may be found. Finally, the amount of active ingredients can vary significantly between capsules in the same bottle. Thus nurses cannot over emphasize the importance of purchasing CAMs from reliable and reputable manufacturers. Second, a variety of dosages and preparations are listed because patients may use CAMs in a variety of ways.

One last comment concerning the CAMs section: The list of uses and indications in this text indicates the conditions for which patients commonly take a particular herbal medicine. This list of indications and conditions are *not* necessarily supported by empirical research. By understanding *why* a patient is taking a CAM, you may be able to better determine his or her health care concerns and needs.

Part Two: Nonpharmacologic Therapies presents 25 of the most commonly implemented CATs. The CATs are further divided into separate sections: "Healing with Physical Power," "Healing with the Mind," and "Healing with Subtle Energy." In each CAT monograph, the "What It IS" section introduces and describes the CAT. "What You NEED TO KNOW" discusses benefits, uses, risks, and precautions. The "What You DO" discussion presents important patient education points and describes the training needed by practitioners of the individual therapy. The "Do You UNDERSTAND" heading refers you to learning activities in Part III.

In Parts I and II, we include many features to help you focus on the most important information needed to succeed in the classroom and in the clinical setting. **Take Home Points** are "pearls of wisdom" designed to assist you in caring for patients. These are drawn from our years of combined academic and clinical experience. The **Key Words** icon indicates where key words or concepts are defined. Content marked with a **Caution** icon is vital and usually involves nursing actions that may have life-threatening consequences or significantly affect patient outcomes. The **Lifespan** icon and the **Culture** icon highlight variations in treatment that may be necessary for specific age or ethnic groups. A **Web Links** icon will direct you to sites on the Internet that specifically help you focus on real-world patient care, the nursing process, and positive patient outcomes.

Part III: Learning Activities contains a variety of questions and exercises that emphasize and reinforce key points and concepts related to each CAM and CAT. Answers are provided for you to test your knowledge. We hope that you will find this section fun *and* educational.

Last, **Part IV: Helpful Cross-References** includes a series of charts and indexes that summarize the important side effects and actions of CAMs and CATs. These resources may be used as a quick reference to refresh your memory of important points of CAMs and CATs and to help integrate these medications and therapies into your nursing education.

We have used our own real-world clinical experiences and the expert experiences of clinicians, current nursing students, and nursing faculty to bring you a text that will help you understand CAMs and CATs and therefore enable you to implement better patient care.

Kathleen R. Wren, CRNA, PhD
Carol L. Norred, CRNA, MHS

Acknowledgments

I would like to thank my co-editor, Carol Norred, who showed me the fascinating field of complementary and alternative medicine. Many thanks to Kristin Geen of Elsevier Science who kept us going and on time—even when we didn't want to be. Cinda, thank you for punting this opportunity our way and for being the magnificent scholar and friend you are! Last, many thanks to my husband and nursing colleagues who wrote chapters, assisted with editing, and were always encouraging. Matt and Leah—the book is done!!!! Let's hit the beach!

Kathy Wren

I would like to thank my co-editor Kathy Wren, CRNA, PhD, for her enduring support of my journey through my doctoral education; for her endearing faith, love, prayer and friendship; and for her joint endeavor in this enterprise. I would also like to thank my husband, Steve, for his guidance, vision, divine love, and protection. I have much gratitude to Kristin Geen of Elsevier Science for supporting our book. I would also like to thank Neil West, PhD, and Nancy Pearson, PhD, of NIH-NCCAM for their support of my doctoral education. My institutional predoctoral training is provided through a National Research Service Award funded by the National Center for Complementary and Alternative Medicine and the National Heart Lung and Blood Institute (HL T32 07085). I am deeply grateful to Thomas Henthorn, MD, and Marvin Schwarz, MD, at the University of Colorado Health Science Center, Denver, Colorado, for facilitating my institutional predoctoral training grant.

Carol Norred

Contents

PART I

Pharmacologic Therapies

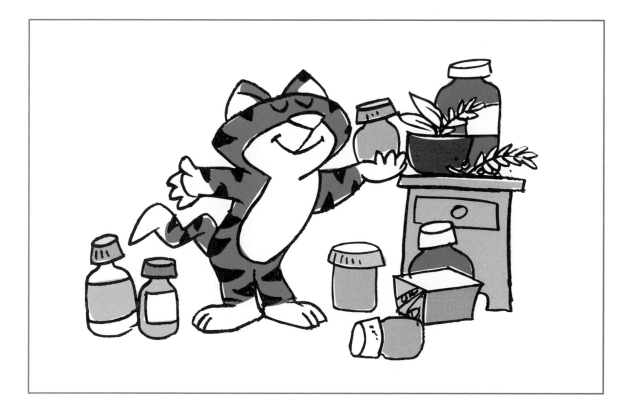

Herbs

ALFALFA

What IS Alfalfa?

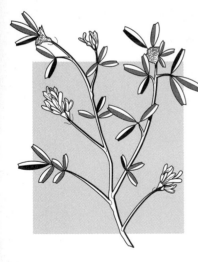

Alfalfa (*Medigo sativa*) is a dark-green plant with blue flowers that grows from spring to fall. Alfalfa's name is derived from the Arabic, *al fal fa*, which means "father of all foods." Other names for alfalfa include Chilean clover, buffalo grass, buffalo herb, Lucerne, and purple medic. Except for the seeds, the entire plant (including roots and blossoms) is used medicinally for human and livestock consumption. Alfalfa is a good source of protein, calcium, magnesium, iron, phosphorous, and potassium. Alfalfa leaves contain eight essential amino acids and high amounts of vitamins A, B_{12}, C, D, E, and K. Beta carotene and chlorophyll are also present in large amounts. Chlorophyll has a similar structure to hemoglobin and will increase the hematocrit. Alfalfa seeds should not be taken because they are toxic and associated with systemic lupus erythematosus (SLE) and **pancytopenia.** The active ingredients in alfalfa are **saponins, coumarins, isoflavonoids,** steroids, and **alkaloids.**

What You NEED TO KNOW

Actions

Alfalfa leaf is rich in vitamins, minerals, and protein. Alfalfa is a natural diuretic, high in fiber, and helpful in reducing serum-cholesterol levels.

Alfalfa possesses antibacterial and antifungal properties. Alfalfa roots contain a small amount of coumarins but is not thought to affect blood clotting because the plant also has large amounts of vitamin K. Root parts have hemolytic properties from decreasing prothrombin factor activity, which may interfere with vitamin E use in the body. However, only the leaf is usually taken. Alfalfa has some small estrogen-like actions. Alfalfa's high-manganese content may help in keeping the blood glucose stable.

Dose

- Dried herb: 5 to 10 gm three times daily
- Oral: two tablets with meals three times daily
- Topical: 4 to 5 oz of juice from pureed alfalfa sprouts to site of infection
- Fluid extract: 1:1 preparation, 5 to 10 ml

Side Effects

Side effects are rare. Preparations containing alfalfa roots may mildly decrease blood clotting. The seeds should not be taken because they may be toxic. Allergic reactions and contact dermatitis have been reported.

Indications and Uses

- Atherosclerosis prevention
- Asthma
- Bladder stones
- Cystitis
- Cerebrovascular accident (CVA) secondary to plaque
- Diabetes
- Diuresis
- Fever reduction
- Fungal infection
- Gram-negative bacteria infection
- Hay fever
- Heart disease
- Hypercholesterolemia
- Kidney stones
- Night blindness
- Nutritional supplementation and protein supplementation
- Tuberculosis infection
- Vitamin K disorders caused by:
  - Diarrhea
  - Lack of dietary Vitamin K
  - Liver insufficiency
  - Over-ingestion of warfarin (Coumadin)
  - Pancreatic insufficiency
  - Vitamin-K deficiency resulting from antibiotic intake
  - Water retention

Contraindications and Precautions

Alfalfa leaves are high in vitamin-K content. Patients taking warfarin should not take alfalfa or other foods with large amounts of vitamin K. Vitamin K works against warfarin (Coumadin), making it less effective.

Decreasing the action of warfarin may promote normal coagulation in patients for whom this may be dangerous (carotid disease, atrial fibrillation heart rhythm). Suddenly stopping alfalfa in patients taking warfarin may result in large increases in clotting times, bleeding, and bruising. The prothrombin time (PT) should be followed closely and the dose changed as needed.

Alfalfa medicine containing alfalfa root should not be taken with warfarin. The anticoagulant effects of alfalfa leaves and the blood-thinning effects of alfalfa root make it difficult to predict what will happen when the patient also takes warfarin. The anticoagulation effects of aspirin, non-steroidal antiinflammatory drugs (NSAIDs), and other anticoagulant medications will be difficult to predict when alfalfa root is also taken.

Alfalfa may increase the metabolism of xenobiotics, which will reduce their effectiveness.

Alfalfa seeds can cause SLE in susceptible patients. Alfalfa seeds can reverse remission, causing acute SLE to occur in patients. Alfalfa has estrogen-like actions. Patients with certain disease states who should avoid estrogen, such as those with some types of breast or uterine cancer, should avoid alfalfa use. Last, alfalfa is contraindicated in pregnancy.

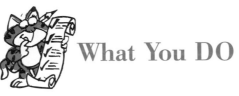

What You DO

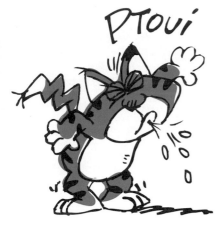

1. Do not take alfalfa with warfarin (Coumadin).
2. Do not take alfalfa with hormone replacement therapy or birth control pills.
3. Hypercoagulable states should be avoided in patients with any of the following: a history of deep vein thrombosis or emboli, peripheral vascular disease, diabetes, mechanical heart valves, and cardiac valve disease.
4. Increased coagulation may lead to increased loss of artificial venous–access devices and renal dialysis–access devices.
5. Alfalfa seeds are toxic.

Patient History

Patients should be questioned about their prescription, over-the-counter, and complementary and alternative medications. Patients' medications should be reviewed for possible interactions. Patients should be asked about autoimmune diseases. If the patient has SLE, the patient should be told to avoid alfalfa.

Potential Drug Interactions

The anticoagulant effects of other herbal medications and blood-thinning medications may be altered. Individuals who are taking warfarin should not take alfalfa because anticoagulation may be inhibited.

Tetracycline absorption can be decreased by foods high in iron, calcium, and magnesium. Thus taking tetracycline antibiotics with alfalfa may decrease tetracycline absorption and effectiveness.

Patient Education

Patients should know about the effects, benefits, and risks of alfalfa. Patients with clotting disorders should be told to avoid alfalfa preparations. Patients should not take alfalfa if they are also taking **xenobiotics**. Patients should stop taking alfalfa 2 weeks before invasive procedures and hospitalizations. The high vitamin-K content can cause the patient to be **hypercoagulable**. Thus alfalfa should be avoided in patients for whom a normal or increase state of coagulability is not wanted. Alfalfa should not be taken by pregnant or nursing mothers.

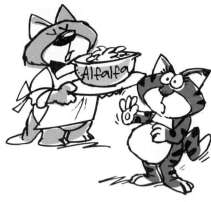

Do You UNDERSTAND?

See pages 218 and 219 for Learning Activities related to this topic.

Key Words

Alkaloids Phytochemicals with potent pharmacologic effects reacting as bases that are alkaline in pH and often have metabolites containing nitrogen. Alkaloids may depress the central nervous system, affect the autonomic system, or have other potent actions. Many plant alkaloids have the ability to cross the blood-brain barrier and interact with neurotransmitters. Plant alkaloids may provide immune stimulation against pathogens.

Contact dermatitis Skin reaction caused by touching an allergy-producing substance.

Coumarins Plant chemicals that may exhibit anticoagulant properties, as well as anticancer, immunostimulant, antifungal, antiinflammatory, vasodilatory, muscle relaxant, hypnotic, central nervous system–stimulant, hypothermal, diuretic, anticholinergic, antiedema, or estrogenic effects.

Hemolytic Causing the blood cells to rupture.

Hypercoagulable Being prone to form clots.

Isoflavonoids Plant constituents that affect estrogen receptors; these substances are often found in soy products. Some isoflavonoids may also have anticarcinogenic or immunostimulatory effects.

Pancytopenia Decrease in all the blood cells, including white blood cells, red blood cells, and platelets.

Older adults often have an increased incidence of vessel plaque development coupled with sedentary lifestyles. Therefore older adults should avoid using alfalfa and the potential hypercoagulable state.

www.holisticonline.com/
Herbal-Med/_Herbs/
h1.htm
www.agric.gov.ab.ca/crops/
special/medconf/ibrahimb.html

Saponins Phytochemical plant constituents that produce foam when dissolved in water. Saponins also reduce surface tension and increase solubility and cell membrane permeability. Saponins may be sugar glycosides or steroidal in composition.

Xenobiotics Ingested or inhaled substances that have biologic effects altering drug metabolism.

ALOE VERA

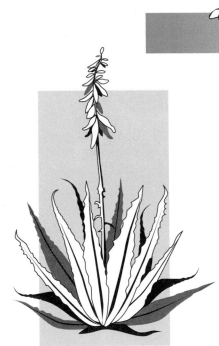

What IS Aloe Vera?

Aloe vera (*Aloe barbadensis*, *Aloe africana*) is a succulent plant from the lily family. The aloe used for medicinal purposes is grown in Africa and the West Indies. Two parts of the aloe vera plant are used: the dried juice from the leaf and the aloe gel. Aloe juice from the leaf comes from cells located just under the leaf's skin. The juice contained within flows out when the leaves are cut. Aloe is also known as latex, burn plant, elephant's gall, lily of the desert, miracle plant, and plant of immortality. Aloe juice is a strong cathartic used to cleanse the intestinal tract. The aloe juice causes the contact dermatologic symptoms. Aloe gel, also known as aloe leaf gel, aloe capensis, and salvia, is harvested from the center of the leaf and is used to promote wound healing. Manufacturing processes greatly alter the amount of active ingredients present in aloe preparations. Heat processing and overexposure of aloe to air (longer than 4 hours) reduces the amount of active ingredients and decreases its effectiveness. *Aloe barbadensis* and *Aloe africana* are considered the best quality of the many aloe vera species.

What You NEED TO KNOW

Actions

Aloe juice contains **phytochemicals** that are changed into **anthrones** in the colon. Anthrones are irritating to intestinal mucosa and increase peristalsis and intestinal fluid secretion in to the bowel. Increased peristalsis causes intestinal contents to move through the gastrointestinal (GI) tract more rapidly. In addition to increased fluid secretions, electrolytes are secreted into the bowel, and fluid reabsorption is inhibited. Thus larger volumes of intestinal contents are moved through the GI tract in less time.

Aloe gel inhibits bradykinin and histamine. Aloe also contains salicylates that decrease pain and inflammation. Aloe gel slows the formation of thromboxane A. Thromboxane A inhibits wound healing. Aloe gel also possesses antibacterial and antifungal actions. Last, aloe stimulates skin cell growth and the production of T cells by the immune system, which helps in wound healing.

Dose

Aloe juice:
- 100 to 200 mg in the evening for laxative effects, or
- 1 to 8 oz of juice daily

Aloe gel:
- 50 to 200 mg capsules orally (PO) every day
- 30 ml by mouth, three times daily
- Topical: liberal application 3 to 5 times daily

Side Effects

Most side effects are from the aloe juice. Side effects of aloe gel are rare and usually relate to contamination with aloe juice. Diarrhea, electrolyte imbalance (especially hypokalemia), and tolerance can occur with chronic use. Abdominal pain and cramping are common complaints. Aloe can lower the blood glucose level. Nephritis, albuminuria, and hematuria have been reported. Muscle weakness, weight loss, and heart disturbances are related to fluid and potassium loss.

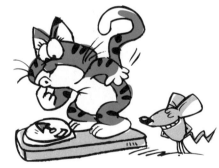

Indications and Uses

Aloe juice:
- Amenorrhea
- Arthritis
- Asthma
- Colds
- Diabetes
- Glaucoma
- Hemorrhoids
- Laxative
- Rectal itching
- Seizures
- Stomach ulcers

Aloe gel:

- Acquired immunodeficiency syndrome (AIDS)
- Analgesia
- Antiinflammatory agent
- Antiseptic
- Cold sores
- Eczema
- Insect bites
- Poison ivy

- Promote burn healing
- Promote wound healing
- Psoriasis
- Skin cancer
- Skin ulcers
- Sunburn
- Topical moisturizer
- Varicose veins

Contraindications and Precautions

Aloe should not be used during menstruation or with dysmenorrhea because increased bleeding may occur. Safety of use in children under age 12 has not been established. Aloe should not be used during pregnancy secondary to uterine stimulation, premature labor, and fluid loss resulting from diarrhea. Aloe should not be used in patients with bowel obstruction or perforation, gangrene colon, or ulcerative colitis. In these situations, bowel stimulation may cause perforation, leakage of bowel contents into the abdomen, and peritonitis. Patients with renal insufficiency, polycystic kidney disease, or other kidney disorders should also avoid aloe.

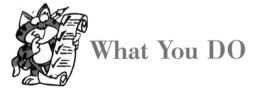

What You DO

Patient History

When obtaining the patient's history, the nurse should review all medications to assess possibilities of interactions with other medications and health problems. Aloe may significantly alter fluid and electrolyte status. The patient's fluid status should be assessed by the following: serum-sodium and serum-potassium levels, blood urea nitrogen (BUN) level, urine concentration, degree of weight loss, and presence of orthostatic hypotension. Patients with fluid deficits are at increased risk during surgery, anesthesia, and invasive procedures. Hypotension in these situations may lead to cardiac, renal, or cerebral ischemia. In cases of severe or prolonged hypotension, cardiac infarction, renal insufficiency or failure, or stroke and neurologic deficit may result. Patients with peripheral vascular disease are especially prone to com-

1. Older adult patients are especially prone to dehydration and electrolyte disturbances.
2. Dehydration and electrolyte disturbances are common causes of mental confusion in older adults.

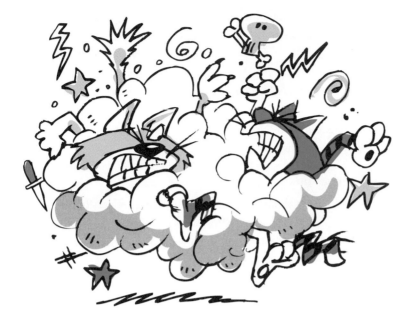

plications from hypotension. Elective surgery, invasive procedures, and studies using radiopaque dye should be delayed until fluid balance is restored.

Aloe may cause hypokalemia resulting from potassium loss in the stool. Hypokalemia during surgery when stress hormones are released is very problematic. During surgery, the body activates the "fight or flight" system, causing release of cortisol, epinephrine, and norepinephrine. Hypokalemia increases the chances of cardiac rhythm problems from epinephrine. Patients will be at increased risk for frequent premature ventricular contractions, ventricular tachycardia, or ventricular fibrillation. Other signs and symptoms of hypokalemia include muscle weakness, lost or decreased deep tendon reflexes, and decreased or inverted T waves, U waves, or flattened ST segments on an electrocardiogram (ECG). The serum-potassium level should be measured and surgery delayed if the potassium level is low.

Potential Drug Interactions

Aloe juice may increase fluid and electrolyte loss when taken with other cathartic medications or herbs, diuretics, and steroids. The toxicity of cardiac glycoside medication, such as digoxin (Lanoxin), is increased in the presence of hypokalemia. Several herbal medications, including hedge mustard or figwort, also contain cardiac glycosides. These herbals may have increased toxicity during hypokalemia.

1. **Individuals with diabetes should monitor their blood glucose levels closely when taking aloe.**
2. **Dehydration can cause premature labor in the parturient.**
3. **Lanoxin and hypokalemia make the patient prone to ventricular dysrhythmias.**
4. **Elective surgery should be postponed in patients with electrolyte or fluid imbalances or both.**

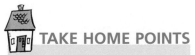

TAKE HOME POINTS

1. Fluid losses from the colon can lead to intracellular and intravascular fluid deficits.
2. Electrolyte losses from the colon will deplete electrolyte levels in the blood and in the tissues.
3. Lymphocyte T cells are the mainstay of the immune system.
4. T cells are the target cells attacked by the AIDS virus.
5. Muscle contraction is dependent on potassium, sodium, and calcium.
6. Dehydration and blood loss decreasing blood flow to the renal tubular membrane can cause renal damage and failure.
7. Increases in BUN indicate dehydration; increases in BUN and creatinine indicate renal insufficiency or renal failure.
8. Dark-colored urine indicates urine concentration in response to a constricted fluid-volume status.
9. Many patients with diabetes have peripheral vascular disease but may not have symptoms yet.
10. Individuals working outside during times of high heat and humidity are more prone to dehydration and heat stroke.

Using aloe juice with licorice, thiazide diuretics, and corticosteroids may increase potassium loss and the chances of side effects and toxicity. Hypokalemia may also be work against the effects of antiarrhythmic agents. Aloe vera improves the blood glucose–lowering effect of glyburnide (Micronase). Patients with diabetes should closely monitor their blood glucose levels when taking these two medicines together. Last, because intestinal contents are moving through the bowel faster, absorption of oral medications may be diminished.

Patient Education

Patients should learn about the fluid and electrolyte effects of aloe. Patients prone to dehydration should avoid using aloe. Also, patients working (and sweating) in hot conditions should avoid using aloe. Patients should not use multiple laxative agents. Aloe should not be used with other medicines that are more toxic with hypokalemia. Patients should report muscle weakness to their health care provider and stop using aloe until their potassium level is assessed. Aloe should not be used for a prolonged period and should be stopped 2 weeks before surgical and invasive procedures.

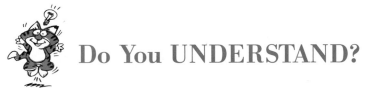

Do You UNDERSTAND?

See pages 220 through 222 for Learning Activities related to this topic.

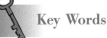

Key Words

Albuminuria Increased amounts of albumin in the urine.

Anthrones Highly irritant plant chemicals that must be oxidized before they are used medicinally. Once oxidized, anthrones become anthraquinones. Anthraquinones are hydrophilic, which accounts for their reduced intestinal absorption and rapid transit to the colon, where they are metabolized into laxatives.

Bradykinin A chemical responsible for pain sensation, vasodilation, and allergic or inflammatory reaction.

Cathartic A substance that stimulates the intestines, causing increased bowel movements.

Cortisol A glucocorticoid hormone secreted from the adrenal cortex that increases the blood glucose level.

Glycosides Plant metabolites that produce sugars through hydrolysis during metabolism. Similar to digoxin, cardiac glycosides, found in plants of the lily family, may increase cardiac output and have toxic effects.

Hematuria Blood in the urine.

Histamine A biochemical mediator of inflammation.

Hypokalemia Low potassium in the blood.

Parturient Pregnant woman.

Phytochemical Chemical of plant origin.

Tolerance When repeated exposure to a medication causes the use of additional medication to obtain the same effect.

www.holisticonline.com/
Herbal-Med/_Herbs/h2.
htm
www.aloe-vera.org/toppage1.
htm
www.herbmed.org/herbs/herb3.
htm

ASTRAGALUS ROOT

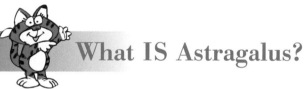

What IS Astragalus?

Astragalus (*Astragalus membranaceus, Astragalus mongholicus*), a member of the pea family, is found only in central and western Asia. Astragalus is also known as buck qi, huang-qi, hwanggi, milk vetch, Mongolian milk, or ogi. Many varieties of astragalus exist, but only the *membranaceus* species is used medicinally. Other varieties may be toxic. The taproots of 4- to 7-year-old plants are used, because other plant parts may be poisonous. Astragalus contains large amounts of selenium, essential oils, amino acids, trace minerals, and **coumarins**. Active ingredients include triterpenoid **saponins** (astragalosides), **flavonoids, polysaccharides**, and **phytosterols**.

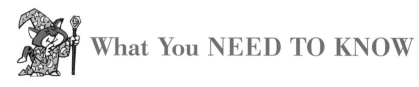

What You NEED TO KNOW

Actions

Astragalus is an **antioxidant** and inhibits free-radical production. Astragalus stimulates the immune system to make immunoglobulin A (IgA) antibodies, IgG antibodies, stem cells, and immune cells. The herb also increases

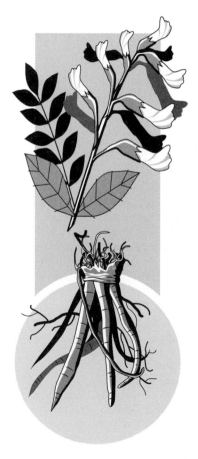

interferon production, stimulates macrophage and T-cell activity, and speeds up immune cell maturation, which is why astragalus is called an immune system stimulant. Astragalus possesses antibiotic and antiviral properties. The herb also causes vasodilation and increases cardiac output because of positive inotropic effects on the heart. Liver function is improved in cases of chronic hepatitis. Astragalus markedly inhibits the formation of thromboxane A2, inhibiting platelet aggregation and blood coagulation. Last, astragalus is a diuretic.

Dose

- 1 to 2 gm dried root by mouth, three times daily
- 4 to 8 ml 1:5 tincture three times daily
- 2 to 4 ml fluid extract 1:1 three times daily
- 100 to 150 mg dry powder three times daily
- 10 to 30 g/day
- Often taken in combination with other herbs

Side Effects

Side effects are mild and rare. Mild GI distress may occur. An allergic response to astragalus is possible. Doses above 28 grams appear to be immunosuppressive.

1. Older adults experience hypertension, peripheral and cardiovascular disease, and arthritis more frequently than younger people. Prescription medications commonly used in these disease states may increase the anticoagulant effects of astragalus.
2. Older adults have coronary artery disease more often than do younger people. Lowered blood pressure from astragalus may decrease blood flow to coronary arteries with blockages. This decrease may lead to myocardial ischemia or infarction.

Indications and Uses

- AIDS
- Antioxidant:
  - Chemotherapy
  - Radiation therapy
  - Steroid therapy
- Asthma
- Bacterial infections
- Cancer patients
- Cardiovascular disease:
  - Angina
  - Heart failure
  - Myocardial ischemia
- Chronic lung disease
- Chronic nephritis
- Diabetes
- Hepatitis
- Herpes type II
- Hypertension
- Immunostimulant
- Influenza
- Insomnia
- Upper respiratory infections
- Viral infections
- Water retention
- Wound healing

Contraindications and Precautions

Astragalus should not be taken during a fever or agitated state. Astragalus should not be used in patients needing immunosuppression, such as post-transplantation patients or those with autoimmune diseases. Safety of use during pregnancy or lactation is unknown.

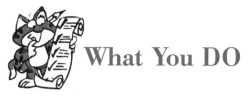 **What You DO**

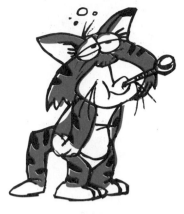

Patient History

The patient's medical history should be reviewed for history of transplant surgery or autoimmune diseases. If these elements are present, the patient should be educated concerning the immune-stimulating actions of astragalus and the need to avoid immune-stimulating herbal medications. Patients should know of the possible immunocompromise seen with doses above 28 grams.

When scheduled for surgery or invasive procedures, patients need to be questioned concerning astragalus use. Further laboratory tests, such as coagulation studies, may be indicated to determine coagulation function.

If taken before surgery, the herb may have additive blood pressure–lowering effects with anesthetics. This instance will make the surgical patient less able to compensate for fluid shifts and blood loss during anesthesia. Astragalus should be discontinued 2 weeks before surgical and other invasive procedures.

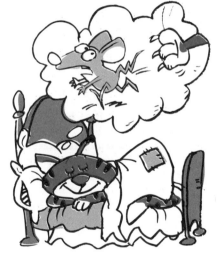

Potential Drug Interactions

Astragalus may increase the blood-thinning effects of anticoagulant medications. The anticoagulant effects of other herbal medications and other blood-thinning medications (NSAIDs) taken on a routine basis may also be increased.

Astragalus may interfere with immunosuppressive medicines such as azathioprine, basiliximab, cyclosporine, daclizumab, muromonab-CD3, tacrolimus, sirolimus, prednisone, or corticosteroids. These medicines are commonly used in patients after transplant surgery.

Astragalus may increase the effects of other antiviral medicines. The effects of interferon-1 and -2, acyclovir, and interlukin-2 may be enhanced.

1. **Do not take astragalus with warfarin (Coumadin) or heparin.**
2. **Do not take astragalus with ginger, gingko, or ginseng.**
3. **Patients taking aspirin, ibuprofen, rofecoxib (Vioxx), or nabumetone (Relafen) on a routine basis should avoid astragalus.**
4. **Surgical patients taking astragalus should not receive ketorolac (Toradol) for postoperative pain management.**
5. **Patients with circulatory disorders such as peripheral vascular disease, carotid artery disease, and diabetes are often taking anticoagulants or blood-thinning agents (aspirin or dipyridamole [Persantine]) for their disorder. These populations may be at increased risk of herb-drug interactions.**
6. **Patients with cardiovascular disease or hypercholesterolemia routinely taking an aspirin a day may be an increased risk population for bleeding complications if they are also taking astragalus.**
7. **Patients taking nifedipine, capoten, captopril, or other antihypertensives may experience increased hypotensive effects when taking astragalus.**

The vasodilating properties of astragalus may enhance the blood pressure–lowering effects of anesthetic agents and antihypertensive medications. Common antihypertensive medications include angiotensin II antagonists, angiotension-converting enzyme (ACE) inhibitors, or calcium channel-blocking agents. A similar increased blood pressure–lowering effect may be expected when taking astragalus with other diuretics. Stopping astragalus after achieving hypertension control may result in increased blood pressure and reemergence of hypertension resulting from the loss of vasodilatory effects from the herb. Last, vasodilation may also be increased when used with other vasodilating medications given for treatment of vascular insufficiency.

Patient Education

Patients should be warned about the possible anticoagulant effects of astragalus. In addition, patients with **thrombocytopenia** and clotting disorders should avoid astragalus. Patients should stop taking astragalus 2 weeks before invasive procedures and inform their surgeon.

Patients should know about the possible increased hypotensive effects of astragalus when used with other blood pressure–reducing agents. Patients should be cautious when using astragalus if they have hypertension. Patients should avoid taking astragalus when taking other medications and herbals that have blood pressure–lowering effects. To avoid the possibility of immunosuppression, patients should not take more than 28 grams of astragalus. Patients with transplanted organs or autoimmune diseases should avoid astragalus use.

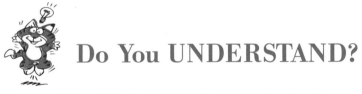

Do You UNDERSTAND?

See pages 223 and 224 for Learning Activities related to this topic.

Key Words

Antioxidant An agent that helps prevent cell damage from oxygen-free radicals or other highly reactive compounds.

Coumarins Plant chemicals that may exhibit anticoagulant properties, as well as anticancer, immunostimulant, antifungal, antiinflammatory, vasodilatory, muscle relaxant, hypnotic, central nervous system–stimulant, hypothermal, diuretic, anticholinergic, antiedema, or estrogenic effects. The anticoagulant Coumadin was derived from the coumarins in the molded sweet clover plant.

Flavonoids Plant pigments responsible for the color of fruits and vegetables. Some flavonoids increase capillary wall stability (decrease capillary fragility) and scavenge free radicals, resulting in antioxidant properties. Other flavonoids have antiarthritis, antiinflammatory, antiviral, or antimutagenic properties.

Inotropic Improving the force of cardiac muscle contraction.

Interferon Proteins with antiviral and immunostimulant properties used in the treatment of cancer.

Phytosterols A sterol from vegetable or plant oil.

Polysaccharides Water-soluble polymer complex carbohydrates that consist of two or more simple sugar molecules joined together. Some polysaccharides stimulate the immune system.

Saponins Phytochemical plant constituents that produce foam when dissolved in water. Saponins also reduce surface tension and increase solubility and cell membrane permeability. Saponins may be sugar glycosides or steroidal in composition.

Thrombocytopenia Decreased number of platelets.

 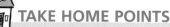
TAKE HOME POINTS

1. Astragalus use during radiation therapy for breast cancer has increased survival rates.
2. Survival rates for lung cancer have been improved when astragalus is given during chemotherapy.

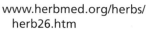 www.herbmed.org/herbs/
herb26.htm

BLACK COHOSH

What IS Black Cohosh?

Black cohosh (*Cimicifuga racemosa, Actaea racemosa, Actaea macrotys*) is a member of the buttercup family. The name comes from the color of its dried roots and the Algonquin Native-American word "cohosh," which means rough. Other names for black cohosh include rattleroot, rattleweed, black snakeroot, squawroot, and bugbane or bugwort. Bugwort refers to the plant's pungent odor and use as an insect repellent. Black cohosh grows wild throughout wooded areas in the eastern United States. The active ingredients in black cohosh are triterpene **glycosides**, **saponins**, **phytosterin**, and **salicylic acid**.

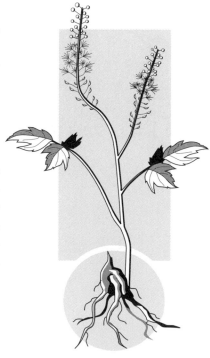

What You NEED TO KNOW

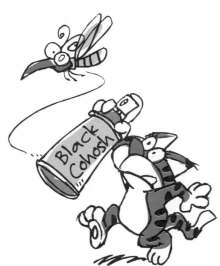

Actions

Black cohosh has estrogen-like actions, but it does not have any effects on estrogen itself. Black cohosh reduces secretion of luteinizing hormone (LH), but not follicle-stimulating hormone (FSH) in menopausal women. Decreases in estrogen production and increases in LH secretion cause the "hot flashes" of menopause. The herb may decrease LH secretion by binding to estrogen receptors. Black cohosh may block the growth of estrogen sensitive tumors by inhibiting estrogen from binding to its receptors. Although black cohosh does not alter blood pressure, it is a vasodilator in animal studies.

Dose

- 1 to 2 mg 27-deoxyacteine every day
- 0.5 to 1.0 g dried root three times daily
- 1.5 to 3.0 ml 1:2 liquid extract every day
- 40 to 200 mg black cohosh herb every day, with use not to exceed 6 months

Side Effects

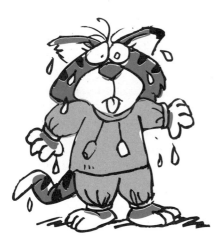

GI side effects are usually rare and mild. Overdoses may produce nausea, vomiting, and dizziness. Black cohosh may slow the heart rate. Large doses of black cohosh can cause sweating, headache, weight gain, hypotension, or joint pains. Black cohosh does not appear to cause cancer or birth defects and is not considered a toxic plant, even at high doses.

Indications and Uses

- Analgesia
- Antiinflammatory
- Antipyretic
- Antispasmodic
- Asthma
- Cardiovascular and circulatory problems
- Cough suppressant
- Diuretic
- Dysmenorrhea
- Expectorant
- Hypertension
- Hypercholesterolemia
- Muscular pain
- Osteoarthritis and rheumatoid arthritis
- Osteoporosis
- Poisonous snakebites

- Premenstrual syndrome (PMS)
- Menopausal symptoms:
  - Anxiety
  - Depression
  - Hot flashes
  - Insomnia
  - Irritability
  - Mood swings
  - Night sweats
  - Palpitations
- Vaginal atrophy
- Vaginal dryness
- Visual disturbances
- Neurologic pain:
  - Neuralgia
  - Sciatic
  - Sedation
- Staphylococcus infections
- Tinnitus

Contraindications and Precautions

Black cohosh stimulates uterine contractions; therefore its use may stimulate premature labor. The herb should not be taken while breast-feeding.

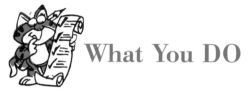 # What You DO

Patient History

Patients should be questioned concerning herbal medicine use to determine potential herb-drug interactions. Administration of black cohosh should be discontinued after 6 months of use.

Potential Drug Interactions

Animal studies of black cohosh report vasodilatory effects. Thus black cohosh may cause increased hypotensive effects with anesthetics during surgery. This may lower the patient's ability to tolerate fluid shifts and blood loss during anesthesia. Black cohosh should be stopped 2 weeks before surgical and other invasive procedures.

Increased hypotensive effects may also occur with patients taking black cohosh and antihypertensive medications. Angiotensin II antagonists, ACE inhibitors, beta blockers, or calcium channel–blocking agents are commonly used antihypertensive medications. A similar effect may occur when taking black cohosh with diuretic agents. Stopping black cohosh after achieving hypertension control may result in increased blood pressure and reemergence of hypertension, which result from the loss of vasodilatory effects from the herb. Last, vasodilation may also be increased when used with other vasodilating medications given for treatment of vascular insufficiency.

1. **Patients who are pregnant or breast-feeding should avoid black cohosh.**
2. **Black cohosh use should not exceed 6 months in duration.**
3. **Black cohosh may increase the vasodilatory and heart rate–slowing actions of clonidine.**
4. **Undesirable hypotension may occur when black cohosh is taken with other vasodilatory agents such as captopril, nifedipine, and losartan.**
5. **Undesirable hypotension may occur when black cohosh is taken with medicines to improve peripheral blood flow. These agents include dipyridamole or papaverine.**
6. **Undesirable hypotension may occur in anesthetized patients who take black cohosh preoperatively.**
7. **Hypotensive states may result in myocardial ischemia or infarction, renal insufficiency or failure, or cerebral ischemia or infarction.**

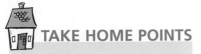

Actual problems when using black cohosh with estrogen or progesterone replacement have not been identified. However, caution is advised.

Black cohosh may help decrease the growth of cancer cells when used with tamoxifen, a medication used in treating estrogen-sensitive cancers. The use of black cohosh with tamoxifen in breast cancer is under investigation.

Patient Education

Patients should learn about the blood pressure–lowering, sedative, and uterine-stimulatory effects of black cohosh. Patients taking antihypertensive medications should be cautioned about the use of herbal medications with blood pressure–lowering effects. Patients with circulatory insufficiency should be cautious in using black cohosh. Black cohosh may increase the blood pressure–lowering effects of other prescription or herbal medications. Large decreases in blood pressure in cases of cardiovascular and peripheral vascular insufficiency may lead to decreased cardiac output. Decreased cardiac output can cause organ ischemia. Patients should not take black cohosh during pregnancy because of the possibility of stimulating labor. Black cohosh should not be taken while breast-feeding.

Do You UNDERSTAND?

See pages 224 through 226 for Learning Activities related to this topic.

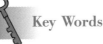

Key Words

Cardiac output The amount of blood ejected from the heart every minute.

Glycosides Plant metabolites that produce sugars through hydrolysis during metabolism. Similar to digoxin, cardiac glycosides, found in plants of the lily family, may increase cardiac output and have toxic effects.

Phytosterin A sterol from plant oil or fat.

Salicylic acid Phytochemical constituents of willow bark are converted into salicin in the bowel and oxidized into salicylic acid by the liver. Salicin is responsible for the herb's antipyretic and antiinflammatory effects. Aspirin is a derivative of salicylic acid obtained from willow bark.

Saponins Phytochemical plant constituents that produce foam when dissolved in water, reduce surface tension, and increase solubility and cell membrane permeability. Saponins may be sugar glycosides or steroidal in composition.

CAPSICUM

What IS Capsicum?

Capsicum or *Capsicum frutescens* is a concentrated extract of the chili or hot pepper plant. Capsicum is also called cayenne, Mexican chilies, African chilies, bird pepper, goat's pod, or grains of paradise. Pepper plants belonging to the *Capsicum* genus include yellow, green, and red (but not black) peppers and paprika. The active ingredients in these plants are called *capsaicinoids*. Of the five capsaicinoids that occur naturally, capsaicin and dihydrocapsaicin are the most abundant and account for the pungency of peppers. Although all pepper plants contain capsaicinoids in varying amounts, the red or "hot" peppers contain the highest concentrations of capsaicin and dihydrocapsaicin. Capsaicin can be obtained in over-the-counter medications containing a standardized, purified form. Capsaicin is also present as cayenne powder or capsules, in hot peppers and their extracts, and in self-defense sprays.

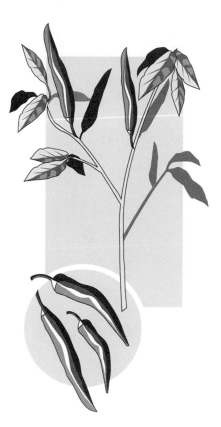

What You NEED TO KNOW

Actions

Capsaicin acts on pain fibers, blood clotting, the respiratory system, and the immune system. Capsaicin both causes and decreases pain. Initially, capsaicin use stimulates specific receptors located on pain neurons (nociceptors) in the skin, thereby causing pain. Stimulation of the neuron results in the release of substance P, a neurotransmitter, to pain-processing centers in the brain and spinal cord. This action accounts for a burning sensation when capsaicin is applied to the skin or ingested. Continued use of capsaicin results in pain relief as pain neurons become desensitized. Desensitization is thought to occur as a result of depletion of substance P and decreased sensitivity of the pain neurons. Capsaicin also has an effect on the immune system, causing a decrease in lymphocyte (white blood cell) and antibody production. Capsaicin is reported to decrease platelet aggregation, thereby stimulating local blood flow and decreasing blood clotting. These effects have not been proven in humans. Capsaicin also stimulates cough receptors in the respiratory tract.

Dose

- Capsicum is available as a topical cream containing 0.025% or 0.075% capsaicin.
- Apply to the affected area 3 to 4 times a day.
- For cluster headaches, apply to the nostril on the same side as the headache.
- Application may need to be continued for several weeks before relief occurs.
- As a tea or infusion: 0.5 to 1.0 tsp cayenne powder in 8 oz of water.

Side Effects

The side effects of capsaicin-containing products are the result of its action on pain receptors and are directly related to the dose and strength. Capsaicin may increase blood flow and decrease blood clotting. Capsaicin causes burning, stinging, pain, and irritation when applied to the skin or mucous membranes. **Contact dermatitis** or "Hunan hand" has been reported after handling of chili peppers without gloves. Contact with the eye can cause severe pain, tearing, blurring of vision, redness, and spasm of the eyelids. Corneal sensitivity is temporarily decreased, which may predispose individuals to corneal abrasions. Breathing pepper spray or the oils of peppers can cause coughing and shortness of breath. Breathing pepper spray can also cause laryngospasm, bronchoconstriction, laryngeal and pulmonary edema, chemical pneumonitis, and even respiratory arrest. Deaths have been reported from pepper spray exposure.

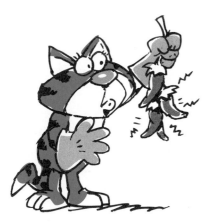

Indications and Uses

- Arthritis
- Bursitis
- Cluster headaches
- Colic
- Diabetic neuropathy
- Diarrhea
- Fever
- Fibromyalgia
- GI cramping
- Improve peripheral circulation
- Neuralgias
- Osteoarthritis
- Pharyngitis
- Postherpetic neuralgia (pain after shingles infection)
- Postmastectomy pain syndrome
- Prevent heart disease
- Pruritus (itching)
- Psoriasis
- Rheumatoid arthritis
- Reflex sympathetic dystrophy
- Seasickness
- Toothache

Contraindications and Precautions

Avoid applying capsicum to open sores, burns, or abrasions. Do not use capsicum for herpes zoster (shingles) pain until the sores have healed. Capsicum should not be used on children under 2 years of age.

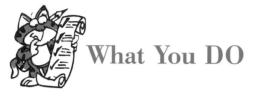 # What You DO

Patient History

When presenting for surgery or invasive procedures, patients need to be questioned concerning their over-the-counter and herbal medication intake. Anesthetics and narcotics may increase the sedative effects of capsicum.

Potential Drug Interactions

No proof exists that capsaicin-containing products affect blood clotting. The use of capsaicin-containing products with other medications that affect blood clotting or platelet aggregation has not been studied. However, considering the known effects of capsaicin, patients should be cautioned about potential interactions with other drugs that inhibit platelet aggregation, such as aspirin and NSAIDs. Patients taking anticoagulants should be cautioned that capsaicin might further decrease blood clotting. Capsicum may increase the anticoagulant effects of herbal medications, which may also decrease clotting. This group would include feverfew, garlic, ginger, gingko, licorice, passionflower, and red clover.

Capsaicin may increase blood levels of theophylline and related drugs, causing an increase in side effects. Side effects of theophylline include increased heart rate, nervousness, and upset stomach.

Capsicum may increase the sedative effects of narcotics, barbiturates, and anesthetics. Capsicum may also increase the sedative effects of sedating herbal medications such as goldenseal, chamomile, hops, kava, and St. John's wort. Last, capsicum may increase the incidence of cough sometimes occurring in patients taking ACE inhibitors.

Patient Education

Patients should report the use of capsaicin to their physician because capsaicin may interact with other medications. Capsaicin must be used regularly to achieve pain relief. Several weeks of use may be necessary to achieve

1. **Individuals with an allergy to hot peppers should not use capsaicin-containing products.**
2. **Individuals with asthma or other respiratory conditions may have an increased sensitivity to the inhalation of pepper spray, ground chili pepper, or chili pepper oils.**
3. **Patients taking theophylline derivatives should talk to their physician before ingesting cayenne powder, capsules, or teas.**
4. **Patients taking anticoagulants should talk to their physician before using cayenne powder, capsules, or teas.**
5. **Capsicum may desensitize the skin to painful stimuli. Hot compresses or heating pads should not be applied to skin areas where capsaicin has been applied.**
6. **Do not take capsicum with captopril.**

www.nlm.nih.gov/
medlineplus/druginfo/
capsaicintopical202626.
html#SXX16
www.holisticonline.com/
Herbal-Med/_Herbs/h43.htm
www.findarticles.com/
cf_dls/g2603/0002/2603000/p1/
article. jhtml
www.cooperfitness.com/ content/
support/pharmaceutical/altmed/
Detail.asp?DocID=1106

the desired effect. Patients should wear gloves or wash hands thoroughly with soap and warm (not hot) water after applying the cream. Individuals using capsaicin ointments should avoid touching the eye or other mucous membranes after applying the ointment. If contact occurs, flush the eye with large amounts of cool water for at least 15 minutes. Hot, moist compresses or heating pads should not be applied to skin areas where capsaicin has been applied.

Patients taking anticoagulants should be cautioned that capsaicin might further decrease blood clotting. Patients taking theophylline should be informed that capsaicin might increase blood levels of theophylline-containing drugs and increase side effects. Patients should not drive or operate heavy equipment until individual sensitivity to the sedation effects of capsicum is determined.

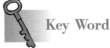

Do You UNDERSTAND?

See pages 226 and 227 for Learning Activities related to this topic.

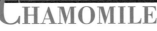 Key Word

Contact dermatitis Skin reaction caused by touching an allergy-producing substance.

CHAMOMILE

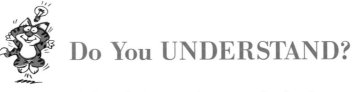

What IS Chamomile?

Chamomile (*Anthemis nobilis* [Roman], *Matricaria chamomilla* [German]) is a plant with strong-smelling foliage. Chamomile is also known as camomilla, Kamillen, Kamille, or pin heads. The daisylike flowers are often dried and used for medicine, tea, and hair products. German chamomile is a tall, erect annual that reaches 2 to 3 feet high. Roman chamomile is a perennial that seldom grows more than 9 inches high. As the herb of choice for Asclepiades, a physician from Bithynia who lived around 90 BC, chamomile is an herb of many uses. Slovakian chamomile specialist, Dr. Ivan Salamon, writes, "Chamomile is the most favored and most used medicinal plant in Slovakia. Our folk saying indicates that an individual should bow when facing a chamomile plant. This respect is the result of 100 years of experience in folk medicine of the country." The active ingredients of chamomile are a volatile oil of pale blue color (becomes yellow with age), anthemic acid (bitter part), tannic acid, coumarins, flavonoids, and terpenoids.

 # What You NEED TO KNOW

Actions

Chamomile has antiallergy, antiinflammatory effects, and peptic ulcer–protecting effects. Chamomile decreases histamine release, which accounts for the antiallergy and antiinflammatory action. Chamomile has antibacterial and antifungal activity. The plant also has antispasm and central nervous system (CNS) depressant effects.

Dose

Internal:
- 1 cup of tea (prepared with 5 oz of boiling water poured over a heaping teaspoon of herb and steeped for 5 to 10 minutes); consumed 3 to 4 times a day between meals
- 1 to 4 ml of 1:1 liquid extract three times daily

External:
- 3% to 10% ointment
- Poultice made from steeped tea

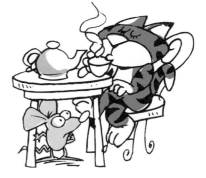

Side Effects

Very few side effects are reported in the literature for chamomile, and it is generally recognized as safe for human consumption. Concentrated tea preparations can cause vomiting. Individuals who are allergic to ragweed, daisies, marigolds, or chrysanthemums may also be allergic to chamomile.

1. Older adults are especially sensitive to the sedative effects of medications and should use caution when taking chamomile.
2. Older adults should not use chamomile with other sedative agents because of the increased sensitivity to sedative medications.

Do not take chamomile with diphen hydramine (Benadryl) or naphazoline hydrochloride (Allerest, Clear Eyes).

Indications and Uses

- Allergies
- Antiinflammatory for skin and mucous membranes
- Bath
- Burns
- Children:
  - Relieves colic
  - Relieves restlessness
  - Relieves teething problems
- Digestion
- Foot bath
- Gastritis
- Hemorrhoids
- Mastitis
- Morning sickness during pregnancy
- Relaxation at bedtime
- Respiratory infections
- Skin ulcers
- Ulcerative colitis
- Wounds

Contraindications and Precautions

Individuals who are allergic to plants that are members of the sunflower or aster family, such as ragweed, should not use chamomile. At least one case of anaphylactic shock has been attributed to chamomile tea use. Chamomile should not be used near the eyes because it is irritating.

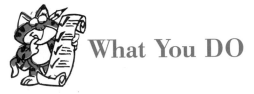

What You DO

Patient History

When presenting for surgery or other invasive procedures, patients need to be questioned concerning their over-the-counter medications and herbal medication intake. Anesthetics and narcotics may increase the sedative effects of chamomile.

Potential Drug Interactions

CNS depressants and anesthetics may have increased effects when used with chamomile. This combination will cause increased levels of sedation or increased length of sedative effects. Sedative effects of other herbal medications, such as catnip, cayenne, chamomile, melatonin, and St. John's wort, may also be increased when used with chamomile. Chamomile may also increase CNS sedation from other CNS-depressant agents, such as sleeping pills, alcohol, or antihistamines.

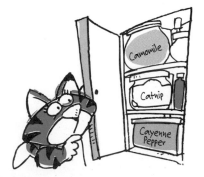

Patient Education

Patients with seasonal allergies, especially to ragweed, should be educated to the possibility of allergies with chamomile.

Increased sedative effects may delay wake up times from surgery, increasing operating room times and postanesthesia care unit (PACU) stays. Severe oversedation problems may result in an overnight hospital stay for what was once a planned outpatient procedure. Patients should avoid driving or using heavy machinery until individual susceptibility to chamomile's sedative effects can be determined. Patients should stop taking chamomile 2 weeks before invasive procedures and inform their surgeon.

Do You UNDERSTAND?

See page 228 for Learning Activities related to this topic.

Key Words

Coumarins Plant chemicals that may exhibit anticoagulant properties, as well as anticancer, immunostimulant, antifungal, antiinflammatory, vasodilatory, muscle relaxant, hypnotic, central nervous system–stimulant, hypothermal, diuretic, anticholinergic, antiedema, or estrogenic effects.

Flavonoids Plant pigments responsible for the color of fruits and vegetables. Some flavonoids increase capillary wall stability (decrease capillary fragility) and scavenge free radicals, resulting in antioxidant properties. Other flavonoids have antiarthritis, antiinflammatory, antiviral, or antimutagenic properties.

Terpenoids Secondary metabolites or phytochemicals in the essential oils of the plant.

Thrombocytopenia Decreased number of platelets.

www.hcrc.org/faqs/
chamom.html
www.hort.purdue.edu/newcrop/
med-aro/factsheets/
CHAMOMILE.html

CRANBERRY

What IS Cranberry?

The American cranberry (*Vaccinium macrocarpon*) is one of only three fruits original to North America. Found in the northeastern United States and eastern Canada, the cranberry plant is a low-growing shrub. The berry, or fruit, is used for medicinal purposes to treat urinary tract infections. Cranberries are commonly used in juice, jellies, jams, and sauce. Cranberries contain ascorbic acid, or vitamin C, other organic acids, **proanthocyanidins**, **flavonoids**, and fructose. Cranberry is also known as trailing swamp, mossberry, moosebeere, and Arandano Americano.

What You NEED TO KNOW

Actions

Cranberry proanthocyanidins and flavonoids prevent bacteria, such as *Escherichia coli* and possibly *Enterococcus facialis*, from sticking to urinary tract lining. Thus bacteria are unable to penetrate and infect urinary tract tissues. Cranberry fructose aids in preventing *E. coli* adhesion to urinary tract tissues. Cranberry may also prevent plaque bacteria from adhering to gum tissues and prevent periodontal disease. Cranberries may also have **antioxidant** and antitumor properties.

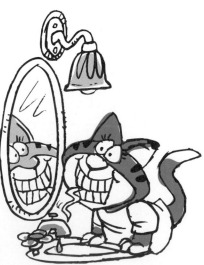

Dose

- 1 to 10 oz juice per day
- 300 to 400 mg dried cranberry powder capsules twice daily (bid)
- 1.5 oz fresh or frozen cranberries

Side Effects

Cranberry does not have any side effects with normal intake. Large doses of cranberries or cranberry juice can cause diarrhea. Prolonged use of large amounts (greater than one liter per day) may contribute to kidney stone formation.

Indications and Uses

- Antipyretic
- Cancer
- Diuretic
- Pleurisy
- Prevention of kidney stones
- Prevention of urinary tract infections
- Promote gastric absorption of vitamin B_{12} in patients with decreased stomach acid
- Scurvy
- Urinary stoma irritation
- Urine deodorizer for urinary incontinence

Contraindications and Precautions

Patients with urinary tract obstruction and problems urinating should not take cranberry.

1. **Do not use cranberry juice if you have prostatic hypertrophy and experience problems with urination.**
2. **Cranberry should not be used in place of an antibiotic when urinary tract infection is already present.**

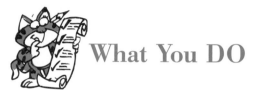 # What You DO

Patient History

Taking large amounts of cranberry may lead to diarrhea. Patients experiencing diarrhea with cranberry use should decrease their intake.

Potential Drug Interactions

Because of its acidic properties, cranberries may interfere with the effectiveness of oral antacids. Patients who take proton pump inhibitors such as lansoprazole, omeprazole, and rabeprazole may have increased absorption of vitamin B_{12} while taking cranberry.

Patient Education

Patients should be told that, although cranberries have demonstrated effectiveness in decreasing the number of urinary tract infections, they have not been shown to cure a urinary tract infection once it has occurred.

Patients with diabetes often have an increased incidence of bladder infections. Patients who are using cranberry juice to help prevent bladder infections should be cautioned to use sugar-free or artificially sweetened juices.

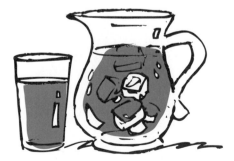

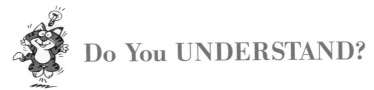

Do You UNDERSTAND?

See page 228 for Learning Activities related to this topic.

Key Words

Antioxidant An agent that helps prevent cell damage from oxygen-free radicals or other highly reactive compounds.

Flavonoids Plant pigments responsible for the color of fruits and vegetables. Some flavonoids increase capillary wall stability (decrease capillary fragility) and scavenge free radicals, resulting in antioxidant properties. Other flavonoids have antiarthritis, antiinflammatory, antiviral, or antimutagenic effects.

Proanthocyanidins Condensed or complex tannins that are astringent and may bind and precipitate large molecules such as proteins from solutions. Tannins have antioxidant, antisecretory, and antiinflammatory effects on mucous membranes.

www.herbmed.org/herbs/
herb131.htm

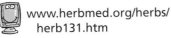

DANDELION

What IS Dandelion?

Dandelion (*Taraxacum officinale*) is a member of the sunflower family. Dandelion's name is thought to arise from the corruption of the French, *dent de lion*. Most people think this name has something to do with the great jagged teeth of the green leaves that somewhat resemble the teeth of a lion. Other names include wet the bed, puffball, swine snout, or wild endive. A common plant in all areas of the Northern Hemisphere, the dandelion is native to Europe and naturalized over North America. The dandelion is able to grow in all areas with a northern temperate climate and is so plentiful that many people consider it a weed. The young green leafs and the roots are used medicinally. The leaves are high in iron, potassium, vitamin A, and other vitamins. The root contains taraxacin, acrystalline, taraxacerin, inulin, gluten, gum, and potash. The active ingredients are sesquiterpene lactones from the root.

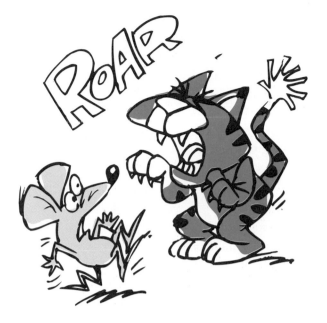

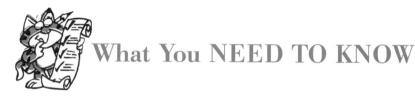 What You **NEED TO KNOW**

Actions

Dandelion has a diuretic effect and also a mild antiinflammatory action. The eudesmanolides, previously called taraxacins, act as an appetite stimulant. Dandelion is a high-nutrient source of vitamins including A (higher than carrots), with small amounts of vitamins B, C, and D. The herb is also a good source of potassium, sodium, phosphorus, and iron. Dandelion is a natural diuretic that does not cause potassium loss because of its high-potassium content. The plant also has mild laxative effects. Dandelion has mild antiinflammatory effects and stimulates bile production as well.

Dose

- 4 to 10 g of the dried leaves three times daily
- 2 to 8 g of dried root three times daily
- Both of these doses can be achieved by brewing in tea
- Tincture dose (1:5) is 5 to 10 ml three times daily

 1. Pregnancy and breast-feeding safety has not been established with dandelion use.

2. Older adults are often prone to heart disease and are taking medications to control blood pressure. Taking dandelion with these medications may cause increased fluid loss, resulting in hypotension and dehydration.

1. **Older adult patients taking diuretics for heart disease and also taking dandelion are at a high risk for developing dehydration.**
2. **Patients with gallbladder disease and obstructive biliary disease should not take dandelion.**
3. **Patients with allergies to the Asteraceae plant family (ragweed, marigolds, chrysanthemums, daisies, and others) should avoid dandelion.**
4. **Patients who are allergic to feverfew should not take dandelion.**

Side Effects

Side effects are usually mild but can be potentially dangerous if not noticed. These effects include diuresis and hypoglycemia. **Contact dermatitis** has been known to occur, as well as allergic reactions from people known to be allergic to plants that are members of the ragweed, chrysanthemum, marigold, or daisy family.

Indications and Uses

- Blood purifier
- Diuretic
- Eczema
- Increase bile production
- Inflammatory skin conditions
- Joint pain
- Indigestion
- Liver disorders (hepatitis, jaundice)
- Mild laxative
- Remove excess estrogen
- Weight loss

Contraindications and Precautions

Dandelion should not be used in patients with acute infections of the gallbladder, biliary obstruction, and intestinal blockages. Information on safe use for lactating women is insufficient; therefore dandelion use should be avoided in this group.

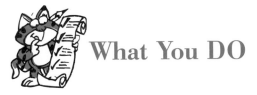

What You DO

Patient History

Patients must be questioned concerning their prescription, over-the-counter, or complementary and alternative medications. Patients with cardiovascular disease who are taking diuretics, as well as patients taking insulin, oral hypoglycemic agents, or both, should be questioned extensively. Patients taking dandelion with other diuretics or herbal medications that also promote diuresis may require further laboratory testing to determine blood-electrolyte levels. Decreased fluid volume from dandelion-induced diuresis may cause increased hypotensive effects with anesthetics during surgery. This increase may lower the patient's ability to compensate for fluid shifts and blood loss during anesthesia. Dandelion should be stopped 2 weeks before surgical and other invasive procedures.

TAKE HOME POINTS

1. Patients taking lithium should avoid dandelion.
2. Patients with diabetes present an increased risk for hypoglycemia if taking dandelion.
3. Herbs such as celery, corn silk, and artichoke also have diuretic effects.
4. Herbs such as ginseng also have glucose-lowering effects.

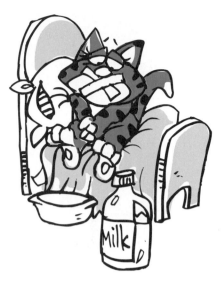

Individuals taking dandelion with other medicines and herbs that also lower blood glucose should have their blood-sugar level tested before "nothing by mouth" (NPO) orders are put into effect.

Potential Drug Interactions

Dandelion may cause **hypoglycemia**, thus diabetic patients need to have blood glucose levels monitored closely. The diuretic effects of dandelion can increase sodium loss if taken with other diuretics; therefore serum-sodium levels will need to be monitored. Patients taking lithium for bipolar disease must be monitored very closely if taking dandelion. Low sodium levels from dandelion diuresis can increase lithium toxicity. Dandelion may increase the effects of medicines that inhibit platelet aggregation and cause anticoagulation.

Patient Education

Patients should be taught that dandelion is a potent diuretic, and use with other diuretics may lead to profound urination, affecting blood pressure and blood-sodium levels. If patients are taking dandelion with lithium, they must have their sodium levels monitored closely. Patients with diabetes must be made aware that dandelion can cause hypoglycemia. If these patients are using other agents to decrease blood glucose, they should conduct more frequent glucose checks. Use of dandelion in pregnancy should probably be avoided because a decreased fluid status can stimulate uterine contractions. Any patient with concerns about dandelion should be encouraged to talk with their health care provider.

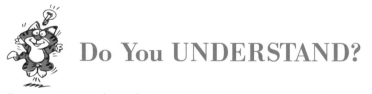

Do You UNDERSTAND?

See pages 228 and 229 for Learning Activities related to this topic.

Key Words

Contact dermatitis Skin reaction caused by touching an allergy-producing substance.
Hypoglycemia Low blood-sugar level.

www.herbmed.org/herbs/
herb125.htm
http://altmed.creighton.edu/end
ometriosis/alternative%5F
therapies.htm
www.holisticonline.com/Herbal-
Med/_Herbs/h48.htm

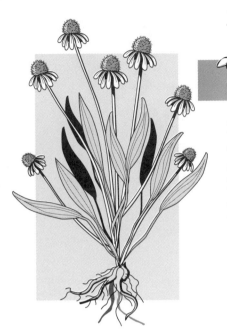

ECHINACEA

What IS Echinacea?

Echinacea (*Echinacea angustifolia*, *E. pallida*, or *E. purpurea*) is a wildflower similar to the plants in the daisy, sunflower, and ragweed family. The name *echinacea* comes from the Greek word *echinos*, meaning sea urchin or hedgehog, which is because of the cone shape of the flower head. Other names for echinacea include purple coneflower and Sampson root. Echinacea has also been called snakeroot because it was traditionally used to treat snakebites. Echinacea grows wild throughout the United States and is a common garden flower. For centuries, Native Americans used echinacea as a medicine. The active ingredients are alkylamides, isobutylamides, and caffeic acid esters (echinasides).

What You NEED TO KNOW

Actions

Echinacea stimulates the immune system to increase resistance to bacterial, fungal, and viral infections. Echinacea is thought to decrease upper respiratory influenza and cold symptoms but not prevent infection. The herb may have antiinflammatory effects by inhibiting hyaluronidase and causes release of cortisol. The herb does not have direct bacteriocidal or bacteriostatic effects. To stimulate the immune system, the herb improves the function of white blood cells (WBCs). Echinacea may promote encapsulation of bacteria and phagocytosis. Echinacea increases the release of tumor necrosis factor and immune cell production. Echinacea promotes tissue granulation to speed wound healing. Echinacea contains flavonoids and may inhibit the hepatic metabolic system cytochrome CYP450 3A4.

Dose

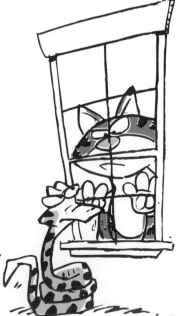

* Expressed juice: 8 to 9 cc every day
* Capsules: 1 to 3 g three times daily
* Tinctures: 3 to 5 cc every day

Side Effects

Echinacea is usually well tolerated but occasionally causes side effects such as nausea, vomiting, diarrhea, fever, sore throat, or dizziness. No acute or chronic toxicity is reported with oral doses, but slight toxicity may exist with intravenous (IV) administration. Because the plant is similar to ragweed, use may cause allergic reactions such as wheezing, edema, urticaria, or anaphylaxis. In high doses, echinacea may diminish both male and female fertility. Echinacea may have decreased effectiveness with prolonged use. Use for more than 6 to 8 weeks has not been shown to have adverse effects. Notwithstanding, the herb should be used for no longer than 3 months.

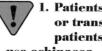

1. **Patients with AIDS or transplant patients should not use echinacea.**
2. **Patients with immune system dysfunction should not use echinacea.**
3. **Women who are pregnant, breast-feeding, or trying to conceive should not use echinacea.**
4. **Patients allergic to ragweed should avoid echinacea.**

Indications and Uses

- Acne
- Bacterial infections
- Bee stings
- Cancer
- Cholecystitis
- Coronary circulation problems
- Digestive tract infections
- Eczema
- Fatigue
- Fungal infections
- Hair loss
- Immune system boost during chemotherapy
- Migraines
- Oncology radiation burns
- Pharyngitis
- Prostatitis
- Rhinorrhea
- Septicemia
- Sinus infections
- Skin wounds and ulcers:
  - Abscesses
  - Boils
  - Carbuncles
- Tonsillitis
- Upper respiratory infections: colds, influenza symptoms
- Urinary tract infections
- Vaginal yeast infections
- Viral infections

Contraindications and Precautions

Echinacea is contraindicated for systemic diseases such as AIDS, tuberculosis, collagen, connective tissue diseases, leukosis, or autoimmune disorders such as multiple sclerosis. Immunosuppressed or transplant patients should not use echinacea. IV echinacea may interfere with glucose control in patients with diabetes. Topical echinacea may cause redness or skin rash. Pregnant women or those who are breast-feeding should not take echinacea. Some echinacea tinctures are alcohol based. These substances should not be given to children, alcoholics, or patients with severe liver disease. Alcohol-based tinctures should not be given to patients on disulfiram (Antabuse) or metronidazole (Flagyl) to avoid abdominal distress, vomiting, flushing, or headache.

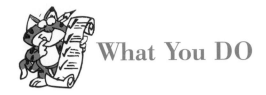

What You DO

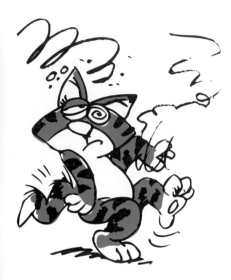

Patient History

Patients should be questioned concerning herbal medicine use to determine potential problems. Patients should stop herbal medication use 2 weeks before surgery or invasive procedures. Some anesthetics, such as midazolam (Versed) or diazepam (Valium), are metabolized by liver enzymes that are inhibited by echinacea, making their actions unpredictable. Decreased metabolism of midazolam may delay wake-up times from surgery, increasing operating room times and PACU stays. Severe oversedation problems may result in an overnight hospital stay for what was once a planned outpatient procedure. Reduced metabolism of lidocaine may result in toxic reactions, such as sedation, altered mental status, convulsions, hypotension, and cardiovascular collapse.

Potential Drug Interactions

Echinacea might counteract immunosuppressive drugs such as cyclosporine and corticosteroids in transplant patients, which may cause increased rejection reactions. Echinacea may cause hepatotoxicity with methotrexate, ketoconazole, cyclosporine, phenytoin, amiodarone, and barbiturates. Echinacea may inhibit hepatic cytochrome CYP450 3A4 activity, which would increase the duration of action of medications that are metabolized by this enzyme system. Medications metabolized by this system include lovastatin, itraconazole, fexofenadine, benzodiazepines (midazolam, diazepam), triazolam (Halcion), and many anesthetic agents. Abruptly stopping echinacea after therapeutic levels have been achieved will allow the metabolic system to return to normal activity, resulting in decreased drug levels, duration of action, and effectiveness. Birth control pills are also metabolized by hepatic cytochrome CYP450 3A4. Whether echinacea affects the metabolism of birth control pills is unknown.

Patient Education

Patients should be educated that echinacea cannot prevent a cold, but it may lessen symptoms of an upper respiratory infection. Patients with hay fever and asthma may be prone to allergic reaction with echinacea. Patients sensitive to ragweed, chrysanthemums, marigolds, or daisies may demon-

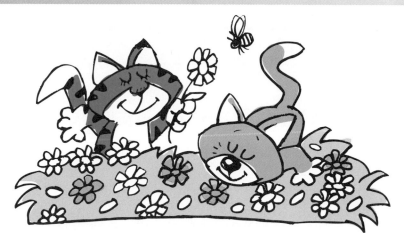

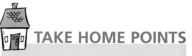

TAKE HOME POINTS

1. Echinacea may not prevent colds or influenza, but it may lessen symptoms.
2. Echinacea may cause adverse effects with anesthetics.
3. Echinacea should be discontinued 2 weeks before surgery.
4. Immunosuppressed patients should not use echinacea.
5. Transplant patients should not use echinacea.

strate increased allergic reactions to echinacea. Infertility patients should avoid using echinacea. Whether echinacea improves the effectiveness of antibiotics is unknown.

Do You UNDERSTAND?

See page 230 for Learning Activities related to this topic.

Key Words

Bacteriocidal The ability to kill bacteria.

Bacteriostatic The ability to prevent bacterial growth.

Cortisol A glucocorticoid hormone secreted from the adrenal cortex that increases the blood glucose level.

Encapsulation The process by which WBCs surround foreign material, such as bacteria.

Flavonoids Plant pigments responsible for the color of fruits and vegetables. Some flavonoids increase capillary wall stability (decrease capillary fragility) and scavenge free radicals, resulting in antioxidant properties. Other flavonoids have antiarthritis, antiinflammatory, antiviral, or antimutagenic properties.

Hepatotoxicity The ability to cause damage to the liver.

Hyaluronidase An enzyme that increases cellular permeability.

Phagocytosis Engulfment and digestion of bacteria and foreign particles by WBCs.

Urticaria An allergic reaction of the skin characterized by wheals or papules and intense itching.

www.herbalgram.org/
  browse.php/echinacea
www.herbmed.org/herbs/
  Echinacea.htm
http://altmed.creighton.edu/ech/

EPHEDRA

What IS Ephedra?

Ephedra is the dried stem of *Ephedra sinica, E. equisetina,* or *E. intermedia* that grows in India, Pakistan, and China. Ephedra is found in products such as "herbal fen-phen," "herbal ecstasy," "Xphoria," "Metabolife," "fatburners," or "Ellsinore pills." Ephedra is also known as ma huang, desert herb, joint fir, popotillo, sea grape, teamster's tea, yellow astringent, and yellow horse. Ephedra has been used for over 5000 years as a traditional Chinese medicine to treat colds, congestion, asthma, bronchitis, edema, and arthritis. In the United States, the herb is often used for "natural" weight loss, as a stimulant, or as an antidepressant. Ephedra's active ingredients are flavonoids, proanthocyanidins, and alkaloids. These ingredients are used to produce ephedrine for raising blood pressure and pseudoephedrine for cold remedies.

What You NEED TO KNOW

Actions

The herb ephedra causes weight loss by decreasing the appetite and increasing the body's metabolic rate. Ephedra causes norepinephrine release, which stimulates the hypothalamus, the body's metabolic control center. Unrestricted metabolic stimulation occurs when ephedra and caffeine are taken together because this combination blocks the negative feedback control of metabolism. Similar to epinephrine, ephedra stimulates the sympathetic nervous system to increase blood pressure, heart rate, and strength of cardiac contraction. Ephedra increases blood flow to the heart, brain, and muscles and decreases flow to the kidneys and liver. The herb is a bronchodilator, stimulates respiration, and is an antitussive. Ephedra has bacteriostatic, antiinflammatory, and diuretic effects. The herb relaxes the smooth muscle of the GI and urinary tracts.

Dose

- U.S. Food and Drug Administration (FDA) recommendations: no more than 8 mg per capsule and no more than 24 mg every day
- Capsules: commonly 15 to 20 mg three times daily
- Tinctures: (1:4) 6 to 8 cc three times daily
- Teas: 1 to 4 gm steeped in 150 cc water for 5 to 10 minutes

Side Effects

In addition to appetite suppression, ephedra may also cause nausea, vomiting, dry mouth and nasal mucous membranes, and bronchodilation. Hyperthermia may result from the increased metabolic rate. Significant cardiovascular side effects include hypertension, tachycardia, and peripheral vasoconstriction. Ephedra has also been linked with chest tightness, palpitations, angina, and coronary artery vasoconstriction and spasm. Use of this herb can cause cardiac dysrhythmias, myocardial infarction, myocarditis, cardiomyopathy, cardiac arrest, and sudden death.

CNS side effects include flushing, tingling, dizziness, restlessness, anxiety, irritability, personality changes, insomnia, headache, agitation, euphoria, psychosis, mania, tremor, vertigo, and headache. Ephedra may cause transient ischemic attack (TIA), cerebral hemorrhage, inflammation of cerebral blood vessels, ischemic stroke, seizure, and loss of consciousness. Ephedra can also cause euphoria, sweating, difficulty urinating, urinary retention, or kidney stones. Ephedra has also caused skeletal muscle destruction, eosinophilia-myalgia syndrome, acute hepatitis, and liver failure.

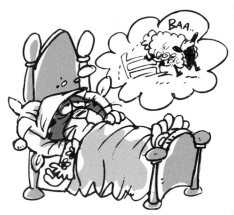

Indications and Uses

- Allergies
- Arthritis
- Asthma
- Athletic performance enhancement
- Bronchitis
- Bronchospasm
- Chills
- Depression
- Edema
- Emphysema
- Fever
- Hay fever
- Headache
- Nasal congestion
- Obesity
- Pertussis
- Rhinitis
- Upper respiratory infections:
  - Colds
  - Influenza
- Weight loss

1. Surgical patients taking diet products containing ephedra have increased anesthetic risks and should have preoperative ECGs.
2. An increased risk of sudden death is possible if ephedra products are taken before exercise.
3. Patients with severe kidney or liver disease should not take ephedra.
4. Patients with diabetes taking ephedra should have vigilant glucose monitoring.

1. Older adult patients with coronary artery or cardiovascular disease may have an increase risk of myocardial infarction, stroke, or death with ephedra use.
2. Obstetric patients may have a risk of hypertension and preterm labor if taking ephedra.

Contraindications and Precautions

Surgical patients should discontinue this herb 2 weeks before surgery to prevent dangerous interactions with anesthetic and cardiovascular drugs. Older adult patients may be more prone to the adverse effects of ephedra compared with the younger population. Patients who have angina, hypertension, coronary artery disease, or peripheral vascular disease should not take ephedra. In addition, patients with cerebral insufficiency, carotid artery disease, tremor, or a history of stroke or transient ischemic attacks should not use ephedra products. Ephedra may worsen glaucoma. Because of the metabolic rate and sympathetic nervous system effects, patients with hyperthyroidism or pheochromocytoma should also avoid this herb. Ephedra may interfere with blood-sugar control in patients with diabetes. Use of this herb may worsen urinary retention in patients, causing problems for patients with benign prostatic hypertrophy. Ephedra may contribute to the formation of kidney stones. Patients who have poor nutritional status from anorexia or bulimia should not use ephedra. Pregnant women should not take ephedra because it may cause preterm labor or hypertension. Ephedra use should be avoided in nursing women and children as well.

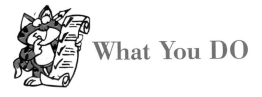

What You DO

Patient History

Surgical patients should be questioned about ephedra use and told to discontinue this herb 2 weeks before surgery. The **sympathomimetic** effects of ephedra may cause problems with anesthetic drugs, leading to dysrhythmias, swings in blood pressure, heart attack, and stroke. A preoperative ECG and assessment of vital signs during positioning changes should be included in the physical examination of patients using ephedra. These tests will help determine cardiac changes and fluid imbalances. Extra diligence in assessing older adult patients and individuals with coronary artery disease is required. These patients present an increased likelihood of experiencing complications from ephedra use. An in-depth cardiac history should be obtained. Important information for the nurse to obtain includes the number and type of angina attacks, exercise tolerance, and shortness-of-breath episodes. Caffeine may increase the problems with ephedrine, such as nervousness, tremors, or palpitations. Patients taking ephedra may develop insomnia. Patients with diabetes taking ephedra may have increased blood-sugar levels and need increased glucose monitoring and insulin intake.

Potential Drug Interactions

Drugs that may cause tachycardia or hypertension should not be used with ephedra (see the list of substances that have a potential ephedra-drug interaction). Patients on antihypertensives or antidepressants, such as monoamine oxidase inhibitors (MAOIs), should not use this herb. Taking caffeine-containing herbs and beverages such as black tea, coffee, cola nut, green tea, guarana, or mate may increase the stimulant effects of ephedra. In addition, the stimulant effects of theophylline may be increased. Cardiac dysrhythmias may result if ephedra is combined with digitalis. Ergotamine or oxytocin use with ephedra may result in hypertension. Amitriptyline might reduce the hypertensive effects of ephedra. Glyburide or other antidiabetic drugs may have decreased effectiveness when used with ephedrine. Dexamethasone may have an increased clearance and decrease effectiveness when taken with ephedrine. In addition, making the urine more acid or more alkaline may alter the excretion of ephedra; acidic urine may increase ephedra excretion, while alkaline urine may decrease urinary excretion of ephedra.

Potential Ephedra-Drug Interactions

- aminophylline
- amitriptyline
- anesthetics
- apomorphine
- beta blockers
- bromocriptine
- bronchodilators
- caffeine
- cardiac glycosides
- decongestants
- dexamethasone
- entacapone
- epinephrine
- ergotamine
- glyburide
- guanethidine
- halothane
- isoprenaline
- marijuana
- MAOIs:
  - phenelzine
  - selegiline
  - tranylcypromine
- methyldopa
- methylphenidate
- methylxanthines
- moclobemide
- oxytocin
- pseudoephedrine
- reserpine
- theophylline
- thyroid hormone
- tricyclic antidepressants

Patient Education

Patients should understand that ephedra or ephedrine is present in many diet aids and cold medications. The ingredient may be listed as pseudo-ephedrine hydrochloride on package inserts. Patients should be educated to not take ephedra with other diet aids, cold medications, and decongestants, which may increase the cardiovascular and CNS stimulation problems seen with ephedra. Patients should not use ephedra and Neo-Synephrine nasal sprays. This combination will compound the vasoconstriction problems. Patients with hypertension, cardiovascular disease, and cerebral vascular disease should not use ephedra. In addition, patients with cardiac dysrhythmia problems should not use ephedra. Patients with aortic and mitral valve problems are especially prone to rapid, cardiac dysrhythmias and should avoid using ephedra.

Ephedra is sometimes included in "natural booster" fruit drinks such as "smoothies." Patients should avoid taking ephedra with coffee, tea, and other caffeinated beverages. Ephedra should also be avoided with "headache" pain relievers and awake aids such as "No-Doz."

Do You UNDERSTAND?

See page 231 for Learning Activities related to this topic.

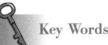 Key Words

Alkaloids Phytochemicals with potent pharmacologic effects reacting as bases that are alkaline in pH and that often have metabolites containing nitrogen. Alkaloids may depress the CNS, affect the autonomic system, or have other potent actions. Conventional drugs such as atropine, curare, cocaine, codeine, and morphine are derived from alkaloid plant constituents. Many plant alkaloids such as those in ephedra or lobelia have the ability to cross the blood-brain barrier and interact with neurotransmitters. Plant alkaloids may provide immune stimulation against pathogens.

Cardiomyopathy Abnormal enlargement of the cardiac muscle.

Eosinophilia-myalgia syndrome A syndrome characterized by increased eosinophils (a type of WBC) with severe muscle pain and edema in the extremities, especially the legs.

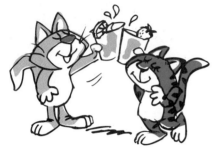

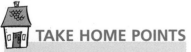

TAKE HOME POINTS

1. Ephedra should be discontinued 2 weeks before surgery.
2. Seizures, strokes, heart attack, and death have been reported with the use of ephedra.

www.mcp.edu/herbal/
ephedra/ephedra.htm

Flavonoids Plant pigments responsible for the color of fruits and vegetables. Some flavonoids decrease capillary fragility and scavenge free radicals, creating antioxidant properties. Other flavonoids have antiatherogenic, antiinflammatory, antiviral, or antimutagenic properties.

Hyperthermia Increased body temperature.

Mania A mental disorder in which an individual exhibits excessive periods of excitement.

Myocarditis Inflammation of the cardiac muscle.

Proanthocyanidins Condensed or complex tannins that are astringent and may bind and precipitate large molecules such as proteins from solutions. Tannins have antioxidant, antisecretory, and antiinflammatory effects on mucous membranes..

Psychosis A mental disorder in which an individual looses contact with reality and with his or her identity.

Sympathomimetic Sympathomimetic agents produce effects that are similar to those seen with stimulation of the sympathetic nervous system. These effects would include increased blood pressure, heart rate, and force of cardiac contraction.

Vertigo The feeling of moving around in space, causing dizziness.

EVENING PRIMROSE

What IS Evening Primrose?

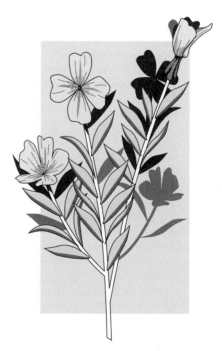

Evening primrose (*Oenothera biennis L., Oenothera biennis*) is grown throughout North America and Europe. The Latin name is derived from Greek word meaning "wine" and "a hunt," indicating its use to minimize hangovers from celebrations during hunting trips. Evening primrose is also known as EPO, fever plant, night willow-herb, or sun drop. The plant leaves, bark, flowers, roots, and seeds are used for medicinal purposes. Evening primrose oil is pressed from seeds to yield many essential, polyunsaturated fatty acids, such as linoleic acid and its metabolite, gamma-linoleic acid (GLA). The seeds have also been used as a coffee substitute during times of war. These essential fatty acids are the active ingredients of evening primrose.

What You NEED TO KNOW

1. **Do not take evening primrose with warfarin (Coumadin) or heparin.**
2. **Do not take evening primrose with antihypertensives, such as clonidine or captopril.**
3. **Patients with chronic and inflammatory conditions such as arthritis or low back pain are often prescribed NSAIDs for pain control. An increased risk of bleeding may occur in these patients if they take evening primrose.**
4. **Patients with circulatory disorders such as peripheral vascular disease, carotid artery disease, and diabetes are often prescribed anticoagulants or blood-thinning agents (aspirin or dipyridamole [Persantine]) for their disorder. The risk of bleeding may be increased in these patients if they take evening primrose.**
5. **Patients with cardiovascular disease or hypercholesterolemia often take an aspirin a day. These patients may have increased risk for bleeding if they are also taking evening primrose.**
6. **Do not take evening primrose with prochlorperazine (Compazine), promethazine (Phenergan), trifluoperazine (Stelazine), or chlorpromazine (Thorazine) because this combination may increase seizure activity.**

Actions

Evening primrose contains GLA, which decreases the production of prostaglandins and leukotrienes. These agents are responsible for inflammation. Thus evening primrose is used to decrease inflammation in many conditions. The herb inhibits coagulation; platelet aggregation can be decreased by 45% and bleeding time increased by 40%. The herb reduces allergy reactions and the blood pressure. Last, evening primrose has some antituberculosis, antimicrobial, and antibacterial actions. Evening primrose is comparable to penicillin in destroying some types of *Staphylococcus*, *Streptococcus*, *Pseudomonas*, and *Diplococcus* bacteria. Evening primrose is also effective against *Escherichia coli* infections.

Dose

- Mastalgia: 3 to 4 g/day
- PMS: 2 to 4 g/day
- Rheumatoid arthritis: 540 mg to 2.8 g per day
- Atopic eczema 6 to 8 g/day
- Children: 2 to 4 g/day

Side Effects

Side effects of evening primrose are usually rare and mild but include headache and GI upset in the form of nausea and diarrhea.

Indications and Uses

- Acne
- Alcoholism
- Alzheimer's disease
- Asthma
- Atopic dermatitis
- Cancer
- Colitis
- Coronary artery disease
- Diabetic neuropathy
- Eczema
- Endometriosis
- Hangovers
- Hyperactivity in children
- Hypercholesterolemia
- Hypertension
- Irritable bowel syndrome
- Mastalgia
- Menopause
- Multiple sclerosis
- Peptic ulcer disease

- Post viral fatigue syndrome
- PMS
- Psoriasis
- Raynaud's phenomenon
- Rheumatoid arthritis

- Schizophrenia
- Sjögren's syndrome
- Ulcerative colitis
- Whooping cough

Contraindications and Precautions

Evening primrose should not be used during pregnancy because it may interfere with the normal progression of labor, which may increase the incidence of oxytocin labor augmentation and vacuum extraction. Seizure activity has been reported in patients with schizophrenia taking phenothiazine medications and evening primrose. Phenothiazines and evening primrose should not be used together. Prochlorperazine (Compazine) and promethazine (Phenergan) are examples of phenothiazine medications. Although uncertainty exists as to whether evening primrose lowers the seizure threshold, patients with epilepsy and individuals prone to seizure activity should not take this herb.

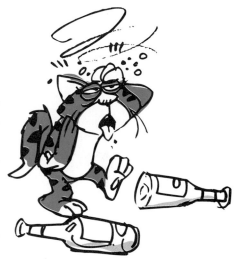

 # What You DO

Patient History

When presenting for surgery or invasive procedures, patients need to be questioned concerning their over-the-counter medications and herbal medication intake. The herb should be discontinued 2 weeks before surgery to prevent interactions with anesthetic drugs. Because evening primrose increases the bleeding time, patients should be questioned about bleeding and bruising tendencies. Further laboratory tests, such as coagulation studies, may be indicated preoperatively. If patients are experiencing bleeding problems, nausea, or diarrhea, the amount of herb taken should be decreased.

The patient's history should be reviewed for schizophrenia or seizure disorders. Patients taking phenothiazines or those being treated for seizure disorders should not take evening primrose.

Potential Drug Interactions

The anticoagulant effects of other herbal medications and other blood-thinning medications taken on a routine basis may be increased. Individuals

Older adults often experience problems with cardiovascular disease and hypertension. Evening primrose may increase the effects of blood-thinning and antihypertensive medications used to treat these disorders.

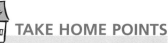 **TAKE HOME POINTS**

Patients who are pregnant may increase the complications of labor and delivery if they take evening primrose.

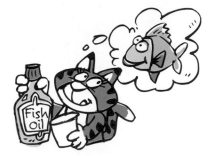

taking warfarin or heparin should not take evening primrose because clotting mechanisms may be inhibited. Patients taking aspirin or NSAIDs may experience increased bleeding or bruising when also taking evening primrose. Many herbs such as gingko and garlic or dietary supplements such as fish oil and vitamin E may increase bleeding times, especially if taken together with evening primrose.

Evening primrose may increase the blood pressure–lowering effects of antihypertensive medications. In addition, evening primrose may cause problems with anesthetic drugs, resulting in severe hypotension.

Patient Education

Patients with hypertension or cardiovascular disease should be cautious when taking evening primrose. Reductions in blood pressure may decrease blood flow across plaque-filled arteries, resulting in ischemia or infarction. Lowered cerebral blood flow may cause decreased alertness and level of consciousness. End-organ damage may occur when blood flow falls to high oxygen–demand tissues, such as the heart, brain, spinal cord, or kidneys.

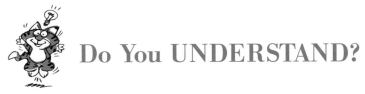

Do You UNDERSTAND?

See page 232 for Learning Activities related to this topic.

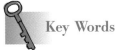

Key Words

Essential Required elements that are not manufactured by the body; they must be obtained in food.

Leukotrienes Metabolites of arachidonic acid with potent bronchoconstriction and vasodilatory effects that increase vascular permeability. Leukotrienes are released by mast cells in response to histamine during allergic or inflammatory reactions.

Polyunsaturated Relating to long carbon chains that do not have their full complement of hydrogen atoms. As such, some of the carbons will have double and triple bonds between each carbon molecule.

Prostaglandins Endogenous chemicals that are derived from arachidonic acid produced through the cyclooxygenase pathway in the allergic or inflammatory response. Prostaglandins promote inflammation, bronchoconstriction, pain, and uterine contraction.

www.agric.gov.ab.ca/
crops/special/medconf/
ibrahimf.html
www.hcrc.org/faqs/
eveprim.html

FEVERFEW

What IS Feverfew?

A member of the daisy, marigold, and dandelion family, feverfew (*Tanacetum parthenium*) is a perennial flower native to Europe. Feverfew gets its name from the Latin *febrifugia*, meaning "fever reducing." Other names for feverfew are featherfew, featherfoil, febrifuge plant, altimisa, bachelor's button, midsummer daisy, and Santa Maria. The leaves and flowers are used medicinally. The active ingredients are parthenolide, sesquiterpenoid lactones, essential oils, melatonin, and flavonoids.

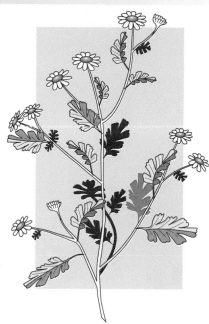

What You NEED TO KNOW

Actions

Feverfew has antiinflammatory properties by inhibiting arachidonic acid and releasing prostaglandins. Feverfew also decreases serotonin and histamine release. Feverfew inhibits platelet aggregation and can also act as a bitter tonic.

Dose

- 0.7 to 2.0 ml 1:1 tincture every day
- 50 to 150 mg dried herb every day
- 0.6 mg standardized parthenolide twice daily
- 2.5 fresh leaves daily

Side Effects

Contact dermatitis has occurred with topical use of feverfew. Oral feverfew can cause mouth sores, irritation, and inflammation, as well as abdominal pain, indigestion, diarrhea, flatulence, nausea, and vomiting. Rare cases of irregular heartbeat, constipation, and dizziness have been reported. Individuals allergic to ragweed, chrysanthemums, marigolds, and daisies may also be allergic to feverfew.

Older adults have cardiovascular, cerebrovascular, and peripheral vascular disease more frequently compared with the general population. Thus these individuals may be on prescription blood-thinning agents more often and may be a special population at risk for herbal-drug interactions.

Indications and Uses

- Allergies
- Antiinflammatory
- Arthritis
- Asthma
- Digestive aid
- Dizziness
- Fever
- Gas, bloating
- Insect bites (external)
- Insect repellent (external)

- Menstrual problems
- Migraine headaches
- Nausea and vomiting
- Pain relief
- Prevention of blood clots
- Psoriasis
- Stomachache
- Tinnitus
- Vertigo

Contraindications and Precautions

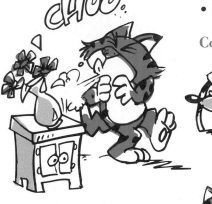

Individuals who are allergic to ragweed, chrysanthemums, marigolds, and daisies should avoid feverfew. Feverfew can induce labor and stimulate uterine contractions and should not be used by women who are pregnant or planning to become pregnant. Children under 2 years of age should also not use feverfew. Surgical patients should stop taking this herb 2 weeks before surgery.

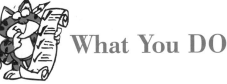

What You DO

Patient History

Patients taking feverfew should have medications reviewed to find other medications that may also cause bruising and bleeding. Surgical patients should not take this herb before surgery because it may increase blood loss or lead to hemorrhage after surgery. The use of feverfew 2 weeks before surgery may cause anticoagulation. Patients should be questioned about their bleeding tendencies. Further laboratory testing, such as coagulation studies, may be needed.

Patients who have hay fever or allergies to chrysanthemums, marigolds, daisies, or ragweed should not take feverfew. A risk of crossover allergic reactions may occur. Patients should not take other herbals such as echinacea that also have crossover allergic reactions with ragweed and members of the daisy family.

1. **Do not take feverfew with warfarin (Coumadin) or heparin.**
2. **Do not take feverfew with gingko, ginseng, fish oil, or vitamin E.**
3. **Do not take feverfew with aspirin, ibuprofen, nabumetone (Relafen), or other NSAIDs.**

Potential Drug Interactions

Other medications such as NSAIDs, aspirin, or Persantine also decrease the patient's ability to clot. Feverfew may add to the anticoagulant effects of these agents. Patients taking warfarin or heparin should avoid using feverfew because it may increase the anticlotting properties. Feverfew should not be combined with other alternative medicines that also decrease clotting. Garlic, ginger, gingko, ginseng, red clover, fish oil, or vitamin E, to name a few, may decrease clotting.

Patient Education

When the leaves are taken orally, feverfew can cause mouth sores or loss of taste. Should this event occur, patients should stop taking the leaf and seek a different form of feverfew preparation after the mouth sores have healed. Allergic reactions and contact dermatitis can occur in sensitive individuals, which is more likely to occur in those who are allergic to ragweed or members of the daisy family.

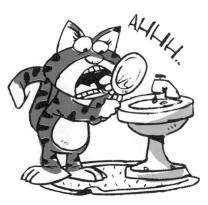

 # Do You UNDERSTAND?

See page 233 for Learning Activities related to this topic.

 ## Key Words

Arachidonic acid A chemical that is part of the inflammatory response.

Bitter Bitter-tasting plant components that are consumed to promote digestion through stimulating gastric motility and acid secretion.

Contact dermatitis Skin reaction caused by touching an allergy-producing substance.

Essential oils Aromatic plant oils isolated by steam distillation often used for perfumes, aromatherapy, or medicinal effects. Many essential oils have antispasmodic, expectorant, sedative, analgesic, or antimicrobial properties.

Flavonoids Plant pigments responsible for the color of fruits and vegetables. Some flavonoids increase capillary wall stability (decrease capillary fragility) and scavenge free radicals, resulting in antioxidant properties. Other flavonoids have antiarthritis, antiinflammatory, antiviral, or antimutagenic properties.

1. Patients with chronic inflammatory conditions such as arthritis, fibromyalgia, bursitis, or low back pain are often prescribed NSAIDs for pain control. The risk of herb-drug interactions may increase in these populations.

2. Patients with circulatory disorders such as peripheral vascular disease, carotid artery disease, and diabetes are often prescribed anticoagulants or blood-thinning agents (aspirin or dipyridamole [Persantine]) for their disorder. The risk of herb-drug interactions may increase in these populations.

3. Patients with cardiovascular disease or hypercholesterolemia routinely taking an aspirin a day may be an at-risk population for bleeding complications if they are also taking feverfew.

Histamine A substance released from injured mast cells in the body that causes flushing of the skin, vasodilation, increased capillary permeability, lowered blood pressure, and bronchial smooth muscle contraction or constriction.

Prostaglandins Endogenous chemicals that are derived from arachidonic acid produced through the cyclooxygenase pathway in the allergic or inflammatory response. Prostaglandins promote inflammation, bronchoconstriction, pain, and uterine contraction.

Melatonin A hormone manufactured by the pituitary gland from serotonin that regulates sleep cycles and has antioxidant properties.

Serotonin A neurotransmitter in the CNS that has strong vasoconstrictor actions.

Sesquiterpenoid lactones Bitter principle ingredients in herbs that have antibacterial, antiparasitic, and antifungal actions.

www.herbmed.org/herbs/
herb124.htm
www.holisticonline.com/Herbal-
Med/_Herbs/h57.htm

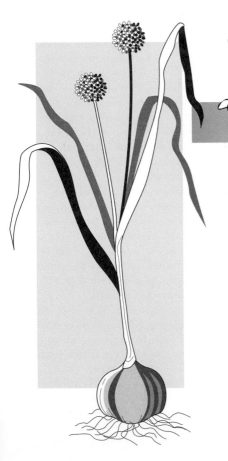

GARLIC

What IS Garlic?

Garlic (*Allium sativum*) is a plant similar to the lily with a bulb encased in white skin. Garlic is also known as Allium, camphor of the poor, clove garlic, and stinking rose. Used for thousands of years in ancient Egyptian and Chinese medicine, garlic is cultivated for use as a spice and medicinal herb. Garlic was used instead of penicillin and applied directly to the wounds of Russian soldiers after antibiotic supplies were gone during World War II. Garlic's smell is produced when garlic cloves are crushed and alliin is converted into allicin, the active ingredient. Fresh garlic contains more alliin. Therefore fresh garlic cloves contain the most active ingredient. Odorless garlic contains a standardized level of alliin.

What You NEED TO KNOW

Actions

Garlic is consumed for prevention of cancer and heart attack and to lower cholesterol. Garlic slows blood clotting, protects against free radicals, and lowers total cholesterol. Garlic also causes moderate decreases in blood pressure and may reduce serum cholesterol and triglycerides, thereby preventing cardiovascular disease. Garlic may slow atherosclerosis and helps keep the aorta elastic. Garlic decreases coagulation by inhibiting platelet aggregation. Garlic may reduce blood sugar by stimulating the release of insulin by the pancreas.

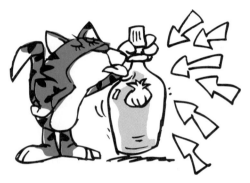

Garlic has antibiotic actions and has been used for treatment of colds, asthma, and yeast infections. Garlic oil may reduce the pain of otitis media but may not be effective in curing the infection. Garlic may increase the activity of WBCs and is an effective antibiotic for *Staphylococcus* and *Streptococcus* bacteria. The herb is also useful against viruses such as herpes and parainfluenza, parasites, and fungi. Garlic's antimicrobial activity may be most effective with topical application.

Dose

- 900 mg of garlic powder with 10 to 12 mg standardized alliin, 1.3%
- One to two cloves of fresh garlic every day

Side Effects

One half of people who consume garlic acquire bad breath. Low blood pressure, allergy, headache, or sweating occurs less frequently when taking garlic. In large doses, headache, facial flushing, rapid pulse, orthostatic

1. **Nondietary or excessive intake of garlic may increase the risk of postoperative bleeding.**
2. **Excessive intake of garlic may contribute to miscarriage in pregnant women.**
3. **Use of garlic by nursing mothers may change the flavor of breast milk.**
4. **Patients with diabetes taking garlic should have close glucose monitoring.**
5. **Patients taking garlic preoperatively should have PT, partial thromboplastin time (PTT), and INR laboratory values.**

hypotension, or insomnia may occur. Garlic may irritate the GI tract and can cause stomach upset, heartburn, nausea, vomiting, diarrhea, gas, and bloating. Skin irritation or blistering may occur with direct skin contact. Excessive consumption of garlic has resulted in prolonged bleeding time, spinal and epidural hematomas, and postoperative hemorrhage.

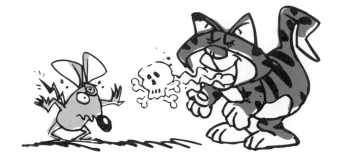

Indications and Uses

- Allergies
- Amoebic dysentery
- Arthritis
- Asthma
- Atherosclerosis
- Athlete's foot
- Cancer prevention
- Candida
- Cardiovascular disease
- Colds
- Diabetes
- Diarrhea
- Fungal infection
- *Helicobacter pylori*

- Hypercholesterolemia
- Hyperlipidemia
- Hypertension
- Myocardial infarction
- Otitis media
- Ringworm
- Snakebites
- Stomachache
- Tick bite prevention
- Traveler's diarrhea
- Tuberculosis
- Vaginitis
- Whooping cough

Contraindications and Precautions

Garlic is generally regarded as safe, but it can thin the blood. Therefore patients should stop taking garlic 2 weeks before surgery or labor and delivery. Pregnant or nursing women, young children, and people with kidney or liver disease should use garlic cautiously. Patients with diabetes should not take garlic because it may affect insulin requirements. Patients with digestive problems should avoid garlic. In addition, patients who have AIDS or human immunodeficiency virus (HIV) infection should not take this herb because of potential drug interactions.

Older adult patients with cardiovascular and peripheral vascular diseases may take anticoagulant medications and may have increased risk of bleeding with garlic.

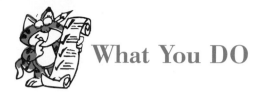

What You DO

Patient History

Preoperative patients should be questioned about herbal medicine use. Patients should be instructed to discontinue the use of garlic at least 2 weeks before surgery. Patients taking garlic should be questioned about their tendencies for bleeding and bruising. If garlic is combined with antiinflammatory analgesics or anticoagulant drugs, laboratory tests, such as coagulation studies, may be indicated preoperatively. In patients exhibiting increased bleeding times, elective surgery should be postponed until clotting returns to normal, which may take 2 weeks.

Potential Drug Interactions

Garlic may increase the anticoagulation seen with anticoagulants and medications that decrease clotting, such as warfarin, pentoxifylline, indomethacin, dipyridamole, aspirin, and ibuprofen. Garlic might also decrease blood clotting when combined with herbs such as gingko, feverfew, red clover, kava kava, ginger, ginseng, or with dietary supplements such as fish oil or vitamin E. Garlic may increase the blood sugar lowering effects of diabetes drugs such as insulin. The herb may prevent **hepatotoxicity** associated with acetaminophen. Garlic may enhance the action of cholesterol-lowering drugs. Because garlic may inhibit the cytochrome CYP450 3A4 in the liver, drugs such as cyclosporine or other immunosuppressants should not be combined with garlic. Protease inhibitor drugs, such as saquinavir or nonnucleoside reverse transcriptase inhibitors or antiretroviral drugs, are also metabolized by this route and should be avoided with garlic.

Other drugs metabolized by CYP450 3A4 include birth control pills, calcium-channel blockers, fexofenadine, chemotherapeutic drugs, losartan, antifungals, glucocorticoids, and cisapride. The metabolism of these drugs may be altered when taking garlic.

Many anesthetics, such as midazolam (Versed) or diazepam (Valium), are metabolized by liver enzymes that are inhibited by garlic. This property would make drug actions unpredictable.

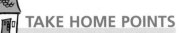

TAKE HOME POINTS

1. Garlic may modestly decrease cholesterol but should not be used as the only treatment for hyperlipidemia.
2. Increased garlic in the diet, but not garlic supplements, may decrease the risk of cardiovascular disease or GI or prostate cancer.
3. Patients should tell their physician or surgeon if they are taking garlic.
4. Garlic should be discontinued before surgery to prevent excessive blood loss.
5. Garlic may prevent tick bites.

Patient Education

Surgical patients should stop taking garlic at least 2 weeks before surgery or invasive procedures and inform their surgeon. Patients should be educated about the anticoagulant effects of garlic. Patients should not combine garlic with other medications that inhibit blood clotting. Patients with thrombocytopenia and clotting disorders should be cautioned against the use of garlic and other herbal medications that have anticoagulant effects. Pregnant women should discontinue taking garlic as they near their delivery date or 2 weeks before a scheduled labor and delivery.

Garlic may interfere with the medical treatment of diabetes. Increased blood glucose monitoring is required to avoid hypoglycemia. Severe or prolonged hypoglycemia can lead to loss of consciousness, coma, seizures, and, eventually, death.

Do You UNDERSTAND?

See pages 233 and 234 for Learning Activities related to this topic.

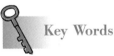

Key Words

Free radicals Reactive molecules with unpaired electrons that may destroy or damage other molecules to accept an electron. Free radicals may interfere with oxidative metabolism of nutrients and cause an increased incidence of cancer, cardiovascular, or cerebrovascular and inflammatory diseases. Antioxidants found in some herbs and vitamins decrease free-radical formation and oxidation of molecules.

Hepatotoxicity The ability to cause damage to the liver.

Hypoglycemia Low blood-sugar level.

Thrombocytopenia Low levels of platelet cells.

www.mcp.edu/herbal/
garlic/garlic.pdf
www.mistral.co.uk/garlic/

GINGER

What IS Ginger?

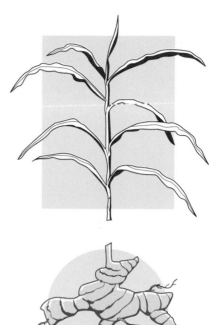

Ginger (*Zingiber officinale*) is a knobby root that grows underground. Preferring a tropical climate, ginger grows in Asia, the West Indies, Jamaica, and Africa. Two different types of ginger are available in stores: black and white. Black ginger is manufactured by scalding ginger roots in boiling water. After boiling, the roots are placed in the sun to dry. White ginger, considered the better type, is scraped clean and then dried, without boiling. The active ingredients in ginger are gingerol, shogaol, and zingerone.

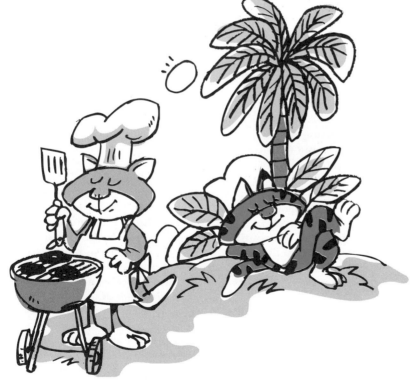

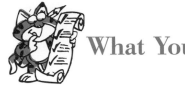

What You NEED TO KNOW

Actions

Ginger increases gastric and intestinal motility, meaning that stomach and intestinal contents move through the GI tract more rapidly. Ginger reduces thromboxane B_2 synthesis, thereby decreasing platelet aggregation. These processes are important in coagulation and clotting. In animal studies, gingerol is a positive **inotrope** by increasing calcium uptake.

Dose

- 1 to 4 g/day, total dose

Motion sickness:

- 1 g 30 minutes before departing
- 500 to 1000 mg after 4 hours if nausea returns

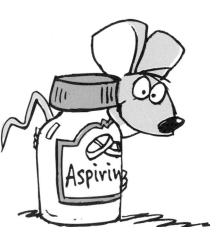

1. **Patients taking warfarin (Coumadin) or heparin should avoid ginger.**
2. **Patients taking nifedipine or diltiazem should avoid ginger.**
3. **Patients with gallstones should not take ginger.**
4. **Patients should not take ginger with gingko, ginseng, garlic, and vitamin E.**
5. **Patients taking aspirin, ibuprofen, or nabumetone (Relafen) on a routine basis should avoid ginger.**
6. **Patients with chronic and inflammatory conditions such as arthritis, fibromyalgia, bursitis, or low back pain are often prescribed NSAIDs routinely for pain control. The risk of herb-drug interactions may be increased in these populations.**
7. **Patients with circulatory disorders such as peripheral vascular disease, carotid artery disease, and diabetes are often prescribed blood-thinning agents for their disorder. Therefore the risk of herb-drug interactions may be increased in these populations.**
8. **Aspirin or dipyridamole (Persantine) decrease blood clotting.**
9. **Patients with cardiovascular disease or hypercholesterolemia routinely taking an aspirin a day may be an at-risk population for bleeding complications if they are also taking ginger.**
10. **Patients taking antacids should avoid ginger because of stomach-irritating effects of ginger.**

Side Effects

Side effects of ginger are usually rare and mild. However, in high doses, ginger has the potential to cause heart palpitations. In addition, ginger may inhibit coagulation.

Indications and Uses

- Alcoholic gastritis
- Atherosclerosis
- Chemotherapy-induced nausea and vomiting
- Dyspepsia
- Flatulent (gaseous) colic
- Ileus (without inflammation)
- Migraine headache
- Motion sickness
- Nausea
- Prevention of postoperative nausea and vomiting
- Rheumatoid arthritis
- Vomiting

Contraindications and Precautions

Ginger should not be used for morning sickness until maternal and fetal risks are determined. Patients with gallstones should not take ginger. The use of ginger for prevention of postoperative nausea and vomiting is currently being studied.

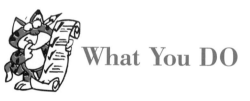 **What You DO**

Patient History

When presenting for surgery or invasive procedures, patients need to be questioned concerning their over-the-counter and herbal medication intake. The patient should be questioned about bleeding and bruising tendencies. Further laboratory tests, such as coagulation studies, may be indicated preoperatively.

Potential Drug Interactions

Ginger may enhance the blood-thinning effects of anticoagulant medications. The anticoagulant effects of herbal medications and other blood-thinning medications taken on a routine basis may also be increased. Stimulation of calcium uptake by ginger may work against the actions of calcium channel–blocking agents.

1. Pregnancy and fetal safety issues may exist with ginger.
2. Ginger may increase heart rate and heart contractility, which may worsen cardiac ischemia in patients with coronary heart disease (CHD). Older adults often have an increased incidence of CHD.

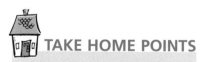 **TAKE HOME POINTS**

1. Because ginger increases intestinal motility, patients with intestinal tumors, obstruction, or perforation should not take ginger.
2. Patients who are pregnant should not take ginger for morning sickness because it might increase the risk of miscarriage.

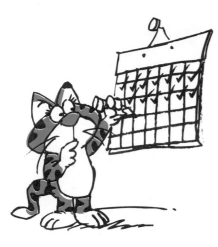

Patient Education

Patients should be educated to the anticoagulant effects of ginger. Patients with thrombocytopenia and clotting disorders should not use herbal medications that have anticoagulation effects. Patients should stop taking ginger 2 weeks before invasive procedures and inform their surgeon. Patients should be educated to avoid taking ginger during pregnancy or lactation. Lastly, patients should be encouraged to talk with their health care provider concerning their use of ginger and other complementary and alternative medications.

Do You UNDERSTAND?

See pages 234 and 235 for Learning Activities related to this topic.

Key Words

Inotrope Pertaining to the contracting ability of the heart.
Thrombocytopenia Low platelet levels.

www.healthlink.com.au/
nat_lib/htm-data/
htm-herb/bhp780.htm

GINGKO

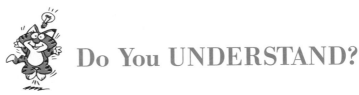

What IS Gingko?

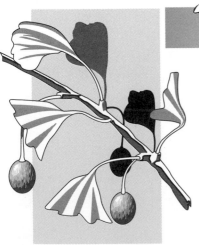

Gingko is made from the leaves of the *Gingko biloba* tree. This tree is one of the oldest surviving tree species. Gingko is also known as Japanese silver apricot, kew tree, maidenhair tree, salisburia, and fossil tree. The leaves have been used as medicine in China for 4000 years. Gingko was brought to Europe and the United States in the 1700s. Common forms of gingko extract include tablets, capsules, and sublingual sprays; it is also available as tea but does not deliver a therapeutic dose in this form. The leaves contain several active ingredients; terpenoids and flavonoids are the most important of the active ingredients. Another ingredient, gingkolic acid, may be toxic and is removed during production.

What You NEED TO KNOW

Actions

Gingko causes arterial and venous vasodilation. This action may result in an increase in cerebral blood flow and tissue perfusion. Gingko may also inhibit arterial spasms and decrease capillary permeability. Erythrocyte aggregation and blood **viscosity** may be lowered as well. These actions are probably the result of **prostaglandins** or the vasoactive effects of catecholamines. Gingko decreases clotting and has antioxidant properties. Gingko's antioxidant properties may help after cardiac infarction or ischemia and postcardiopulmonary bypass.

Gingko may help mental function by its effects on nerve cells. Gingko appears to stimulate nerve cells and helps protect nerve cells from damage caused by harmful **free radicals**. Gingko may also increase cerebral blood flow and may help protect against ischemia from vascular accidents and strokes.

Dose

- 120 to 240 mg/day (may divide doses) for dementia
- 120 to 160 mg/day in 2 to 3 doses for peripheral vascular disease (PVD) and vertigo

Side Effects

The side effects of gingko include GI irritation, headache, dizziness, and bleeding. An allergic reaction may occur if contact is made with gingko fruit, pulp, or leaves. A **cross-sensitivity** may occur in individuals who are allergic to poison ivy, poison oak, or poison sumac. The seeds and pulp may be toxic if swallowed.

Indications and Uses

- Acute mountain sickness
- Alzheimer's disease
- Arterial occlusive disease
- Attention-deficit hyperactivity disorder (ADHD)
- Cardiac disease
- Dementia
- Depression
- Dysentery
- Headache
- Hypercholesterolemia
- Improve overall brain function

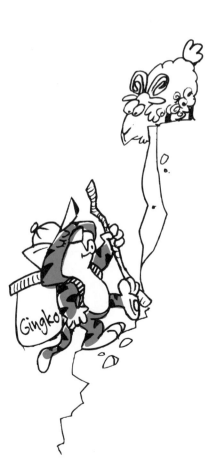

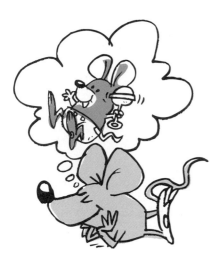

- Improve systemic circulation
- Increasing mental alertness
- Intermittent claudication
- Macular degeneration
- PMS
- Potent antioxidant
- PVD

- Reverse sexual dysfunction caused by selective serotonin reuptake inhibitors (SSRIs)
- Thrombosis
- Tinnitus
- Vertigo

Contraindications and Precautions

Because of its anticoagulant properties, gingko should not be taken with aspirin, warfarin, and heparin. Patients with epilepsy should avoid gingko because the anticonvulsive effects of treatment medications may be reduced. Taking large amounts of gingko may reduce fertility in both men and women. Thus those desiring to conceive should not take gingko.

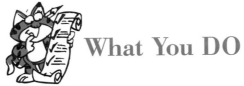 # What You DO

Patient History

The nurse should assess any over-the-counter, herbal, or prescriptive drug use. Patients taking gingko should be asked about their bleeding and bruising tendencies. Further laboratory testing, such as coagulation studies, may be needed before invasive procedures.

Potential Drug Interactions

Gingko may decrease the effects of anticonvulsants. Gingko appears to lower the seizure threshold, thereby increasing the risk of seizures.

Gingko use may cause bleeding problems in patients taking aspirin, warfarin, heparin, NSAIDs, or other antiplatelet drugs. Garlic, feverfew, ginger, red clover, and passionflower also affect coagulation. These herbs should not be taken with gingko.

Gingko may increase blood pressure when taken with thiazide diuretics. Gingko use in hypertensive patients who are also taking thiazide diuretics may make blood pressure control and management more difficult.

Patient Education

Patients should be educated to the anticoagulative effects of gingko. Patients should stop taking ginger 2 weeks before invasive procedures and inform their surgeon. Patients with thrombocytopenia or other clotting disorders should be advised against using gingko.

Patients with a history of epilepsy should be cautioned against using gingko with anticonvulsant medications because gingko decreases the seizure thresholds. Gingko is not for use in pregnant or breast-feeding patients.

Do You UNDERSTAND?

See page 236 for Learning Activities related to this topic.

Key Words

Cross-sensitivity When allergies to one agent increase the likelihood that another related agent will also cause an allergic reaction.

Flavonoids Plant pigments responsible for the color of fruits and vegetables. Some flavonoids increase capillary wall stability (decrease capillary fragility) and scavenge free radicals, resulting in antioxidant properties. Other flavonoids have antiarthritis, antiinflammatory, antiviral, or antimutagenic properties.

Free radicals Reactive molecules with unpaired electrons that may destroy or damage other molecules to accept an electron. Free radicals may interfere with oxidative metabolism of nutrients and cause an increased incidence of cancer, as well as cardiovascular or cerebrovascular and inflammatory diseases. Antioxidants found in some herbs and vitamins decrease free-radical formation and oxidation of molecules.

Prostaglandins Endogenous chemicals that are derived from arachidonic acid produced through the cyclooxygenase pathway in the allergic or inflammatory response. Prostaglandins promote inflammation, bronchoconstriction, pain, and uterine contraction.

1. **Patients taking warfarin or aspirin should avoid gingko.**
2. **Patients taking anticonvulsive medications should avoid gingko.**
3. **Patients should not take gingko with other herbs such as ginger or ginseng that decrease clotting.**
4. **Gingko should not be taken if pregnant or breast-feeding.**
5. **Patients should report any bruising or bleeding to their health care provider.**
6. **An occasional allergic reaction may be seen with gingko use, especially in patients who are also allergic to poison ivy.**

http://altmed.creighton.
edu/migraine/herbal.htm
www.personalhealthzone.com/
gingko.html
www.herbmed.org/herbs/herb1.
htm

Seizure threshold The lowest point at which a seizure can be made to occur.

Terpenoids Secondary metabolites or phytochemicals in the essential oils of the plant.

Thrombocytopenia Low platelet levels.

Viscosity Referring to the tendency to stick together or clump.

GINSENG

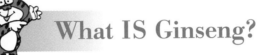

What IS Ginseng?

Ginseng is one of the most expensive and most popular herbs in the world. Although several types exist, the two most popular are Asian or Chinese ginseng (*Panax ginseng*). The second type of ginseng is American ginseng (*Panax quinquefolius*). The name *panax* comes from the Greek word for panacea meaning "cure all." American ginseng is also known as red berry, sang, and Wisconsin ginseng. Asian ginseng is also known as ginseng root, Japanese ginseng, Korean ginseng, Korean red, Oriental ginseng, and Panax ginseng. Although ginseng has become popular in the United States only recently, it has been used in Oriental cultures for over 2000 years. The American type is the most common and is sought after mainly for its root system. The Asian variety is usually dried, while the American version usually undergoes less preparation. The active ingredients in ginseng are ginsenosides. Ginseng also contains saponins, polysaccharides, and essential oils.

What You NEED TO KNOW

Actions

The ginsenosides are the active ingredients in ginseng. About 12 ginsenosides have been found, but their small amounts make them hard to separate. The different ginsenosides sometimes work against each other. Because of these opposing features, ginseng is called an adaptogen. As an adaptogen, ginseng balances bodily functions, improves stamina, and increases resistance to stress. Ginsenoside actions include antiarrhythmic activity, anticoagulation, and an increase in fibrinolysis. Ginseng has analgesic, antiinflammatory, immune stimulation, and antitumor properties. Ginseng may help to prevent wide swings in the blood glucose level. Ginseng has negative inotropic and chronotropic effects on the heart.

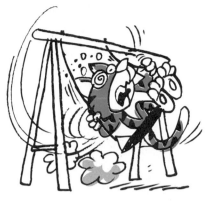

Dose

- 1 to 2 g of the root every day
- 100 to 200 mg of the extract three times daily

Note: Contents of commercial preparations vary.

Side Effects

Side effects of ginseng vary by preparation and dosage. Adverse reactions include chest pain, headache, hypertension, impotence, epistaxis, insomnia, nausea, nervousness, palpitations, and vomiting. Ginseng abuse syndrome is characterized by hypertension, insomnia, anxiety, agitation, and diarrhea. Large doses of ginseng or prolonged use can cause symptoms of estrogen excess. These symptoms include mastalgia, vaginal break-through bleeding, nausea, and bloating. These reactions are uncommon.

Indications and Uses

- Anemia
- Antidepressant
- Aphrodisiac
- Asthma
- Cancer
- Depression
- Diuretic
- Dysentery
- Hangover
- Headache
- Healing
- Immune stimulation
- Improve concentration
- Improve stamina
- Inflamed tissues
- Insomnia
- Menopause
- Mental fatigue
- Reduce activity of thymus gland
- Sedative
- Sleep aid
- Soothe inflammation of internal organs
- Stress resistance
- Type 2 diabetes
- Vomiting

1. **Do not take ginseng with hypoglycemic agents or insulin.**
2. **Do not take ginseng with MAOIs.**
3. **Do not take ginseng with anticoagulants.**
4. **Do not take ginseng with gingko, ginger, or other medications that also decrease clotting.**
5. **Do not take ginseng with propranolol or metoprolol.**
6. **Do not take ginseng with nifedipine.**

Contraindications and Precautions

Use this herb cautiously in patients with heart conditions, hypertension, or diabetes. Patients receiving steroid therapy should also be cautious when taking ginseng. Ginseng appears to be excreted into breast milk and should be avoided in pregnant women or those who are breast-feeding.

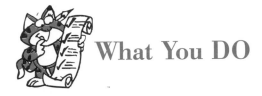

What You DO

Patient History

Patient history should be obtained concerning the use of over-the-counter or prescription drugs, as well as the use of other herbal medication. Patients should be cautioned that ginseng preparations vary in their form and dosage. Also, some products have been found to contain other ingredients as well. Caution should be used because ephedrine, caffeine, and other herbal stimulants may be added to some preparations to meet the label promises of an energy boost.

Potential Drug Interactions

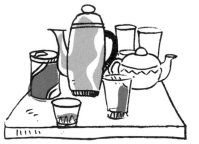

Ginseng may decrease blood glucose, and its use with oral hyperglycemic agents or insulin should be avoided. Using ginseng with MAOIs may result in headaches, tremors, and mania. Ginseng may also increase the anticoagulant effects of warfarin and aspirin.

Ginseng should not be used with estrogens or corticosteroids because of the possibility of additive effects and increased actions of both medicines. Ginseng appears to increase the effect of digoxin. Last, ginseng increases the stimulant effects of coffee, tea, other caffeine-containing beverages, and herbal stimulants.

Ginseng may add to the negative inotropic and chronotropic effects of other medications. Calcium-channel blockers and many anesthetic agents have negative inotropic effects. Beta-blocking agents, calcium-channel blockers, and many narcotics have negative chronotropic effects.

Patient Education

Instruct patients to watch for symptoms such as nervousness and palpitations because these may be signs of toxicity. Teach patients with diabetes the signs and symptoms of hypoglycemia, and advise them on daily blood-sugar monitoring.

Any patient with a preexisting medical condition should check with their physician before beginning ginseng. Patients with heart failure may experience worsening of their condition because of depressed cardiac contractility.

Warn patients that, when ginseng is used with stimulants, hypertension, insomnia, diarrhea, and appetite suppression may occur. Patients with schizophrenia should avoid ginseng because cases of insomnia, agitation, and **mania** have been reported.

Ginseng should be stopped 2 weeks before surgery to avoid possible additive cardiac depressant effects with ginseng and anesthetic agents. Increased cardiac depression during anesthesia might cause severe hypotension and cardiovascular collapse during surgery.

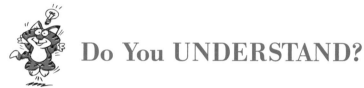 # Do You UNDERSTAND?

See pages 236 and 237 for Learning Activities related to this topic.

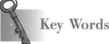 ## Key Words

Adaptogen Herbal medicine that improves or supports adaptation to the stress response.

Chronotropic Pertaining to heart rate. Negative chronotropic agents would reduce the heart rate, while positive chronotropic agents would increase the heart rate.

Essential oils Aromatic plant oils isolated by steam distillation often used for perfumes, aromatherapy, or medicinal effects. Many essential oils have antispasmodic, expectorant, sedative, analgesic, or antimicrobial properties.

Fibrinolysis Breaking down the fibrin strands that form a clot.

Inotropic Pertaining to the contracting ability of the heart. A negative inotropic agent would decrease the heart's ability to contract and pump blood out of the left ventricle. A positive inotropic agent would increase cardiac contractility and output.

Mania A mental disorder in which an individual exhibits excessive periods of excitement.

Mastalgia Pain in one or both breasts.

Polysaccharides Water-soluble polymers containing plant sugars. Some polysaccharides stimulate the immune system, as found with echinacea and aloe vera.

Saponins Phytochemical plant constituents that produce foam when dissolved in water, reducing surface tension and increasing solubility and cell membrane permeability. Saponins may be either sugar glycosides or steroidal in composition. Saponins are easily dissolved in the bloodstream and have antiinflammatory, adaptogenic, and aldosterone-like effects. Although saponins may lower cholesterol or affect estrogen metabolism, some saponins may be toxic and cause hemolytic reactions with red blood cells or may cause GI upset.

www.personalhealthzone.
com/ginseng.html
www.herbmed.org/herbs/
herb108.htm

GOLDENSEAL

What IS Goldenseal?

Goldenseal (*Hydrastis canadensis*), a native North American plant of the buttercup family, grows well in moist, mountainous, wooded areas. Goldenseal is also called eye balm, eye root, ground raspberry, Indian dye, jaundice root, orange root, yellow paint, yellow root, or tumeric root. Previously abundant in the eastern United States, goldenseal has been over-harvested to the point of near extinction, which has drastically increased the price. The so-called "goldenseal" sold at moderate or decreased prices is most likely curry or another yellow powder. Goldenseal is named for its bright, yellow root and stem that, when broken, resembles a gold letter wax seal. The root rhizomes contain the medicinal parts of the plant. The active ingredients are the alkaloids berberine and hydrastine.

What You NEED TO KNOW

Actions

Goldenseal has antibacterial and amebicidal actions with direct application. However, when taken orally, berberine is not absorbed well and may not reach the needed concentration for antimicrobial actions. Berberine is a cardiovascular vasodilator and stimulates the heart, although higher doses can depress the heart. The hydrastine component is a peripheral vasodilator in lower doses but can cause vasoconstriction in higher doses. Goldenseal stimulates the immune system, increases levels of IgM antibodies, and can act as an antiinflammatory agent. The herb is a CNS depressant but stimulates the respiratory center, uterus, and bladder. Goldenseal also has antitumor actions.

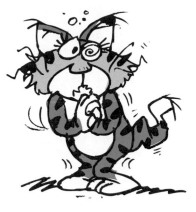

Dose

- 250 to 500 mg PO three times daily
- Liquid extract 1:1, 0.3 to 1.0 ml PO three times daily
- Tincture 1:10, 2 to 4 ml PO three times daily
- Mouthwash, 6 gm steeped in 150 ml water for 5 to 10 min, strained, three to four times daily
- Teas for topical use, 2 tsp (6 g) in 150 ml water steeped

Side Effects

Goldenseal has many side effects that may be severe, depending on dose and duration of use. When used longer than the recommended 2 weeks, goldenseal may cause GI problems, nervousness, excitation, hallucinations, and delirium. In large doses, goldenseal may cause GI upset, nervousness, depression, dyspnea, slowed heart rate, cardiac failure, respiratory failure, hypotension, paralysis, and convulsions. Respiratory or cardiac failure may result in death.

Indications and Uses

- Acne
- Analgesia
- Athlete's foot
- Bronchitis
- Cancer
- Colitis
- Conjunctivitis
- Dandruff
- Dysmenorrhea
- Eczema
- Gastritis
- Herpes
- Infections of mucous membranes
- Influenza
- Itching
- Jaundice
- Menorrhagia
- Nasal congestion
- Peptic ulcers
- Postpartum hemorrhage
- Psoriasis
- Ringworm
- Sedation
- Sore gums
- Upper respiratory tract inflammation
- Urinary tract infection

1. Goldenseal is harmful to infants who may be exposed to goldenseal through the breast milk.
2. Do NOT take goldenseal when breast-feeding.
3. Goldenseal is harmful to the fetus.
4. Goldenseal crosses the placenta and should NOT be taken by the parturient.
5. Older adults are especially sensitive to the sedative effects of medications and should use caution when taking goldenseal.

1. Do not take goldenseal with antihypertensive medications, such as captopril or nifedipine.

2. Patients with coronary artery disease should use caution when taking goldenseal to avoid (a) higher doses that may cause harmful vasoconstriction or (b) hypotension that might cause reduced perfusion and cardiac ischemia.

3. Goldenseal may increase sedative effects of diphenhydramine (Benadryl), naphazoline hydrochloride (Allerest, Clear Eyes), or other antihistamines.

4. Do not drink alcohol when taking goldenseal.

5. Do not take goldenseal with diltiazem, propranolol (Inderal), metoprolol, digoxin (Lanoxin), or other medications that slow the heart rate.

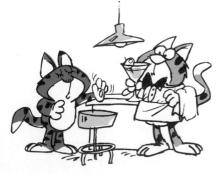

Contraindications and Precautions

Goldenseal should not be used during pregnancy, lactation, or childhood. Kernicterus in the newborn and breast-feeding infant have been reported. This condition occurs because goldenseal crosses the placenta and is transferred through breast milk. Fetal and neonatal deaths from kernicterus have occurred during goldenseal use. In addition, goldenseal may demonstrate oxytocin-like effects, which can cause uterine contractions and premature labor during pregnancy.

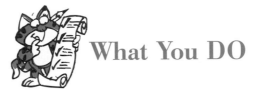

What You DO

Patient History

Pregnant patients, women planning on becoming pregnant, and breast-feeding mothers should not use goldenseal. Parents should be warned against goldenseal use in infants and children. When presenting for surgery or invasive procedures, patients need to be asked about their herbal medication use. Anesthetics and narcotics may increase the hypotensive and sedative effects of goldenseal. In large doses, goldenseal may worsen angina.

Potential Drug Interactions

CNS depressants and anesthetics may have increased effects when used with goldenseal. This combination will cause increased levels of sedation or increased lengths of sedative effects. Catnip and goldenseal increase barbiturate sleep time in mice. Sedative effects of other herbal medications, such as catnip, cayenne, chamomile, melatonin, and St. John's wort, may also be increased when used with goldenseal. Goldenseal may also increase CNS sedation from other CNS-depressant agents, such as sleeping pills, alcohol, or antihistamines. The gastric irritating effects of goldenseal may work against the actions of antacids, hydrogen (H_2) blockers, or proton-pump inhibitors.

Goldenseal may alter the hypotensive effects of antihypertensive agents. Larger doses may work against these agents because of the vasoconstrictive effects of larger doses. The bradycardic effects of berberine may be increased by beta-blocking agents, calcium-channel blockers, and digoxin (Lanoxin).

Drugs metabolized by hepatic enzyme cytochrome CYP450 3A4, such as lovastatin, ketoconazole, cyclosporine, itraconazole, fexofenadine, triazolam, or midazolam, may have altered drug action if taken with goldenseal. Decreased metabolism of midazolam or fentanyl may delay wake-up times from surgery, increasing operating room times and PACU stays. Severe oversedation problems may result in an overnight hospital stay for what was once a planned outpatient procedure. Reduced metabolism of lidocaine may result in elevated levels and toxic reactions, such as sedation, altered mental status, convulsions, hypotension, and cardiovascular collapse.

Patient Education

Patients should stop goldenseal use 2 weeks before surgery to avoid sedative, blood-thinning, and cardiovascular problems. Increased sedative effects may delay wake-up times from surgery. This delay will increase surgical times and PACU stays. Severe oversedation problems may result in an overnight hospital stay for what was once a planned outpatient procedure. Patients should avoid driving or operating heavy machinery until individual susceptibility to the sedative effects can be determined.

Do You UNDERSTAND?

See page 237 for Learning Activities related to this topic.

Key Words

Amebicidal　The ability to kill ameba organisms.

Alkaloids　Phytochemicals with potent pharmacologic effects reacting as bases that are alkaline in pH and often have metabolites containing nitrogen. Alkaloids may depress the CNS, affect the autonomic system, or have other potent actions. Many plant alkaloids have the ability to cross the blood-brain barrier and interact with neurotransmitters. Plant alkaloids may provide immune stimulation against pathogens.

Bradycardic　Describing a heart rate less than 60 beats per minute.

Dyspnea　Rapid, labored breathing.

Kernicterus　Accumulation of bilirubin in the brain and spinal cord of newborns.

Parturient　Pregnant woman.

Rhizomes　Roots growing horizontal to the ground that send out other roots and shoots.

 www.botanical.com/
botanical/mgmh/g/
golsea27.html

HAWTHORN

What IS Hawthorn?

Hawthorn (*Crataegus oxyacantha*) is a shrublike hedge that grows in temperate climates of North America, Asia, and Europe. The Latin name refers to the shrub's sharp thorns. Hawthorn is also known as haw, hedgethorn, may, may tree, maybush, maythorn, oneseed, thorn-apple tree, and whitethorn. The plant's medicinal parts include the leaves, fruit, and blossoms. Hawthorn has also been used as a flavoring for liquor. Hawthorn's active ingredients are flavonoids and oligomeric procyanidins, as well as vitamin C.

What You NEED TO KNOW

Actions

Hawthorn has many actions on the heart muscle. Hawthorn is a positive inotrope. By increasing calcium entry into the heart muscle cells, hawthorn improves the force of cardiac contraction. Hawthorn inhibits phosphodiesterase, which helps metabolize cyclic adenosine monophosphate (cAMP). Increased cAMP increases the amount of intracellular calcium. Increased intracellular calcium causes enhanced muscle contraction. When cardiac muscle contraction is improved, cardiac output increases and blood flow to tissues is improved. Increasing the cardiac output decreases the amount of blood left in the heart at the end of systole. This quantity is called left ventricular end-diastolic volume (LVEDV). Decreasing LVEDV in the heart that is too full decreases the amount of oxygen the heart needs to work. The heart get too full in congestive heart failure or cardiomyopathy.

Hawthorn's calcium effects also help prevent dysrhythmias. Hawthorn vasodilates coronary vessels, which increases coronary blood flow and oxygen delivery to the cardiac muscle. However, some coronary vessels may be stenotic and unable to dilate because of hardening or plaque formation. Blood flow to these vessels may actually decrease when the other cardiac vessels dilate. This vasodilatory effect will cause decreased blood flow and oxygen delivery to tissues supplied by the stenotic vessels. These areas will become ischemic. If ischemia is severe, infarction can result.

Hawthorn also causes vasodilation in the peripheral blood vessels and may decrease blood pressure. Peripheral vasodilation decreases afterload. Decreasing afterload may help increase cardiac output, especially in patients with hypertension or congestive heart failure (CHF). These patients typically have increased afterload and peripheral vasoconstriction. Hawthorn is useful in treating CHF because it increases cardiac contraction, decreases dysrhythmias and afterload, and dilates coronary and peripheral vessels. Hawthorn decreases blood-cholesterol levels and blood coagulation. The herb is an antioxidant. Antioxidants may help limit tissue damage by free radicals after ischemia. Hawthorn has varying effects on uterine tone and contraction; it also possesses antibacterial, antispasmodic, and analgesic actions.

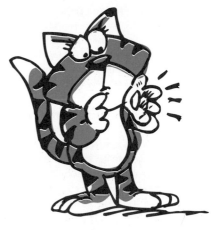

Dose

- Powder: 300 to 1000 mg three times daily
- 1:1 liquid extract: 0.5 to 1.0 ml three times daily
- 1:5 liquid tincture: 1 to 2 ml three times daily
- Fruit syrup: 1 tsp two to three times daily

Side Effects

Side effects have rarely been reported with the fruit, but the leaf and flower preparations may cause nausea. Headache, dizziness, fatigue, insomnia, agitation, palpitations, circulatory disturbances, sweating, hand rash, and allergic reactions have been reported with hawthorn use.

Indications and Uses

- Abdominal distention
- Abdominal pain
- Acute bacillus dysentery
- Amenorrhea
- Angina
- Antioxidant
- Arteriosclerosis
- Bradycardic dysrhythmias
- Buerger's disease
- Cerebral insufficiency
- Coronary artery disease
- Cor pulmonale
- Decreased cardiac output states
- Diarrhea
- Diuresis
- Enteritis
- Frost bite
- Gastric infection
- Heart failure
- Hyperlipidemia
- Hypertension
- Hypertriglyceridemia

 1. Older adults are especially sensitive to the sedative effects of medications and should use caution when taking hawthorn.
2. Older adults should not use hawthorn with other sedative agents because of the increased sensitivity to sedative medications.
3. Older adults often have cardiac or vascular disease and are taking prescription medications that increase bleeding time. They may be a population at increased risk for prolonged bleeding when taking herbs that also have anticoagulant effects.
4. Older adults being treated with pharmaceuticals for hypertension or cardiovascular disease should not take hawthorn.

1. **Do not take hawthorn with nifedipine or propranolol (Inderal).**
2. **Do not take hawthorn with warfarin (Coumadin).**
3. **Do not take hawthorn with digoxin (Lanoxin).**
4. **Do not take hawthorn with triazolam (Halcion).**
5. **Do not take hawthorn with diphenhydramine (Benadryl) or naphazoline hydrochloride (Allerest, Clear Eyes).**
6. **Patients should seek medical advice for their heart disease.**
7. **Do not take hawthorn with aspirin or ibuprofen.**
8. **Patients with chronic and inflammatory conditions such as arthritis, fibromyalgia, bursitis, or low back pain are often prescribed NSAIDs routinely for pain control. The risk of herb-drug interactions may be increased in these populations.**
9. **Patients with circulatory disorders such as PVD, carotid artery disease, and diabetes are often prescribed anticoagulants or blood-thinning agents (aspirin or dipyridamole [Persantine]) for their disorder. The risk of herb-drug interactions may be increased in these populations.**
10. **Patients with cardiovascular disease or hypercholesterolemia routinely taking an aspirin a day may be an at-risk population for bleeding complications if they are also taking hawthorn.**

- Increased effects of cardiac glycosides
- Indigestion
- Ischemic heart disease
- Itching
- Menopause
- Paroxysmal tachycardia
- Sedation
- Tapeworm

Contraindications and Precautions

Hawthorn may cause uterine contractions and should not be used by pregnant individuals or those desiring to become pregnant. Children and lactating mothers should not use hawthorn. Hawthorn is best used for mild congestive heart disease and is contraindicated in severe cardiac disease. Hawthorn should not be used in severe liver or kidney disease.

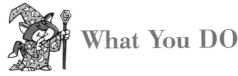 # What You DO

Patient History

The use of hawthorn 2 weeks before surgery may decrease coagulation. The nurse should ask the patient about bruising and bleeding tendencies. Further laboratory testing, such as coagulation studies, may be indicated.

The patient's history should be reviewed for signs and symptoms of CHD and CHF. Problems for which to look include fatigue, peripheral edema, shortness of breath, and chest pain. CHD and CHF should not be self-diagnosed or self-managed. Patients should be encouraged to seek medical consultation for their disease management, herbal medication use, and conventional medication intake.

Potential Drug Interactions

Hawthorn has several drug and herbal interactions. Hawthorn may increase the effects and toxicity of other herbals that have cardiac-stimulating effects. Digitalis leaf, goldenseal, ginseng, and ginger all have cardiac effects. Similarly, hawthorn may increase the effects of digoxin. The effects of related cardiac medications used in treating CHF, high blood pressure, angina, and dysrhythmias may also be increased.

Many CNS depressants and anesthetics may have increased effects when used with hawthorn. This combination may lead to increased sedation or longer duration of sedative effects. Sedative effects of other herbals may be increased. Herbals with sedative effects include catnip, cayenne, chamomile, melatonin, St. John's wort, valerian, or kava kava. Hawthorn may increase the sedative action of sleeping pills, alcohol, or antihistamines. Hawthorn may have added hypotensive effects with antihypertensive and anesthetic agents. The antiarrhythmic actions of hawthorn may be unpredictable when used with beta-blocking agents, calcium-channel blockers, or digoxin (Lanoxin).

Hawthorn may increase the blood-thinning effects of anticoagulant medications. The anticoagulant effects of other herbal and blood-thinning medication may also be increased, which would increase risks of bruising, bleeding, and hemorrhage.

Patient Education

Patients should stop hawthorn use 2 weeks before surgery to avoid the sedative, blood-thinning, cardiovascular, and peripheral vascular effects of hawthorn. Increased sedative effects may delay wake-up times from surgery, increasing operating room times and PACU stays. Severe oversedation problems may result in an overnight hospital stay for what was once a planned outpatient procedure. Patients should not use hawthorn with alcohol, diphenhydramine (Benadryl), and other antihistamines that also have sedative effects. Hawthorn should not be used with St. John's wort, kava kava, hops, and other herbals that also have sedative effects. Patients should avoid driving or operating heavy machinery until individual susceptibility to hawthorn's sedative effects can be determined.

Patients should be educated about the anticoagulant effects of hawthorn. Prolonged bleeding times may result in spontaneous or surgical hemorrhage. Patients with **thrombocytopenia** and clotting disorders should avoid hawthorn. Patients should not use hawthorn with warfarin. Patients should not use hawthorn with aspirin, ibuprofen, and other NSAIDs that also decrease blood clotting.

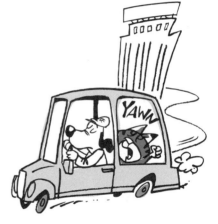

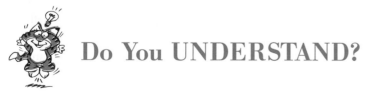

Do You UNDERSTAND?

See pages 238 and 239 for Learning Activities related to this topic.

TAKE HOME POINTS

1. Hawthorn should be discontinued 2 weeks before surgery to prevent interaction with anesthetics.
2. Hawthorn should be discontinued before surgery to prevent potential for excessive blood loss.

www.herbmed.org/herbs/
herb97.htm
www.herbalgram.org/
browse_site.php/herbal_e_
hawthorn/

Key Words

Afterload The resistance against which the heart has to pump to move blood through the body.

Antioxidant An agent that helps prevent cell damage from oxygen free radicals or other highly reactive compounds.

Cardiac output Amount of blood ejected from the heart every minute.

Flavonoids Plant pigments responsible for the color of fruits and vegetables. Some flavonoids increase capillary wall stability (decrease capillary fragility) and scavenge free radicals, resulting in antioxidant properties. Other flavonoids have antiarthritis, antiinflammatory, antiviral, or antimutagenic properties.

Inotrope Pertaining to the contracting ability of the heart.

Intracellular Inside the cell.

Oligomeric procyanidins Agents with astringent properties that may prevent cardiovascular disease through antioxidant effects.

Phosphodiesterase Enzyme needed for breakdown of cAMP.

Systole The time during which the left ventricle is contracting and ejecting blood out of the heart.

Thrombocytopenia Decreased platelet levels.

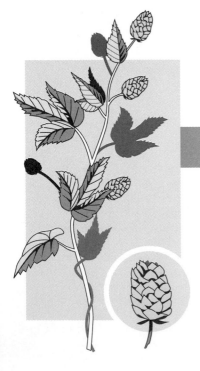

HOP

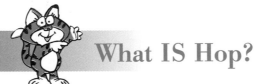

What IS Hop?

Hop (*Humulus lupulus*) is a climbing vine native to Europe, Asia, and North America. Other names for hop include hopfenzafen and houblon. The cone-shaped flower from the female plant is used for medicinal purposes. Since the ninth century, hop has been used medicinally. Pillows were once filled with hop flowers to reduce anxiety and promote restful sleep. Hop is also used for the brewing of beer. Hop harvesters seem to tire easily at their job, probably because of the hop on their hands. Hop is a good source of vitamin C and vitamin B complex. The active ingredients are **flavonoids**, **terpenoids**, **volatile oils**, and **bitter** acid ingredients (lupulone and humulone).

What You NEED TO KNOW

Actions

Hop has sedative, hypnotic, anticonvulsant, and antimicrobial activities. Hop also demonstrates pain- and fever-reducing actions. The herb has estrogen-like actions and reduces the secretion of LH. The bitter acid ingredients are responsible for the sedative and antimicrobial properties of hop. The bitter acids also scavenge free radicals and act as antioxidants. Hop is a diuretic. Hop is active against types of *Bacillus subtilis*, *Staphylococcus aureus*, and *Trichophyton mentagrophytes* (fungus).

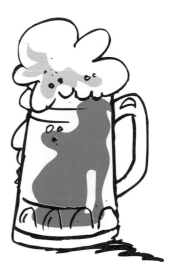

Dose

- 0.5 to 1.0 g 1 to 3 times daily
- 1:5 tincture: 1 to 2 ml two or three times daily
- Teas: 0.5 to 1.0 gm in 150 cc water steeped for 10 min twice daily
- Topical as a poultice

Side Effects

Sedation and decreased mental acuity may occur from hop. Hop can also cause allergic reactions such as contact dermatitis, airway irritation, and bronchitis. Breathing in the hop dust may cause chest tightness, wheezing, hives, itching, anaphylaxis, and respiratory failure.

Indications and Uses

- Analgesia
- Antiinflammatory
- Anxiety
- Appetite stimulant
- Boils
- Constipation
- Crohn's disease
- Digestive aid
- Dysentery
- Dysmenorrhea
- Excitability
- Headache
- Hypnotic
- Insomnia
- Irritable bowel syndrome
- Irritability
- Leprosy
- Muscle relaxant
- Neuralgia
- Osteoporosis
- Rheumatic pain
- Toothache
- Tuberculosis
- Urinary tract infection

1. **Do not take hop with diphenhydramine (Benadryl), naphazoline hydrochloride (Allerest, Clear Eyes), or other antihistamines.**
2. **Using alcohol with the herb hop may increase the sedative properties of both agents.**
3. **Pregnant women and nursing mothers should avoid hop.**
4. **Infertile men should not take hop.**

Contraindications and Precautions

Hop may increase depression and should be avoided in depression disorders. Hop should be avoided during pregnancy and in patients with estrogen-sensitive tumors. The estrogen effects of hop may also decrease male sexual drive. Hop has been known to cause gynecomastia with prolonged exposure. Men experiencing problems with infertility should not take hop.

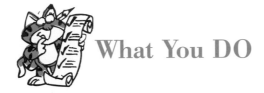

What You DO

Patient History

Patients should be questioned concerning their medication intake, including prescription, over-the-counter, and herbal medications. Patients presenting for surgical and invasive procedures should discontinue their use of hop 2 weeks before their procedure to avoid problems with anesthesia, sedative, and pain-relieving medications.

Potential Drug Interactions

Many CNS depressants and anesthetics may have increased effects when used with hops. This combination may lead to increased or prolonged sedative effects. Other sedative herbal medications, such as catnip, cayenne, chamomile, melatonin, goldenseal, and St. John's wort may also cause increased sedation when used with hops. Hop may increase depressant effects of alcohol, allergy medications, cold remedies, and narcotics.

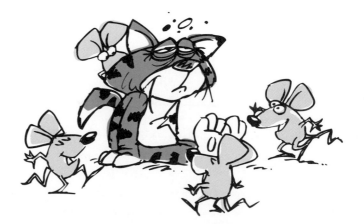

Patient Education

Patients should stop herbal medication use 2 weeks before surgery. Combining sedating herbal medicines with anesthetics may delay wake-up times from surgery. This combination may increase operating room times and PACU stays. Severe oversedation problems may result in an overnight hospital stay for what was once a planned outpatient procedure. Patients taking hop should be cautioned to avoid alcohol intake because the sedative actions of alcohol may be enhanced. Patients should avoid using other CNS-depressant agents such as sleeping pills, antianxiety drugs, or antihistamines with hops.

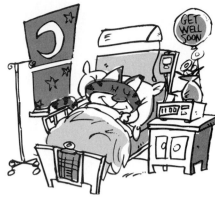

Do You UNDERSTAND?

See pages 239 and 240 for Learning Activities related to this topic.

Key Words

Bitters Bitter-tasting plant components that are consumed to promote digestion through stimulating gastric motility and acid secretion.

Contact dermatitis Skin reaction caused by touching an allergy-producing substance.

Flavonoids Plant pigments responsible for the color of fruits and vegetables. Some flavonoids increase capillary wall stability (decrease capillary fragility) and scavenge free radicals, resulting in antioxidant properties. Other flavonoids have antiarthritis, antiinflammatory, antiviral, or antimutagenic properties.

Gynecomastia Enlargement of the breasts.

Terpenoids Secondary metabolites or phytochemicals in the essential oils of plant.

Volatile oils Also known as essential oils, aromatic plant oils isolated by steam distillation often used for perfumes, aromatherapy, or medicinal effects. Many essential oils have antispasmodic, expectorant, sedative, analgesic, or antimicrobial activity.

 www.herbmed.org/herbs/
herb44.htm

KAVA KAVA

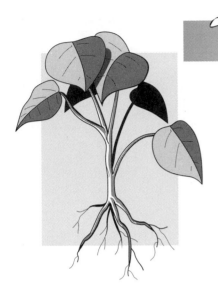

What IS Kava Kava?

Kava kava, also known simply as kava (*Piper methysticum*), is a member of the pepper family. Kava is also known as ava, ava pepper shrub, awa, kawa, intoxicating pepper, sakau, tonga, and yagona. Kava is native plant of the Pacific Islands and has been used since ancient times by the islanders. The plant has large heart-shaped leaves and may grow as tall as 6 feet. Captain James Cook discovered kava during his explorations and named the plant "intoxicating pepper" because of its sedative and relaxing effects that are similar to those of alcohol. The root and rhizome systems are used for making the medicinal product. These roots contain the active ingredients called kavalactones.

What You NEED TO KNOW

Actions

Sedation is kava's most well-known action. The effect may be a result of action on the limbic system of the brain. The limbic system is responsible for emotions and serves as a control center for the body's vital, life-sustaining functions. Kava also acts as an anxiolytic, anticonvulsant, antispasmodic, anticoagulant, and analgesic. The analgesic activity occurs through nonopiate pathways. The anticonvulsant properties are caused by kava's effect on the sodium and calcium channels of nerves. Kava can produce local anesthesia when it comes in contact with mucous membranes. In summary, little is actually known about the way that kava works or about the way it interacts with other medicines.

Dose

- Anxiety disorders: 100 mg three times daily
- Nervousness, stress, restlessness: 60 to 120 mg three times daily
- Tea made from boiling 2 to 4 g of root in 150 ml water and strained 1 cup three times daily
- Poultice for infections

Side Effects

Sedation is the most common side effect of kava. Headache, dizziness, motor impairment, or allergic reaction may also occur. Long-term use of high doses can cause kava dermopathy, which results in yellowing of the skin, hair, and nails. Red eyes, GI problems, decreased appetite, **ataxia**, and visual disturbances occur as well. Rarely, kava can cause damage to the eyes, skin, liver, and spinal cord after prolonged use. Long-term use may lead to problems with serum blood levels of albumin, protein urea, and bilirubin. **Liver failure requiring transplantation has also been reported.** Hypertension, **hematuria**, shortness of breath, **thrombocytopenia**, and **leukopenia** have also been reported. Currently, sales of kava have been suspended in Switzerland and Britain. Germany is acting to make kava a prescription medication. In the United States, the National Institutes of Health (NIH) has suspended two NIH-funded studies of kava because of its serious side effects.

 1. Older adults are sensitive to CNS-depressant effects of medications. These individuals should avoid kava.
2. Older adults frequently have cardiovascular, cerebrovascular, and peripheral vascular disease. Thus these older adults may often be on prescription blood-thinning agents and represent a special population at risk for herbal-drug interactions.
3. Because of age-related changes in kidney and liver function, older adults should avoid kava until safety and dose issues are resolved.

Indications and Uses

- Abscess
- Analgesic
- Anticonvulsant
- Anxiety
- Asthma
- Benzodiazepine withdrawal
- Canker sores
- Chronic cystitis
- Diuretic
- Epilepsy
- Fungal infections
- Gonorrhea
- Headaches
- Insomnia
- Irritable bladder
- Leprosy
- Menstrual problems
- Nervousness
- Psychosis
- Otitis media
- Rheumatism
- Sedative
- Sore gums
- Sore throat
- Tooth ache
- Tuberculosis
- Urinary infections
- Vaginal infections
- Worms

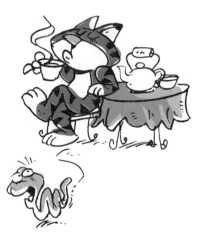

Contraindications and Precautions

Kava should not be used longer than 1 month. Kava may decrease uterine tone and is contraindicated in pregnancy. Kava use when breast-feeding is contraindicated because toxic ingredients may be found in breast milk. Kava interferes with the action of dopamine and should not be used by individuals with Parkinson's disease. Because of its sedative actions, kava should not be used with depressive disorders or when operating heavy machinery or

1. **Patients taking warfarin (Coumadin) or heparin should not take kava.**
2. **Do not take kava with gingko, ginseng, fish oil, vitamin E, or any other herbals that also decrease blood clotting.**
3. **Patients taking aspirin, ibuprofen, nabumetone (Relafen) or other NSAIDs on a routine basis should avoid kava.**
4. **Patients with chronic and inflammatory conditions such as arthritis, fibromyalgia, bursitis, or low back pain are often prescribed NSAIDs for pain control. Therefore the risk of herb-drug interactions may be increased in these populations.**
5. **Patients with circulatory disorders such as PVD, carotid artery disease, and diabetes are often prescribed anticoagulants or blood-thinning agents (aspirin or dipyridamole [Persantine]) for their disorder. Therefore the risk of herb-drug interactions may be increased in these populations.**
6. **Patients with cardiovascular disease or hypercholesterolemia routinely taking an aspirin a day may be an at-risk population for bleeding complications if they are also taking kava.**
7. **Patients should not take kava with diphenhydramine (Benadryl) or other antihistamine agents to avoid oversedation problems.**
8. **Kava is currently under investigation for problems with liver and kidney failure.**

driving. Patients with liver disease, renal disease, alcoholism, hepatitis, or jaundice should not take kava. Transplant patients should not take kava. Nursing or pregnant women, as well as children, should not take kava.

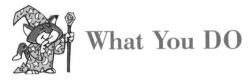

What You DO

Patient History

Patients taking kava should have medications reviewed to determine interactions with other medications that may cause bruising and bleeding. Surgical patients, including those undergoing dental procedures, should not take this herb preoperatively because it may increase surgical blood loss. Kava may also lead to hemorrhage during the postoperative period. Further laboratory testing of the clotting system may be needed before surgery or other invasive procedures. In addition, liver function tests may be needed in patients who take kava longer than 1 month or have jaundice, fatigue, or dark urine.

Potential Drug Interactions

Drugs such as alcohol, barbiturates, or antianxiety agents may increase the sedative effects of kava, thus these drugs should not be taken with kava. Many medications given during anesthesia and the perioperative period, such as midazolam, diazepam, narcotics, antinausea medications, and inhalational-anesthetic agents, demonstrate CNS depression. Kava may increase the sedative properties of these medications when given together. The sedative effects of other herbal medications, such as St. John's wort or hops, may also be increased by kava and should not be taken at the same time. Kava may increase the depressant effects of allergy medications and cold remedies. Kava may also increase the intoxicating effects of alcohol.

Other medications such as NSAIDs, aspirin, or dipyridamole (Persantine) also decrease the patient's ability to clot. Kava may add to the anticoagulant effects of these agents. Patients taking warfarin or heparin should avoid using kava. Kava should not be combined with other herbals that also decrease clotting ability. Herbals such as garlic, ginger, gingko, ginseng, red clover, fish oil, or vitamin E also decrease clotting.

Kava interferes with the action of dopamine and should not be taken with levodopa (L-dopa, Sinemet) and other Parkinson's medications. Also, kava should not be taken with other agents that interfere with dopamine's actions, such as droperidol or metoclopramide. Drugs that may cause hepatotoxicity—amiodarone, ketoconazole, methotrexate, nitrofurantoin, pravastatin, and tamoxifen—may increase the risk of liver damage if taken with kava.

Patient Education

Patients should be educated to avoid the use of other CNS-depressant agents such as sleeping pills, pain pills, alcohol, or antihistamines with kava. Patients should stop herbal medication use 2 weeks before surgery to avoid the sedative and blood-thinning effects of kava. Increased sedative effects may delay wake up times from surgery, increasing operating room times and PACU stays. Severe oversedation problems may result in an overnight hospital stay for what was once a planned outpatient procedure. Patients should avoid driving or operating heavy machinery until individual susceptibility to kava's sedative effects can be determined.

Patients with **thrombocytopenia** or clotting disorders should not take kava. Patients should not take kava with other medications that may lead to liver damage. Yellowing of the skin with itching and dark urine are late signs of extensive liver damage.

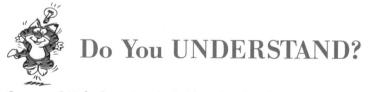

Do You UNDERSTAND?

See page 241 for Learning Activities related to this topic.

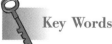

Key Words

Ataxia A neurologic disorder causing gait impairment, slurred speech, blurry vision, hand tremor, and problems with coordination.

Hematuria Blood in the urine.

Leukopenia Low level of WBCs.

Thrombocytopenia Low level of platelets.

 http://altmed.creighton.
  edu/kava/default.htm
www.herbmed.org/herbs/
  herb110.htm
www.personalhealthzone.com/
  kavakava.html

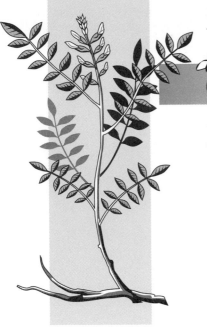

LICORICE

What IS Licorice?

Licorice (*Glycyrrhiza glabra*) is a perennial shrub grown mainly in Russia, Turkey, Syria, Iran, Iraq, Spain, Italy, Greece, and India. Other names for licorice include sweet root or alcacuz. Licorice has been used since ancient times for medicinal purposes. Because of its extremely sweet taste (reportedly 50 times sweeter than is sugar), glycyrrhizin is used as a flavoring agent in many medicines. Although many candies overseas are flavored with licorice, in the United States, licorice candies are actually flavored with anise oil. Licorice also contains magnesium, silicon, thiamine, lecithin, protein, and vitamin E. Glycyrrhizin, isoflavonoids, and coumarins are the active ingredients found in the plant's yellow-colored roots.

What You NEED TO KNOW

Actions

Glycyrrhizin is responsible for licorice's many actions. This ingredient is a mild laxative and is used to control gastric hyperacidic diseases, such as peptic or duodenal ulceration. The use of glycyrrhizin in hyperacidic diseases is probably based on decreased prostaglandin metabolism. Glycyrrhizin binds directly to mineralocorticoid receptors and decreases the metabolism of cortisol. This action is responsible for many side effects, such as hypertension, edema, hypokalemia, and cardiac dysrhythmias. Because of its antitussive and expectorant actions, glycyrrhizin increases production and transport of bronchial mucus.

Licorice also demonstrates antiinflammatory, antispasmodic, antiviral, antimicrobial, antioxidant, and antitumor effects. Licorice promotes estradiol- and estrogen-receptor binding, which accounts for its estrogenic activity. At higher doses, licorice actually blocks estrogen receptors and may work against estrogen. Licorice decreases testosterone production. Coumarins are responsible for the blood-thinning effects of licorice. Last, other constituents may demonstrate MAOI properties.

1. Licorice use may worsen water retention during pregnancy.
2. Licorice may cause hypertension during pregnancy.

Dose

- GI ulcers: 2 to 6 ml per day of 1:1 liquid extract
- Respiratory ailments: 1 to 2 g powdered root three times daily for no longer than 1 week
- Topical: twice daily application

Side Effects

Prolonged use or use of large doses can result in pseudoaldosteronism. Because of its mineralocorticoid activity, licorice may cause edema, weight gain, headache, CHF, pulmonary edema, hypertension, cardiac dysrhythmias, and muscle weakness. As a result of decreased testosterone production, licorice may cause decreased libido and sexual dysfunction. Licorice may inhibit coagulation.

1. **Patients taking warfarin (Coumadin) or heparin should avoid licorice.**
2. **Patients taking hydrochlorothiazide should avoid licorice.**
3. **Patients using birth control pills or hormone replacement therapy should avoid licorice.**
4. **Patients prone to ankle and pedal edema should avoid licorice.**

Indications and Uses

- Addison's disease
- Adrenocortical insufficiency
- Arthritis
- Asthma
- Autoimmune deficiency syndrome
- Bronchitis
- Chronic fatigue syndrome
- Cough
- Duodenal ulcer
- Eczema
- Gastritis
- Heartburn
- Hepatitis B and C
- HIV
- Influenza
- Laryngitis
- Lung congestion
- Menopause
- Peptic ulcer
- Prostate cancer, combination therapy
- Psoriasis
- Respiratory tract infections
- Shingles

Contraindications and Precautions

Patients with diabetes should not use licorice because it can interfere with blood glucose control. Patients with CHF or hypertension should not use licorice because of its mineralocorticoid activity. Licorice may cause hypertension or stimulate uterine contractions, thus the herb should not be used during pregnancy. Patients with cirrhosis or liver or renal failure may have increased problems with the mineralocorticoid actions of licorice. Safety of licorice use during lactation or childhood has not been determined; therefore these populations should avoid licorice intake.

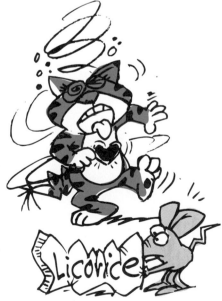

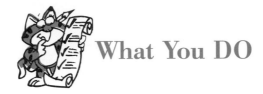

What You DO

Patient History

Because of the anticoagulation effects of licorice, patients should discontinue use 2 weeks before surgery or invasive procedures. Further assessment of bleeding tendencies and laboratory testing, such as coagulation studies, may be indicated preoperatively.

Licorice may cause **hypokalemia** because of increased renal excretion of potassium in the urine. Hypokalemia during surgery combined with the stress response of surgery and release of stress hormones is especially problematic. The body's stress response to surgery activates the "fight or flight" system, causing release of **cortisol**, epinephrine, and norepinephrine. The **dysrhythmic** effects of epinephrine are increased by hypokalemia, which increases the risk of ventricular tachyarrhythmias (frequent premature ventricular contractions, ventricular tachycardia, or ventricular fibrillation). Ventricular fibrillation and death have been reported with licorice-induced hypokalemia. Laboratory determination of preoperative serum-potassium level may be needed. Elective surgery should be delayed to bring the potassium level up to normal. Licorice may contribute to kidney stone formation.

Potential Drug Interactions

By causing decreased potassium levels, licorice may increase the toxicity of digoxin (Lanoxin). Other herbals possessing cardiac **glycosides**, such as hellebore, pheasant's eye, broom, lily of the valley, pleurisy root, wintersweet, figwort, or squill, should be avoided with licorice use. The hypokalemic effects of licorice may be increased when used with diuretic or steroid medications. This combination may result in severe decreases of fluid and electrolytes. Other herbs such as aloe, celery, chamomile, or horseradish also affect electrolyte levels and may increase electrolyte loss when taken with licorice.

Licorice may help protect against **gastritis** from medications. On the other hand, licorice may increase the sodium- and fluid-retention actions of NSAIDs agents. Licorice should also not be used with aspirin, NSAIDs, or anticoagulants such as warfarin or heparin to prevent severe anticoagulation. Licorice may also enhance the GI-protective effects of cimetidine.

Licorice should not be taken with other MAOIs. These agents are sometimes used for depressive disorders and parkinsonism. Similarly, medications such as meperidine, atropine, or ephedrine that also demonstrate severe reactions when taken with MAOIs should be avoided.

Licorice may inhibit hepatic cytochrome CYP450 3A4 activity, which may increase the action of medications metabolized by this system. These medications include cyclosporine, lovastatin, itraconazole, fexofenadine, benzodiazepines (midazolam and diazepam), triazolam (Halcion) and many anesthetic agents. Decreased metabolism of midazolam or fentanyl may delay wake-up times from surgery, increasing operating room times and PACU stays. Severe oversedation problems may result in an overnight hospital stay for what was once a planned outpatient procedure. Reduced metabolism of lidocaine may result in elevated levels and toxic reactions such as sedation, altered mental status, convulsions, hypotension, and cardiovascular collapse.

Licorice use with insulin administration may worsen hypokalemia as a result of two mechanisms: (a) when insulin causes glucose to enter the cell, potassium will follow; this action will decrease the amount of potassium in the blood; and (b) licorice causes urinary potassium loss. Depending on the dose, licorice may increase or interfere with estrogen therapy, potentially causing drug toxicity or decreased action of the drug. Last, grapefruit juice may increase the mineralocorticoid actions of licorice.

Patient Education

Patients with hypertensive or cardiovascular disease should be cautioned to avoid using licorice. Increases in **intravascular** volume may worsen hypertension and volume overload in patients with cardiovascular disease, possibly leading to cardiac failure. To avoid toxicity, patients should not use licorice for more than 4 weeks or in large doses. Patients with diabetes should be cautioned to avoid licorice because the mineralocorticoid effects may cause **hyperglycemia**. Women with PMS may experience increased bloating and water retention when taking licorice before menses. Fluid retention caused by licorice may worsen fluid problems in renal insufficiency.

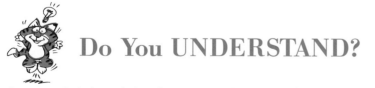

Do You UNDERSTAND?

See pages 242 through 244 for Learning Activities related to this topic.

TAKE HOME POINTS

1. Licorice may raise the blood glucose level and increase insulin requirements of patients with diabetes.
2. Discontinuing licorice use in the patient with diabetes requires increased attention to blood glucose testing to avoid **hypoglycemia**.
3. Patients with cardiovascular disease should avoid licorice.
4. Licorice should be discontinued 1 week before an expected menses in patients who are prone to PMS, water weight gain, engorgement, and bloating.
5. Patients taking licorice may want to increase their dietary intake of potassium.
6. Bananas and orange juice are good sources of potassium.

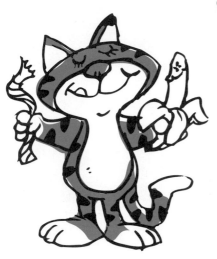

Key Words

Addison's disease A disease resulting from inadequate secretion of adrenal cortex hormones.

Antioxidant An agent that helps prevent cell damage from oxygen free radicals or other highly reactive compounds.

Antitussive An agent that decreases coughing.

Cortisol A glucocorticoid hormone secreted from the adrenal cortex that increases the blood glucose level.

Coumarins Plant chemicals that may exhibit anticoagulant properties, as well as anticancer, immunostimulant, antifungal, antiinflammatory, vasodilatory, muscle-relaxant, hypnotic, CNS-stimulant, hypothermal, diuretic, anticholinergic, antiedema, or estrogenic effects.

Dysrhythmic Pertaining to an abnormal heart rhythm.

Expectorant An agent that helps in transport and removal of bronchial secretions.

Gastritis Inflammation of the stomach.

Glycosides Plant metabolites that produce sugars through hydrolysis during metabolism. Similar to digoxin, cardiac glycosides, found in plants of the lily family, may increase cardiac output and have toxic effects.

Hyperglycemia High blood glucose level.

Hypoglycemia Low blood glucose level.

Hypokalemia Low potassium level in the blood.

Intravascular Within the blood vessels.

Isoflavonoids Plant constituents that affect estrogen receptors, often found in soy products. Some isoflavonoids may also have anticarcinogenic or immunostimulatory effects.

Mineralocorticoid Hormonal or medicinal activities resulting in sodium and water retention and potassium excretion.

Pseudoaldosteronism A condition mirroring the symptoms seen in elevated levels of aldosterone: sodium retention, urinary potassium loss, and alkalosis.

www.herbmed.org/herb/
herb101.htm
www.herbmed.org/herbs/
Glycyrrhiza1.htm

PASSIONFLOWER

What IS Passionflower?

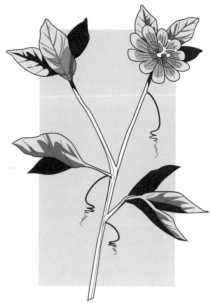

Passionflower (*Passiflora incarnata*) is a climbing vine that grows in tropical and subtropical areas. Passionflower obtained its name from the shape of the flowers. The flowers resemble objects from Christ's crucifixion. Other names for passionflower include apricot vine, Corona de Cristo, Fleur de la Passion, and water lemon. Some varieties of passionflower are flowering, while others produce edible fruits. The plant, flower, and fruit are used for medicinal purposes. Active ingredients of passionflower include coumarins and phytosterols.

What You NEED TO KNOW

Actions

Passionflower has many actions; it is a sedative, hypnotic, antispasmodic, and analgesic. Passionflower binds to central benzodiazepine receptors. This action causes passionflower's antianxiety properties. Passionflower possesses some antibacterial and antifungal actions as well. Passionflower reduces skeletal muscle contraction and activity and corneal reflexes. Passionflower contains coumarins, which may affect coagulation.

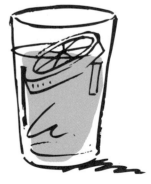

Dose

- 0.25 to 2.0 gm three times daily
- 1:1 extract: 0.5 to 1.0 ml three times daily
- 1:8 tincture: 0.5 to 2.0 ml three times daily
- Topically, as hemorrhoid rinse

Side Effects

The primary side effect of passionflower is sedation. Less frequently, passionflower may cause vasculitis, nausea, vomiting, and cardiac dysrhythmias.

1. **The sedative effects of diphenhydramine (Benadryl), naphazoline hydrochloride (Allerest, Clear Eyes), or other antihistamines may be enhanced by passionflower.**
2. **Passionflower should not be used with alcohol.**
3. **Passionflower may increase the sedative effects of narcotics, antispasmodic muscle relaxants, and other sleeping agents.**
4. **Passionflower should not be taken with warfarin (Coumadin) or heparin.**
5. **Passionflower should not be taken with gingko, ginseng, or other herbals that also decrease clotting.**
6. **Passionflower should not be taken with ibuprofen.**

Older adults are especially sensitive to the sedative effects of medications and should use caution when taking passionflower.

Indications and Uses

- Analgesia
- Antianxiety
- Burns
- Cardiac dysrhythmias
- Hemorrhoids
- Inflammation
- Insomnia
- Nervous stomach
- Neuralgia
- Palpitations
- Pediatric attention disorders
- Pediatric nervousness

Contraindications and Precautions

Passionflower should not be taken during pregnancy, lactation, or childhood. Patients with liver or kidney disease or depression should avoid passionflower.

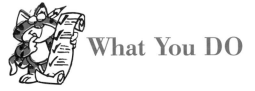

What You DO

Patient History

Pregnant patients and women planning on becoming pregnant should be counseled against passionflower use. When facing surgery or invasive procedures, patients need to be questioned concerning their herbal medication intake. The sedative effects of passionflower may be increased by medications used during the perioperative period.

Patients undergoing surgery or other procedures should be questioned about their use of herbal medications. Patients taking passionflower should be asked about their tendencies for bleeding and bruising. Further laboratory testing, such as coagulation studies, may be needed preoperatively. Elective surgery for patients with increased clotting times should be delayed until their clotting times return to normal levels.

Potential Drug Interactions

Many CNS depressants and anesthetics may have increased effects when used with passionflower, causing increased or longer sedative effects. Passionflower has been shown to increase barbiturate sleep time in mice. Sedative effects of other herbal medications, such as catnip, cayenne, chamomile, melatonin, and St. John's wort, may also be increased when used with passionflower. Patients should be educated to avoid using other CNS-depressant agents such as sleeping pills, benzodiazepines, alcohol, or antihistamines with passionflower.

Passionflower may increase the action of monoamine oxidase inhibiting (MAOI) agents. Thus these pharmaceuticals should not be used at the same time.

Because passionflower contains coumarins, it may increase the blood-clotting effects of anticoagulants such as warfarin (Coumadin) and heparin. The anticoagulant effects of other herbal medications, such as ginger, garlic, vitamin E, or red clover, may be increased. Other medications that have blood-thinning action may also enhance the blood-thinning properties of passionflower. These medications include aspirin or NSAIDs.

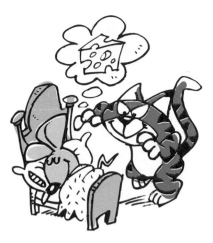

Patient Education

Patients should stop passionflower use 2 weeks before surgery to avoid increased sedative effects. Increased sedative effects may delay wake-up times from surgery, increasing operating room times and PACU stays. Severe oversedation problems may result in an overnight hospital stay for what was once a planned outpatient procedure. Patients should avoid driving or operating heavy machinery until individual susceptibility to passionflower's sedative effects can be determined.

Patients should be educated about the potential for blood-thinning effects with passionflower. Patients should not use passionflower with other medications that decrease blood clotting.

Do You UNDERSTAND?

See pages 244 and 245 for Learning Activities related to this topic.

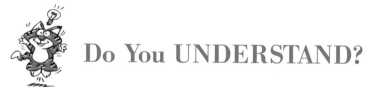

Key Words

Coumarins Plant chemicals that may exhibit anticoagulant properties, as well as anticancer, immunostimulant, antifungal, antiinflammatory, vasodilatory, muscle-relaxant, hypnotic, CNS-stimulant, hypothermal, diuretic, anticholinergic, antiedema, or estrogenic effects.

Phytosterols A sterol from plant oil or fat.

www.herbmed.org/herbs/
herb109.htm

RED CLOVER

What IS Red Clover?

Red clover (*Trifolium pratense*) is a wild plant used both medicinally and for livestock fodder.

The Irish shamrock is also a member of the clover family. Red clover is also known as cleaver grass, honeysuckle clover, meadow clover, wild clover, cow clover, cow grass, marlgrass, and purple clover. Red clover is common throughout the United States, Canada, Europe, and parts of Asia. The flowers—which can be white, red, or purple—are used for medicinal purposes. Red clover contains calcium, chromium, iron, magnesium, niacin, phosphorus, potassium, thiamine, and vitamin C. Active ingredients of red clover include **isoflavonoids**, **coumarins**, **salicylates**, and **saponins**.

What You NEED TO KNOW

Actions

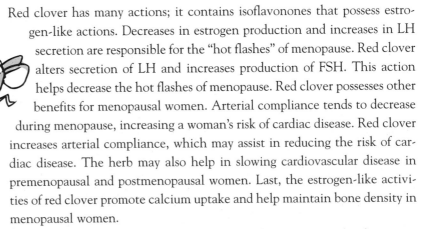

Red clover has many actions; it contains isoflavonones that possess estrogen-like actions. Decreases in estrogen production and increases in LH secretion are responsible for the "hot flashes" of menopause. Red clover alters secretion of LH and increases production of FSH. This action helps decrease the hot flashes of menopause. Red clover possesses other benefits for menopausal women. Arterial compliance tends to decrease during menopause, increasing a woman's risk of cardiac disease. Red clover increases arterial compliance, which may assist in reducing the risk of cardiac disease. The herb may also help in slowing cardiovascular disease in premenopausal and postmenopausal women. Last, the estrogen-like activities of red clover promote calcium uptake and help maintain bone density in menopausal women.

Red clover may inhibit estrogen-sensitive breast cancers by decreasing the "sticking together" of cancer cells and preventing growth of new blood vessels that feed the cancerous tumor. However, because estrogen-like agents can promote growth of breast tumors, further studies are needed before red clover is used in the treatment for breast cancer.

In large doses, red clover also decreases coagulation. Red clover has expectorant and antispasmodic action. This property makes red clover useful in dry, hacking coughs, such as those seen in whooping cough. Red clover has moderate antiinflammatory actions because of its salicylates. Red clover may show mild antibiotic activity.

Red clover is also known as an alternative or an agent that is useful in cleansing the blood of impurities.

Dose

- 2 to 4 g flowers three times daily
- Capsules and tablets: 2 to 6/day (500 mg)
- 2 to 4 ml 1:1 (in 25% alcohol) tincture three times daily
- Topical ointment

Side Effects

Side effects from red clover are usually caused by its estrogen-like activities and include breast enlargement and tenderness, menstrual changes, and weight gain. Urticaria has also been reported in sensitive individuals.

Indications and Uses

- Acne
- Analgesia
- Antispasmodic
- Arthritis
- Asthma
- Bronchitis
- Burns
- Conjunctivitis
- Dermatitis
- Eczema
- Expectorant
- Gout
- Menopause
- Pharyngitis
- Psoriasis
- Sexually transmitted diseases
- Skin cancer
- Skin poultice
- Whooping cough

Contraindications and Precautions

Women who are pregnant, planning on becoming pregnant, or breast-feeding should not take red clover. Women who have a history of breast or uterine cancer should not take red clover. Interactions with other hormonal-replacement therapies have not been identified. However, red clover may have additive effects or interfere with hormone-replacement therapy. Therefore women on prescription hormone-replacement therapy or birth

1. Do not take red clover with warfarin (Coumadin) or heparin.
2. Do not take red clover with gingko, ginseng, and other herbals that also decrease blood clotting.
3. Do not take red clover with ibuprofen.
4. Patients with chronic and inflammatory conditions such as arthritis, fibromyalgia, bursitis, or low back pain are often prescribed NSAIDs for pain control. Therefore the risk of herb-drug interactions may be increased in these populations.
5. Patients with circulatory disorders such as PVD, carotid artery disease, and diabetes are often prescribed anticoagulants for their disorder. Therefore the risk of herb-drug interactions may be increased in these populations.
6. Patients with cardiovascular disease routinely taking an aspirin a day may be an at-risk population for bleeding complications if they are also taking red clover.

control pills should not take red clover. Patients with estrogen-sensitive tumors, such as breast, ovarian, or uterine cancer, should avoid red clover. Patients with liver or kidney disease should also avoid red clover. Safety of use in children has not been determined and should be avoided.

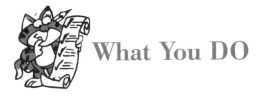

What You DO

Patient History

Patients having surgery or other invasive procedures should be questioned about their herbal medication use. Patients taking red clover should be questioned about their tendencies for bleeding and bruising. Further laboratory testing, such as coagulation studies, may be needed preoperatively. Testing is especially needed if red clover is also taken with antiinflammatory analgesics or anticoagulant medications. Elective surgery should be delayed in patients with increased clotting times until clotting times return to normal.

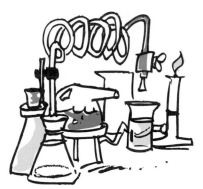

Potential Drug Interactions

Coumarins were originally discovered in spoiled red clover plants. As such, not surprisingly, red clover may increase the blood-thinning effects of warfarin (Coumadin) and heparin. The anticoagulant effects of other herbal medications, such as ginger, garlic, gingko, or vitamin E, may also be increased. Other medications that have blood-thinning action may also enhance the blood-thinning properties of red clover. These medications include aspirin, NSAIDs, or dipyridamole (Persantine).

The estrogen-like activities of red clover may increase the action of other steroid-based medications, such as **corticosteroids**. Red clover may enhance the action of other antituberculosis agents. In addition, red clover inhibits cytochrome CYP450 3A4 hepatic enzyme. By inhibiting this system, red clover has the potential to increase serum levels of drugs such as lovastatin, ketoconazole, itraconazole, fexofenadine, triazolam, or other benzodiazepines. Decreased metabolism of midazolam or fentanyl may delay wake-up times from surgery, increasing operating room times and PACU stays. Severe oversedation problems may result in an overnight hospital stay for what was once a planned outpatient procedure. Reduced metabolism of lidocaine may result in elevated levels and toxic reactions such as sedation, altered mental status, convulsions, hypotension, and cardiovascular collapse. Last, red clover has the potential to interfere with drug absorption in the intestinal tract.

Older adults often have cardiovascular and PVD for which they take anticoagulant medications. The risks of herb-drug interactions may be increased in these older adults.

Patient Education

Patients should be educated about the anticoagulant effects of red clover. Patients should not use red clover with other medications that decrease blood clotting. Patients with **thrombocytopenia** and clotting disorders should be cautioned against using red clover. Patients should stop taking red clover 2 weeks before invasive procedures and inform their surgeon.

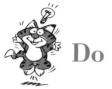

Do You UNDERSTAND?

See pages 245 and 246 for Learning Activities related to this topic.

Key Words

Alterative An ingredient that stimulates elimination that is meant to change an unhealthy state into a healthy one. An alterative is also known as a blood purifier.

Corticosteroid Hormones secreted from the adrenal cortex.

Coumarins Plant chemicals that may exhibit anticoagulant properties, as well as anticancer, immunostimulant, antifungal, antiinflammatory, vasodilatory, muscle-relaxant, hypnotic, CNS-stimulant, hypothermal, diuretic, anticholinergic, antiedema, or estrogenic effects.

Isoflavonoids Plant constituents that affect estrogen receptors often found in soy products. Some isoflavonoids may also have anticarcinogenic or immunostimulatory effects.

Salicylates Phytochemical constituents that are converted into salicin in the bowel and oxidized into salicylic acid by the liver. Salicin is responsible for the herbal antipyretic and antiinflammatory effects. Aspirin is a derivative of salicylic acid obtained from willow bark.

Saponins Phytochemical plant constituents that produce foam when dissolved in water. Saponins reduce surface tension and increase solubility and cell membrane permeability. Saponins may be sugar glycosides or steroidal in composition. Saponins are easily dissolved in the bloodstream and have antiinflammatory, adaptogenic, and aldosterone-like effects. Although saponins may lower cholesterol or affect estrogen metabolism, some saponins may be toxic and cause hemolytic reactions with red blood cells or cause GI upset.

Thrombocytopenia Low levels of platelet cells.

Urticaria An allergic skin reaction, resulting in wheels or papules and intense itching.

TAKE HOME POINTS

Gynecologic patients should remind their physician that they are taking red clover. A good time to convey this information is during their yearly gynecologic examination.

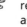

www.consumerlab.com/
results/phytoestrogens2.
asp

St. John's Wort

What IS St. John's Wort?

St. John's wort (*Hypericum perforatum*) is a native wildflower of North America, Europe, and Asia. This type of wildflower is a perennial weed that has yellow flowers with reddish-brown dots. The red color symbolizes the blood of St. John after his beheading. Wort is Old English for "plant." The herb's name also comes from the Greek meaning "over an apparition" because the herb was thought to protect a person from evil spirits. Other names for St. John's wort include demon chaser, goatweed, hardhay, klamath weed, rosin rose, SJW, and tipton weed. St. John's wort has been used for centuries to treat depression. The plant has also been used for trauma, snakebites, gastroenteritis, bruises, menstruation, and hysteria. St. John's wort is prescribed in Germany more often than are other traditional antidepressants. The potency of St. John's wort may vary greatly between products. The active ingredient in St. John's wort is hypericin.

What You NEED TO KNOW

Actions

St. John's wort has been found to be as effective as some standard pharmaceutical antidepressants such as imipramine. The antidepressant activity of St. John's wort is related to the action of several plant constituents such as hypericin, **flavonoids** or hyperforin. St. John's wort stimulates many **neuroreceptors**. Hypericin works at 30 different types of neuroreceptor sites. St. John's wort inhibits uptake of serotonin, dopamine, and norepinephrine. Serotonin and norepinephrine are potent vasoconstrictors. Dopamine readily increases heart rate and is a vasoconstrictor at higher levels. St. John's wort inhibits binding of naloxone to opioid receptors. St. John's wort induces hepatic cytochrome CYP450 3A4, which will increase the metabolism of many drugs. St. John's wort has also demonstrated antiviral and antibacterial activity.

Dose

- Capsules: 5% hyperiforin 300 mg or 300 mg hypericin three times daily
- Liquid extract: 1:1 in 25% alcohol 2 to 4 cc three times daily
- Teas: 2 to 4 gm dried herb steeped 10 minutes in 150 cc water
- The dose should not exceed 1800 mg/day because of phototoxic skin reactions

Side Effects

St. John's wort is generally well tolerated and has fewer side effects than other prescription antidepressants. St. John's wort may rarely cause GI upset, allergic reaction, tiredness, restlessness, or sensitivity to sunlight, resulting in sunburn. Use of St. John's wort may cause abnormal menstrual bleeding. Other infrequent side effects include headache or skin rash. St. John's wort is less likely to cause insomnia if taken in the morning. Rarely, the herb may cause neuropathy. A single case report described possible serotonin syndrome symptoms with hypertension, tachycardia, anxiety, and nausea when St. John's wort was consumed. Withdrawal symptoms may be possible when abruptly stopping the herb.

Indications and Uses

- Anorexia
- Anxiety
- Cancer
- Depression
- Diuretics
- Dysthymia
- Exhaustion
- Fatigue
- Fibrositis
- Headache
- HIV and AIDS
- Indigestion
- Insomnia
- Menopausal symptoms
- Muscle pain
- Neuralgia
- Obsessive compulsive disorder
- Palpitations
- Sciatica
- Seasonal affective disorder
- Sleep disorders
- Topical:
  - Bruises
  - Burns
  - Hemorrhoids
  - Inflammation
  - Neuralgia
  - Wound healing
- Vitiligo

Contraindications and Precautions

Patients with bipolar disease or major depression may possibly experience mania if St. John's wort is consumed. A mild case of mania may occur if severely depressed patients take this herb; schizophrenic patients may

1. St. John's wort should be discontinued 2 weeks preoperatively to prevent interactions with anesthetic drugs.
2. St. John's wort should not be taken by women on birth control pills, by those trying to conceive, or by pregnant or breast-feeding women.
3. Transplant patients may reject organs if they are taking St. John's wort.
4. Patients with HIV and AIDS may have failure of antiviral protease inhibitor drugs when taking St. John's wort.
5. Patients on medications for high blood pressure, angina, or high cholesterol should not take St. John's wort.
6. Chemotherapy may be rendered ineffective if St. John's wort is consumed.
7. The effectiveness of anticoagulants may be decreased by St. John's wort.
8. Patients taking St. John's wort should wear extra sunscreen or clothing to prevent burning on exposure to sunlight.
9. St. John's wort may enhance the sedative effects of diphenhydramine (Benadryl), naphazoline hydrochloride (Allerest, Clear Eyes), or other antihistamines.
10. Patients taking antihypertensive medications, such as diltiazem or nifedipine, should not take St. John's wort because of serotonin uptake inhibition and the resultant vasoconstriction.
11. Patients with coronary artery disease should avoid St. John's wort because the herb may worsen their condition.

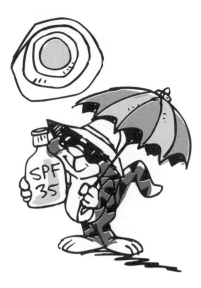

become increasingly psychotic with St. Johns' wort use. Patients with Alzheimer's disease and dementia should avoid this herb because it may provoke psychotic delirium.

St. John's wort may decrease oocyte and sperm formation; therefore patients desiring to have children should not take this herb. Pregnant women should not take St. John's wort because it may stimulate uterine contractions. Infants of breast-feeding mothers who are taking St. John's wort have experienced colic, drowsiness, and lethargy. Thus breast-feeding women should avoid St. John's wort. In addition, fair-skinned individuals should avoid sunlight if taking this herb.

Because St. John's wort affects neurotransmitters, surgical patients should discontinue the use of St. John's wort at least 2 weeks before surgery. St. John's wort has been associated with hypotension and cardiovascular collapse on induction of general anesthesia. St. John's wort may increase narcotic actions.

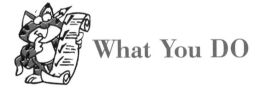

What You DO

Patient History

Nurses should obtain a complete history of herbal medicine use; herbal history is vital to prevent adverse herb-drug interactions. Patients should also be encouraged to discuss herbal medicine use with their physician. Patients with a history of depression or bipolar disease should not take their prescription antidepressants with St. John's wort. Patients requiring surgery should be questioned about their herbal medication use. Many anesthetic agents may interact with St. John's wort, causing adverse cardiovascular or sedative effects and patient compromise. If preoperative surgical patients are taking St. John's wort, elective surgery should be delayed for 2 weeks and St. John's wort use discontinued.

Potential Drug Interactions

St. John's wort increases drug metabolism by the cytochrome CYP450 3A4 enzyme system in the liver, resulting in lowered serum drug levels and decreased actions of many pharmaceutical agents. When drug metabolism is increased, medication action and duration are decreased. When a patient stops taking St. John's wort, the metabolic enzyme system will return to normal. This action may result in toxic drug reactions with medications in that the drug is no longer being metabolized as rapidly as it once was, causing the drug to increase and accumulate in the blood.

Hepatic cytochrome CYP450 3A4 metabolizes many drugs, such as anesthetic agents, anticonvulsants, barbiturates, benzodiazepines, steroids, and narcotics (see list of "Potential Drug Interactions with St. John's Wort). Increased metabolism by cytochrome CYP450 3A4 may account for the decreased action of theophylline in patients taking St. John's wort. St. John's wort also increases drug transportation, which further reduces serum drug levels for medications such as digoxin and cyclosporine.

 1. Older adults are especially sensitive to the sedative effects of medications and should use caution when taking St. John's wort.

2. Older adults should not use St. John's wort with any other sedative agents because of the increased sensitivity to sedative medications.

Potential Drug Interactions with St. John's Wort

- Adriamycin
- alcohol
- alfentanil
- amitriptyline
- amoxapine
- amprenavir
- benzodiazepines
- birth control pills
- carbamazepine
- ciprofloxacin
- citalopram
- clozapine
- cyclophosphamide
- cyclosporin
- delavirdine
- desogestrel
- dextromethorphan
- digoxin
- diltiazem
- doxorubicin
- efavirenz
- ephedrine
- ethinylestradiol
- etoposide
- fenfluramine
- fentanyl
- fexofenadine
- fluoxetine
- fluvoxamine

- frovatriptan
- gatifloxacin
- imipramine
- indinavir
- levofloxacin
- lithium
- local anesthetics
- lomefloxacin
- losartan
- Marplan
- meperidine
- midazolam
- mitoxantrone
- naloxone
- naratriptan
- Nardil
- nefazodone
- nelfinavir
- Neo-Synephrine
- nevirapine
- nicardipine
- nifedipine
- norfloxacin
- nortriptyline
- Olanzapine
- ofloxacin
- omeprazole
- ondansetron
- paclitaxel

- paroxetine
- phenobarbital
- phenprocoumon
- phenytoin
- piroxicam
- propofol
- rapamycin
- reserpine
- ritonavir
- rizatriptan
- saquinavir
- selegiline
- sertraline
- sparfloxacin
- steroids
- sulfa drugs
- sumatriptan
- tacrolimus
- tamoxifen
- taxol
- teniposide
- tetracycline
- theophylline
- tramadol
- trazodone
- verapamil
- vinblastine
- warfarin
- zolmitriptan

The metabolic implications of St. John's wort are far reaching. For example, St. John's wort increases the metabolism of birth control pills. Increased metabolism of birth control pills decreases the effectiveness of birth control pills and increases the risks of pregnancy in women taking St. John's wort and oral contraceptives together.

St. John's wort increases the metabolism of immunosuppressive agents. Thus transplant patients may experience organ rejection if taking both St. John's wort and immunosuppressant drugs. Similarly, St. John's wort increases the metabolism of anticoagulant agents, reducing the anticoagulation effects of these agents. The presence of normal coagulation in patients with a history of deep vein thrombosis or atrial fibrillation can lead to pulmonary or cerebral emboli, stroke, and even death. The effects of cholesterol-lowering drugs may be reduced if taken with St. John's wort. Bronchodilator action is reduced in patients taking St. John's wort, resulting in increased bronchial constriction and asthmatic episodes. Anticonvulsant medications demonstrate less of an effect when taken with St. John's wort, resulting in increased seizure activity in patients with epilepsy and patients who are prone to seizures. St. John's wort decreases the activity of antiviral protease inhibitor drugs prescribed for the treatment of HIV infections and AIDS. Chemotherapeutic agents are also less effective in patients also taking St. John's wort. Thus patients with cancer who are on chemotherapy should not take this herb.

St. John's wort may decrease the effectiveness of cardiovascular drugs, such as beta blockers, or drugs that affect the sympathetic nervous system, resulting in decreased cardiac protection in patients with angina and coronary artery disease.

St. John's wort may work against other antihypertensive agents. First, St. John's wort increases the metabolism of these agents, thereby decreasing their duration and action. Second, the herb's effect on serotonin reuptake promotes vasoconstriction, which is directly counterproductive to the vasodilation effects of many antihypertensive agents.

St. John's wort is a potent serotonin reuptake inhibitor and may cause serotonin surge when taken with nefazodone, sertraline, or other SSRIs. Combined with paroxetine, St. John's wort may cause confusion and agitation, hypertension, or sedative-hypnotic reaction. St. John's wort may increase **photosensitivity** side effects of some antibiotics. St. John's wort increases the action of sedative drugs. Patients should not take St. John's wort with other medications, such as antihistamines, that also cause sedation. Also, patients should not take St. John's wort with other herbal medications (e.g., goldenseal, hops, kava, valerian) that can cause sedation. Patients should not operate heavy equipment until individual sensitivity to the herb's sedative effects is determined.

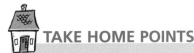

TAKE HOME POINTS

1. St. John's wort should not be combined with prescription antidepressant medications.
2. Patient populations at high risk for drug interactions (those with AIDS, cancer, transplant surgery, and cardiovascular disease) should be informed of the risks of herb-drug interactions with St. John's wort.

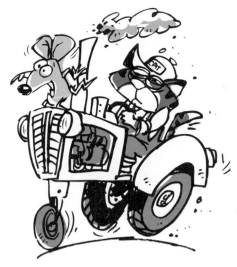

Patient Education

Nurses should educate patients of the many drug interactions with St. John's wort. Surgical patients should be informed to discontinue St. John's wort 2 weeks before surgery. Identification of groups at high risk for adverse herb-drug interactions is important to prevent complications of drug or treatment failure, such as patients with cancer, AIDS, and asthma, as well as transplant and cardiac patients.

If patients on warfarin or heparin therapy are taking St. John's wort, coagulation tests such as PT or PTT must be followed closely because the herb may prevent the anticoagulant from working effectively. Women on birth control pills should understand that they may become pregnant if taking St. John's wort and should be counseled to obtain another form of birth control.

Patients who are depressed should be encouraged to seek medical treatment and not to self-prescribe with herbal medicines because of the many drug interactions with the herb St. John's wort.

Patients taking St. John's wort should avoid alcohol intake because the sedative actions of alcohol may be enhanced.

Patients taking St. John's wort have experienced neuropathies after sunlight exposure. Thus patients taking St. John's wort should avoid direct sunlight exposure and use sun blocking creams with high sun protection factors (SPF 35) when outside.

Do You UNDERSTAND?

See pages 246 through 248 for Learning Activities related to this topic.

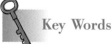

Key Words

Bipolar A mental disorder characterized by manic or hyperexcitable episodes.

Flavonoids Plant pigments responsible for the color of fruits and vegetables. Some flavonoids decrease capillary fragility and scavenge free radicals, creating antioxidant properties. Other flavonoids have antiatherogenic, antiinflammatory, antiviral, or antimutagenic properties.

Mania A mental disorder in which an individual exhibits excessive periods of excitement.

Neuroreceptors Receptors that bind with neurotransmitters for the transmission of nerve impulses.

Photosensitivity Increased sensitivity to light.

 http://nccam.nih.gov/
health/stjohnswort/
index.htm
www.fda.gov/cder/drug/
advisory/stjwort.htm

Vitamins and Dietary Supplements

CHONDROITIN

What IS Chondroitin?

Chondroitin (Chondroitin sulfate), a long-chain polymer of disaccharide units, contains a mixture of intact or partially hydrolyzed glycosaminoglycans found in joint cartilage. Chondroitin sulfate is derived from bovine and calf cartilage. Absorption after oral intake is limited, with only approximately 10% of chondroitin absorbed as a result of its large molecular size. Theories suggest that low–molecular-weight chondroitin may be better absorbed and more effective than is chondroitin sulfate, but this assertion has not been adequately tested to date. Although chondroitin is sold in health food stores, the purity, bioactivity, and equivalent doses of chondroitin differ between manufacturers.

What You NEED TO KNOW

Actions

Chondroitin may be beneficial (e.g., improvements in joint pain and function) to individuals with osteoarthritis. In osteoarthritis, proteoglycan production decreases, leading to a loss of cartilage in the joints. Antiinflammatory effects of chondroitin sulfate have been demonstrated. Chondroitin also increases proteoglycan concentration and reduces collagen breakdown. Some research has suggested that glucosamine and chondroitin are similar in antiinflammatory actions. Chondroitin is often given with glucosamine. Consequently, few studies are available on the effectiveness of chondroitin alone. One recent study, however, indicated that chondroitin with glucosamine had greater reductions in joint pain than when either one was taken by itself.

Dose

The often recommended dose of chondroitin sulfate is:
- 1200 mg/day, and
- May be taken in divided doses; dose response studies are needed.

Side Effects

When taken orally, chondroitin appears to be safe. No adverse effects or very mild side effects (usually mild gastrointestinal symptoms) occur. However, long-term safety and efficacy have not been adequately tested.

Indications and Uses

- Osteoarthritis
- Reduce joint pain and tenderness

Contraindications and Precautions

Purity, bioavailability, and dose of chondroitin may differ by manufacturer.

Individuals taking warfarin (Coumadin) should not take chondroitin.

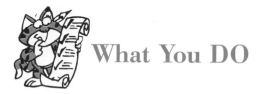

What You DO

Patient History

Patients should be questioned concerning supplement or natural product use. If the patient is taking chondroitin, the nurse should determine the dose per day and the duration of use.

Potential Drug Interactions

Chondroitin may increase the action of hyaluronic acid. This action may be of benefit during cataract surgery.

Patient Education

Patients should be taught to monitor the effects of chondroitin, such as reductions in joint pain and tenderness. Patients should be told that the effectiveness of chondroitin alone or in combination with glucosamine has not been thoroughly studied. Thus whether the addition of chondroitin (with its added costs) to glucosamine preparations increases the effectiveness is unclear.

Do You UNDERSTAND?

See pages 249 and 251 for Learning Activities related to this topic.

Key Words

Glycosaminoglycans Building blocks of connective tissue, such as the cartilage found in joints.
Proteoglycan A protein polysaccharide compound.
Thrombocytopenia Low levels of platelet cells.

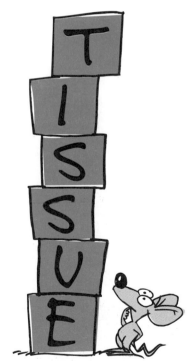

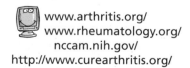

www.arthritis.org/
www.rheumatology.org/
nccam.nih.gov/
http://www.curearthritis.org/

COENZYME Q10

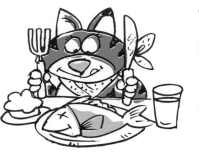

What IS Coenzyme Q10?

Coenzyme Q10 is a fat-soluble essential nutrient found in the mitochondria of the body's cells. High amounts of coenzyme Q10 are present in the liver, kidney, heart, and pancreas. Mitochondria are the powerhouse of the cell that use coenzyme Q10 to make adenosine triphosphate (ATP). Mitochondria also store energy for cell use in maintaining homeostasis and performing cellular functions. Coenzyme Q10 is similar in structure to vitamin K. Coenzyme Q10 is also known as vitamin Q, ubiquinone, and mitoquinone. Coenzyme Q10 is found in meats, seafood, and plants (especially soybeans), and is also manufactured by the body. The name ubiquinone comes from ubiquitous, which describes something that is present everywhere, and quinone, which refers to its biochemical structure. "Q10" refers to the 10-unit side chain of its molecular structure that is present in humans. Decreased levels of coenzyme Q10 have been associated with hypertension, heart failure, periodontal disease, some types of muscular diseases, some types of breast cancer, and poor nutritional states.

What You NEED TO KNOW

Actions

Coenzyme Q10 works as an antioxidant, scavenging free radicals that can be harmful to cell membranes and integrity. Coenzyme Q10 is used in to make ATP, acts as an immune-system stimulator, and may be administered for treating cancer. Coenzyme Q10 is also used for treating heart failure, cardiomyopathy, hypertension, angina, and dysrhythmias. Coenzyme Q10 has positive inotropic effects similar to but less potent than those of digoxin. This effect increases the pumping ability of the heart. Coenzyme Q10 improves heart failure by increasing cardiac output and stroke volume. Coenzyme Q10 also reduces cardiac depression during angina, and it reduces peripheral resistance and decreases the blood pressure in essential hypertension.

 Older adults often have an increased incidence of vessel plaque development coupled with sedentary lifestyles. They should avoid hypercoagulable states.

Dose*

- Heart failure: 100 mg/day in two to three divided doses
- Angina: 50 mg three times daily
- Chemotherapy cardiotoxicity: 50 mg/day
- Acquired immunodeficiency syndrome (AIDS) and human immunodeficiency virus (HIV): 200 mg/day
- Muscular dystrophy: 100 mg/day
- Hypertension: 60 to 120 mg bid

Side Effects

Side effects from coenzyme Q10 are usually rare and mild; they include mild gastric distress, loss of appetite, nausea, and diarrhea. Taking large doses (larger than 100 mg/day) in two to three doses throughout the day can minimize side effects. If doses exceed 300 mg/day, coenzyme Q10 may cause asymptomatic elevations in the liver enzymes lactic dehydrogenase (LDH) and serum glutamic-oxaloacetic transaminase (SGOT) or aspartate aminotransferase (AST).

Indications and Uses

- AIDS
- Atherosclerosis
- Angina
- Cancer
- Cardiac dysrhythmias
- Cerebrovascular accident
- Chemotherapy-induced cardiomyopathy (treatment and prevention)
- Dyspnea
- Heart failure
- Immune system stimulation
- HIV
- Hypertension
- Liver congestion
- Mitral valve prolapse
- Muscular dystrophy
- Myocardial infarction
- Obesity
- Peripheral edema
- Periodontal disease
- After open-heart surgery reperfusion injury syndrome
- Pulmonary edema

1. Coenzyme Q10 may increase the hypotensive actions of clonidine or other anti-hypertensive agents.
2. Undesirable hypotension may occur when coenzyme Q10 is taken with other hypotensive agents, such as captopril, nifedipine, and losartan.
3. Undesirable hypotension may occur when coenzyme Q10 is taken with agents targeted to improve peripheral blood flow, such as dipyridamole or papaverine.
4. Undesirable hypotension may occur in anesthetized patients who take coenzyme Q10 preoperatively.
5. Patients taking warfarin (Coumadin) should avoid coenzyme Q10.
6. Hypercoagulable states should be avoided in patients with a history of deep vein thrombosis or emboli, peripheral vascular disease, diabetes, cardiac valve disease, or those with mechanical heart valves.
7. Increased coagulation may lead to increased loss of artificial venous access devices and renal dialysis access devices.

Contraindications and Precautions

The safety of using coenzyme Q10 in pregnancy or lactation has not been established and therefore should be avoided. Cardiovascular and cerebrovascular diseases should not be self-treated. Trained medical personnel should direct the management of these disease conditions.

*It is recommended that doses exceeding 100 mg be taken in divided doses to minimize side effects.

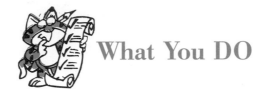

What You DO

Patient History

The patient's medication history should be reviewed for compatibility with their other medications and disease state. Patients with coronary or cerebral vascular disease should seek the advice of trained health care personnel. Coenzyme Q10 is not effective in cases of severe heart failure. Patients should discontinue coenzyme Q10 use 2 weeks before surgery and anesthesia.

Potential Drug Interactions

Coenzyme Q10 may increase the hypotensive effects with intravenous and inhalational anesthetics during surgery, rendering the patient less able to compensate for fluid shifts and blood loss during anesthesia. Coenzyme Q10 should be stopped 2 weeks before surgical and other invasive procedures.

Increased hypotensive effects may also occur with patients taking coenzyme Q10 and antihypertensive medications, such as angiotensin II receptor blockers, angiotension-converting enzyme (ACE) inhibitors, or calcium channel–blocking agents. A similar effect may be expected when taking coenzyme Q10 with other diuretic agents. Stopping coenzyme Q10 after achieving hypertension control may result in increased blood pressure and reemergence of hypertension. This result is caused by the loss of vasodilatory effects from coenzyme Q_{10}. Last, vasodilation may also be increased when coenzyme Q10 is used with other medications given for treatment of vascular insufficiency.

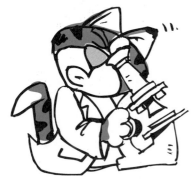

Laboratory testing has shown that cancer cells may increase their resistance to chemotherapy in the presence of antioxidant medications. Patients with cancer should consult with their oncologist before taking coenzyme Q10.

Patients taking warfarin should not take coenzyme Q10. Coenzyme Q10 may have actions similar to those of vitamin K. Vitamin K works against the actions of warfarin (Coumadin), reducing its effectiveness. Taking coenzyme Q10 may decrease the anticoagulant actions of warfarin. This decrease would allow normal coagulation to occur in patients in whom this is undesirable (those with carotid disease or atrial fibrillation heart rhythm). Abruptly stopping coenzyme Q10 intake in patients taking warfarin may result in drastic increases in clotting times, bleeding, and bruising. The prothrombin time should be followed closely and warfarin dose adjusted accordingly in this situation.

When taken with aspirin, nonsteroidal antiinflammatory drugs (NSAIDs), and other anticoagulant medications, the anticoagulation effects of coenzyme Q10 may work against the blood-thinning effects of these agents.

Herbal preparations of red yeast, beta-blocking medications, cholesterol-lowering agents (lovastatin, simvastatin, and fluvastatin), and some oral hypoglycemic agents (glyburide and tolazamide) may reduce blood levels of coenzyme Q10. The meaning of this interaction has not been determined.

Patient Education

Coenzyme Q10 levels increase during biliary obstruction or liver insufficiency. Patients with these complications should avoid or stop using coenzyme Q10.

Patients should be educated about the vasodilatory effects of coenzyme Q10. Patients receiving antihypertensive therapy should not use alternative medications with vasodilatory effects. Patients with circulatory insufficiency should also be cautious in using coenzyme Q10 because it may increase the effects of their other prescription. Excessive vasodilation in patients with cardiovascular and peripheral vascular insufficiency may lead to decreased cardiac output, decreased blood flow, and organ ischemia.

Do You UNDERSTAND?

See pages 249 and 250 for Learning Activities related to this topic.

 Key Words

Free radicals Reactive molecules with unpaired electrons that may destroy or damage other molecules to accept an electron. Free radicals may interfere with oxidative metabolism of nutrients and cause an increased incidence of cancer, cardiovascular or cerebrovascular, and inflammatory diseases. Antioxidants found in some herbs and vitamins decrease the formation of free radicals and oxidation of molecules.

Inotropic Pertaining to the contracting ability of the heart.

Cardiac output The amount of blood pumped out of the heart in a minute.

Stroke volume The amount of blood pumped out of the heart during one heartbeat.

 www.vvv.com/
healthnews/dq10rewb.
html
http://cis.nci.nih.gov/fact/9_16.htm
www.cancer.gov/cancerinfo/pdq/
cam/coenzymeQ10

FISH OIL

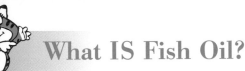

What IS Fish Oil?

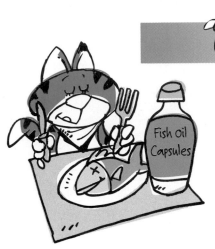

Fish oil (also known as omega-3 fatty acid, n-3 fatty acid, n-3 polyunsaturated fatty acid [PUFA], eicosapentaenoic acid [EPA], and docosahexaenoic acid [DHA]) is abundant in shellfish, marine mammals, and fish. The highest concentration of n-3 PUFAs is found in herring, cod liver, salmon, mackerel, and sardines. Most fish oil supplements contain between 300 and 500 mg of omega-3 fish oil per 1-g capsule; therapeutic levels may require 15 to 30 capsules per day.

What You NEED TO KNOW

Actions

Fish oils have antiinflammatory and antiembolus effects. Fish oils promote vasodilation and reduce platelet stickiness. Fish oils may be similar to lithium in slowing nerve conduction.

Fish oils reduce the production of very low–density lipoproteins, the so-called "bad" cholesterol. Fish oils also reduce fatty acid production, cholesterol absorption from the gastrointestinal (GI) tract, and cholesterol production. Last, fish oils may also have some anticancer actions.

Dose

- 5 to 15 g of fish oil per day
- Study doses range from 3 g of fish oil per day to 18 g per day
- 4 to 6 months possibly required to obtain benefits

Side Effects

Fish oils may cause belching, bad breath, heartburn, and nosebleeds. A review found that 10 capsules of fish oil per day or 25 ml of cod liver oil per day was associated with long-term safety. Long-term studies of potentially adverse effects have not been published, however. Starting with lower doses and then increasing the dose over time can decrease side effects.

Indications and Uses

- Angina
- Asthma
- Atherosclerosis
- Autoimmune diseases
- Cachexia
- Coronary heart disease
- Diabetes
- Dysmenorrhea
- Hyperlipidemia
- Hypertension
- Hypertriglyceridemia
- Inflammatory bowel disease
- Myocardial infarction
- Nephrotic syndrome
- Rheumatoid arthritis
- Psoriasis
- Migraines
- Malaria
- Some cancers
- Thrombosis

Contraindications and Precautions

Fish oils may increase bleeding time, thus caution should be used in patients on anticoagulants, pregnant women, anyone with bleeding disorders, or patients on medications that increase bleeding time.

Eating large quantities of fish may increase the risk of toxicity, depending on the source of the fish.

Fish oil taken for many months may deplete the body of vitamin E and contribute to cardiac necrosis.

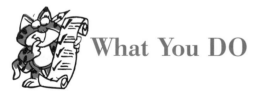 **What You DO**

Patient History

Patients taking aspirin or other anticoagulants should limit fish oil intake and have their clotting time monitored. Pregnant women, although often

1. **Do not take fish oil with warfarin (Coumadin) or heparin.**
2. **Do not take fish oil with ginger, ginkgo, or ginseng.**
3. **Patients taking aspirin, ibuprofen, rofecoxib (Vioxx), or nabumetone (Relafen) on a routine basis should avoid fish oil.**
4. **Surgical patients taking fish oil should not receive ketorolac (Toradol) for postoperative pain management.**
5. **Patients with circulatory disorders such as peripheral vascular disease, carotid artery disease, and diabetes are often taking anticoagulants or blood-thinning agents (aspirin or dipyridamole [Persantine]) for their disorder. These populations may be at increased risk of herb-drug interactions.**
6. **Patients with cardiovascular disease or hypercholesterolemia routinely taking an aspirin a day may present an increased risk for bleeding complications if they are also taking fish oil.**
7. **Patients taking nifedipine, captopril, or other antihypertensives may experience increased hypotensive effects when taking fish oil.**

1. Older adults frequently experience hypertension, peripheral and cardiovascular disease, and arthritis. Prescription medications commonly used in these disease states may increase the anticoagulant effects of fish oil.

2. Older adults are often have coronary artery disease. Lowered blood pressure from fish oil may decrease blood flow to coronary arteries with blockages. This decrease may lead to myocardial ischemia or infarction.

deficient in EPA and DHA, should use caution because of potentially prolonged bleeding times. When presenting for surgery or invasive procedures, patients need to be questioned concerning fish oil use. Further laboratory tests, such as coagulation studies, may be indicated to determine coagulation function.

If taken before surgery, fish oil may have additive blood pressure–lowering effects with anesthetics. This effect will make the surgical patient less able to compensate for fluid shifts and blood loss during anesthesia. Fish oil should be discontinued 2 weeks before surgical and other invasive procedures.

Fish oil may increase blood-sugar levels in patients with diabetes. Patients with diabetes who are using fish oil should closely monitor their blood-sugar level and adjust insulin dose as needed.

Potential Drug Interactions

Fish oil taken for many months may cause a deficiency of vitamin E. Fish oil may increase the anticoagulation seen with anticoagulants and medications that decrease clotting, such as warfarin, pentoxifylline, indomethacin, dipyridamole, aspirin, and ibuprofen. Fish oil might also decrease blood clotting when combined with herbs such as ginkgo, feverfew, red clover, kava kava, ginger, or ginseng.

The vasodilating properties of fish oil may enhance the blood pressure–lowering effects of anesthetic agents and antihypertensive medications. Common antihypertensive medications include angiotensin II receptor antagonists, ACE inhibitors, and calcium channel–blocking agents. A similar increased blood pressure–lowering effect may be expected when taking fish oil with other diuretics. Stopping fish oil use after achieving hypertension control may result in increased blood pressure and reemergence of hypertension resulting from the loss of vasodilatory effects from the oil. Vasodilation may also be increased when used with other vasodilating medications given for treatment of vascular insufficiency. Last, increased hypotension may occur when fish oil is used with other herbs that also cause vasodilation. Herbs and dietary supplements that also lower blood pressure include astragalus, black cohosh, coenzyme Q10, evening primrose, garlic, ginkgo, goldenseal, and hawthorn. Niacin, or vitamin B3, has been recommended for lowering lipids. Niacin may also cause vasodilation and flushing. Thus it should not be taken with fish oil.

Patient Education

Taking large doses of fish oil can be a significant source of calories (9 cal/g of oil). Patients should be warned about the possible anticoagulant effects of fish oil. In addition, patients with **thrombocytopenia** and clotting disorders should avoid fish oil. Patients should stop taking fish oil 2 weeks before invasive procedures and inform their surgeon.

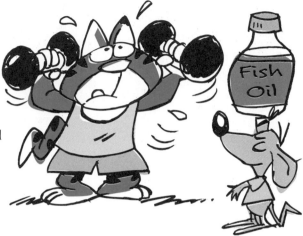

Patients should know about the possible increased hypotensive effects of fish oil when used with other blood pressure–reducing agents. Patients should be cautious when using fish oil if they have hypertension. Patients should avoid taking fish oil when taking other medications and herbals that have blood pressure–lowering effects.

Patients with any disease that may effect blood-sugar levels (e.g., diabetes mellitus, polycystic ovarian syndrome) should be cautioned in using fish oil because blood-sugar levels may be increased.

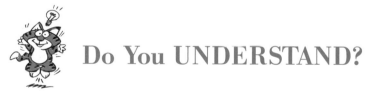

Do You UNDERSTAND?

See pages 250 and 251 for Learning Activities related to this topic.

Key Word

Thrombocytopenia Low levels of platelet cells.

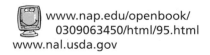
www.nap.edu/openbook/
0309063450/html/95.html
www.nal.usda.gov

GLUCOSAMINE

What IS Glucosamine?

Glucosamine is an aminomonosaccharide that stimulates the manufacture of **glycosaminoglycans** and **glucoprotein,** which form cartilage. Found in joint cartilage, glycosaminoglycans are used in replacing losses to cartilage structure as individuals age. Thus glucosamine may be used in the treatment of osteoarthritis. Glucosamine is made by humans through the addition of an amino group to glucose. About 90% of glucosamine is absorbed when taken orally. Various forms of glucosamine are available, and the purity, sodium content, bioactivity, and the equivalent doses of glucosamine differ. Glucosamine sulfate is the form that most clinical studies have tested for effectiveness.

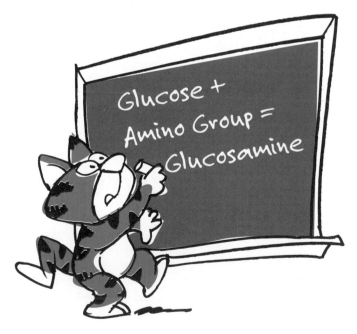

Glucose +
Amino Group =
Glucosamine

What You NEED TO KNOW

Actions

Many studies have demonstrated improvements in joint pain and function after individuals with osteoarthritis received glucosamine. In osteoarthritis, proteoglycan production decreases, leading to loss of cartilage structure in the joints. Although the exact mechanism of action remains unknown, research suggests that glucosamine stimulates proteoglycan production in joint cartilage, which reduces the overall loss of cartilage. The antiinflammatory effects of glucosamine are different from those of NSAIDs (e.g., ibuprofen) that inhibit prostaglandins. Because glucosamine stimulates proteoglycan production, cell membranes appear to be stabilized. This action leads to an antiinflammatory effect. Additionally, glucosamine may decrease the amount of superoxide radicals produced by macrophages. Glucosamine is slow acting, thus a person may have to take it for a long period (perhaps as long as 2 months) before realizing any benefits.

Dose

- 1500 mg/day
- May be taken in divided doses

Side Effects

When taken orally, glucosamine appears to be safe. No adverse effects or very mild side effects occur with glucosamine. These side effect include mild GI complaints such as gas, bloating, and cramps. Side effects may be decreased by taking glucosamine with food. The long-term safety has not been established through clinical studies.

Indications and Uses

- Osteoarthritis
- Reduce joint pain and tenderness

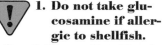

1. **Do not take glucosamine if allergic to shellfish.**
2. **Carefully monitor blood sugar when taking glucosamine, especially if patient has diabetes mellitus, polycystic ovarian syndrome, or other diseases with hyperinsulinemia.**
3. **Purity, bioavailability, and dose of glucosamine may differ by manufacturer.**

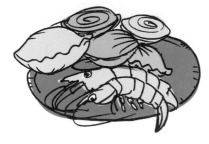

Contraindications and Precautions

Glucosamine should not be taken by individuals who have allergies to shellfish. Glucosamine may raise blood-sugar levels. Therefore patients with diabetes mellitus, polycystic ovarian syndrome, or other diseases with hyperinsulinemia should discuss glucosamine use with their physician. Patients should also continue careful blood-sugar monitoring if taking this supplement.

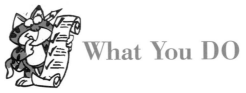

What You DO

Patient History

Patients should be questioned concerning supplement or natural product use. If taking glucosamine, determine the dose per day, the duration of use, and the patient's assessment of its effectiveness. The nurse should also ask whether other arthritis or antiinflammatory medication use has been reduced after taking glucosamine. Blood-sugar levels should be monitored if the patient has diabetes mellitus, prediabetes factors (e.g., weight gain or obesity, high normal fasting blood sugars, sedentary lifestyle), polycystic ovarian syndrome, or other conditions that influence glucose metabolism.

The nurse should caution patients about using glucosamine preparations that also contain manganese. These preparations of glucosamine may contain large amounts of manganese, even when taken according to manufacturer directions. Taking more than 11 mg of manganese a day can result in serious central nervous system (CNS) problems.

Potential Drug Interactions

If glucosamine is effective for the patient, reducing NSAID use may be possible. Glucosamine may decrease the blood sugar–lowering effects of insulin or oral hypoglycemic agents. However, this property has not been studied clinically.

Patient Education

Patients should be taught to monitor the effects of glucosamine, such as reductions in joint pain and tenderness. If joint pain is decreased after glucosamine use, patients should discuss the possibility of reducing NSAID use with their physician. Patients with any disease that may affect blood-sugar levels (e.g., diabetes mellitus, polycystic ovarian syndrome) should be cautioned in using glucosamine because it may increase blood-sugar levels.

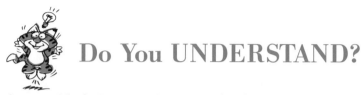

Do You UNDERSTAND?

See page 251 for Learning Activities related to this topic.

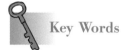

Key Words

Glycosaminoglycans and glucoproteins Building blocks of connective tissue, such as the cartilage found in joints.

Prostaglandins Released after tissue injury, these proinflammatory substances sensitize nerve cells, which increases sensation of pain. Aspirin and NSAIDs decrease the amount of prostaglandins, resulting in decreased inflammation and pain sensations.

Superoxide A highly reactive form of oxygen that can damage tissues.

www.arthritis.org/
www.rheumatology.org/
http://nccam.nih.gov/
www.curearthritis.org/

VITAMIN C

What IS Vitamin C?

Vitamin C (*ascorbic acid*) is an essential nutrient, abundantly found in many fruits. The herbal form of vitamin C comes from the fruit of the rose plant, also called rose hips (*Rosa canina*). Rose hips are also known as dog rose, wild

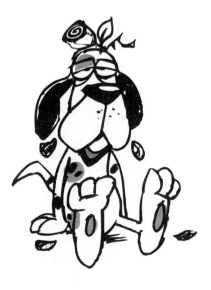

boar fruit, or rose hip with seed. Vitamin C is also known as sodium ascorbate and ascorbic acid. The Greeks called roses the "Queen of Flowers," Ancient Christians considered rose hips sacred; they created rosary beads from the fruit of the rose plant. The petals, fruits, seeds, and leaves are used medicinally. Rose hips also contain vitamins E, B, and K, as well as pectin, carotene, citric acid, flavonoids, oils, and proteins. Processing of rose hips destroys much of the vitamin C. Commercial preparations of rose hips are usually enhanced with laboratory-manufactured vitamin C, even though product labeling does not state this fact.

 # What You NEED TO KNOW

Actions

Vitamin C is needed for collagen and tissue formation, hormone production, carbohydrate metabolism, production of lipids and proteins, iron metabolism, cellular metabolism, and immune-system function. Vitamin C acts as an antioxidant, scavenging free radicals that can cause cellular damage; it is also used in red blood cell production and bone development. Taking high doses of vitamin C may decrease the duration of cold symptoms. Vitamin C may decrease the risk of gall bladder disease in women but not men. Topical vitamin C may decrease the appearance of skin wrinkles. The pectin and citric acid components of rose hips have laxative and diuretic actions.

Dose or Recommended Daily Allowance (RDA)

- Tea from steeping 2.0 to 2.5 g of crushed rose hips in 150 ml boiling water and strained
- RDA for vitamin C is 80 to 150 mg

Older adults have an increased incidence of cardiovascular and peripheral vascular disease. These individuals represent an at-risk population that should be cautioned to avoid large doses of vitamin C.

Side Effects

Vitamin C rarely causes side effects in adults. Vitamin C or rose hips may cause nausea, vomiting, diarrhea, heartburn, and intestinal cramping. Taking large amounts of vitamin C may lead to deep vein thrombosis. Breathing in rose hip dust has caused allergic reactions in individuals processing rose hips.

 Consuming large amounts of vitamin C may be harmful.

Indications and Uses

- Aids
- Alcoholism
- Allergies
- Alzheimer's disease
- Antioxidant
- Arthritis
- Asthma
- Burns
- Cataracts
- Chest congestion
- Colds
- Collagen development
- Depression
- Diabetes
- Diarrhea
- Diuretic
- Fever
- Fractures
- Gallbladder ailments
- Gallstones
- Gastric spasms
- Gastric ulcers
- Gout
- Hematuria
- Hepatitis
- Herpes
- Hypertension
- Hypercholesterolemia
- Influenza
- Immune system stimulation
- Increasing peripheral circulation
- Inflammatory bowel disease
- Kidney disorders
- Laxative
- Lower urinary tract disorders
- Male infertility
- Menopause
- Morning sickness
- Myocardial infarction
- Parkinson's disease
- Periodontal disease
- Rheumatoid arthritis
- Sciatica
- Scurvy
- Sore throats
- Total parenteral nutrition
- Uric acid disorders
- Wound healing

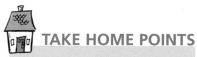

TAKE HOME POINTS

1. Foods high in vitamin C include citrus fruits, strawberries, tomatoes, broccoli, bell peppers, and green leafy vegetables.
2. Vitamin C is lost from food when food is heated. Foods rich in vitamin C should be eaten raw for maximal vitamin C content.
3. The RDA of vitamin C is 150 mg for adults.

Contraindications and Precautions

Side effects from taking vitamin C are rare when taken in amounts normally found in food or as found in the RDA. Vitamin-C toxicity is rare because of the water solubility and renal excretion of vitamin C. Taking large amounts is to be avoided and may cause diarrhea. Infants of pregnant or breast-feeding women who take large quantities of vitamin C may develop scurvy. Pregnant and breast-feeding women should not consume more than 2 grams of vitamin C per day. Large doses of vitamin C may increase the risk of kidney stone formation.

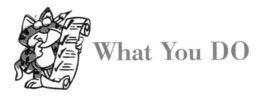

What You DO

Patient History

The patient's medical and medication history should be reviewed for herbal and alternative medication intake to determine interactions between medications and disease processes.

Potential Drug Interactions

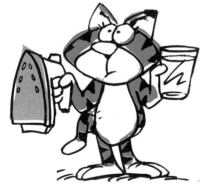

Taking vitamin C with anticoagulants such as heparin or warfarin (Coumadin) may decrease the effect of the anticoagulant. Coagulation studies should be followed closely so that appropriate levels of anticoagulation are maintained. Taking vitamin C with iron may increase the absorption of iron. Chronic use of estrogen hormone therapy, birth control pills, tetracyclines, and salicylic acid (aspirin) increases the daily requirements of vitamin C. Taking large doses of vitamin C may decrease the elimination of acetaminophen and aspirin. Taking large amounts of vitamin C interferes with many laboratory tests. Cigarette smoking may increase the elimination of vitamin C.

Patient Education

Patients should be educated to avoid consuming large amounts of vitamin C. Taking large amounts of vitamin C during cancer therapy has not been proven to be helpful. Patients with peripheral vascular and cardiovascular disease should avoid taking large amounts of vitamin C. This excess may lead to increased risks of thrombosis. Taking large doses of vitamin C may be harmful in patients with cardiac disease and cancer. Patients should inform their health care provider about their vitamin C intake before laboratory testing.

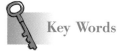 # Do You UNDERSTAND?

See pages 252 and 253 for Learning Activities related to this topic.

 ## Key Words

Flavonoids Plant pigments responsible for the color of fruits and vegetables. Some flavonoids increase capillary wall stability (decrease capillary fragility) and scavenge free radicals, resulting in antioxidant properties. Other flavonoids have antiarthritis, antiinflammatory, antiviral, or antimutagenic properties.

Free radicals Reactive molecules with unpaired electrons that may destroy or damage other molecules to accept an electron. Free radicals may interfere with oxidative metabolism of nutrients and cause an increased incidence of cancer, cardiovascular, or cerebrovascular and inflammatory diseases. Antioxidants found in some herbs and vitamins decrease free-radical formation and oxidation of molecules.

 www.usda.gov
www.realtime.net/anr/
vitamins.html

VITAMIN E

What IS Vitamin E?

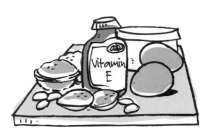

Vitamin E is an essential fat-soluble vitamin that includes eight naturally occurring ingredients in two classes designated as tocopherols and tocotrienols. D-alpha-tocopherol has the highest biologic activity and is the most widely available form of vitamin E found in food. However, gamma-tocopherol accounts for 75% of vitamin E in Western diets. Levels of vitamin E in the body depend on proper levels of zinc. Vitamin E can be found in beans, eggs, almonds, apricot oil, cottonseed oil, hazelnuts, margarine, peanut oil, safflower nuts, walnuts, wheat germ and whole-wheat flour, and assorted fruits and vegetables.

What You NEED TO KNOW

Actions

Vitamin E is an antioxidant, meaning that it binds with free radicals to neutralize their harmful effects. Vitamin E is responsible for proper functioning of the immune system and for maintaining healthy eyes and skin. Vitamin E protects polyunsaturated fats in the body from oxidation, maintains the integrity of the body's membranes, and promotes normal clotting of the blood. Vitamin E also has some antitumor capabilities. Vitamin E taken with vitamin C may help prevent preeclampsia.

Vitamin E is absorbed through the GI tract and is stored in tissues and organs throughout the body, its major site of storage being adipose tissue. Some conditions may cause vitamin E depletion. These conditions include liver disease, celiac disease, and cystic fibrosis. Patients with end-stage renal disease who are undergoing chronic dialysis may also be at risk for vitamin E deficiency.

Older adults are a special population who may be taking vitamin E (for prevention of dementia), as well as other medications for heart and vascular diseases that decrease blood clotting.

Dose or RDA

- Men: 10 mg or 15 international units (IU)
- Women: 8 mg or 12 IU
- Pregnant women: 10 mg or 15 IU
- Requirement dependent on intake of polyunsaturated fatty acids, intake of other antioxidants, age, environmental pollutants, and physical activity

Side Effects

Vitamin E deficiency may cause fatigue, concentration problems, weakened immune system, anemia, and low thyroid levels. Low serum levels of vitamin E have also been linked to depression. Vitamin E is well tolerated, and side effects of high intakes are rare; however, daily doses should not exceed 1000 to 1200 IU. In some individuals who are deficient in vitamin K, vitamin E may increase the risk of hemorrhage or bleeding. Ointments, oils, and creams that contain vitamin E may cause contact dermatitis. Individuals considering using these topical preparations should try it on a small patch of skin before use.

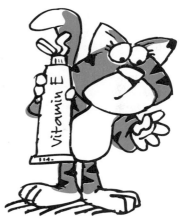

Indications and Uses

- AIDS
- Alzheimer's disease
- Asthma
- Cancer prevention
- Cystic fibrosis
- Diabetes
- Duodenal ulcers
- Eye disease prevention
- Fibrocystic breast disease
- Gallstones
- Gastric ulcers
- Gout
- Heart disease prevention
- Huntington's chorea
- Immune system protection
- Inflammatory bowl disease
- Liver disease
- Male infertility
- Memory loss prevention
- Menopause
- Multiple sclerosis
- Neuromuscular disorders
- Osteoarthritis
- Pain relief
- Parkinson's disease
- Periodontal disease
- Preeclampsia
- Premenstrual syndrome
- Skin disorders
- Tardive dyskinesia

1. **Patients taking warfarin (Coumadin) or heparin should avoid vitamin E.**
2. **Patients should not take vitamin E with ginkgo, ginseng, garlic, and ginger.**
3. **Patients taking aspirin, ibuprofen, or nabumetone (Relafen) on a routine basis should avoid vitamin E.**
4. **Patients with chronic and inflammatory conditions such as arthritis, fibromyalgia, bursitis, or low back pain are often prescribed NSAIDs routinely for pain control. The risk of herb-drug interactions may be increased in these populations.**
5. **Patients with circulatory disorders such as peripheral vascular disease, carotid artery disease, and diabetes are often prescribed blood-thinning agents for their disorder. Therefore the risk of herb-drug interactions may be increased in these populations.**
6. **Aspirin and dipyridamole (Persantine) decrease blood clotting.**
7. **Patients with cardiovascular disease or hypercholesterolemia routinely taking an aspirin a day may be an at-risk population for bleeding complications if they are also taking vitamin E.**
8. **Patients with liver dysfunction and vitamin-K deficiencies should not take vitamin E.**

Contraindications and Precautions

Individuals taking anticoagulant or antiplatelet medications should consult their health care provider before taking vitamin E because it may increase the anticoagulation seen with these drugs. Patients with decreased vitamin K should not take vitamin E because bleeding problems may increase. Patients with retinitis pigmentosa should not take vitamin E (400 IU dose), which has been reported to cause worsening of the condition.

Some iron supplements (nonheme, inorganic) destroy vitamin E. Patients taking vitamin E supplements and iron should space out their doses. Alcohol, mineral oil, and large doses of vitamin A can decrease vitamin E absorption. Dosage adjustments may be necessary in patients who fall into these categories.

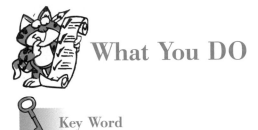

What You DO

Key Word

Alkaloids Reactive molecules with unpaired electrons that may destroy or damage other molecules to accept an election. Free radicals may interfere with oxidative metabolism of nutrients and cause an increased incidence of cancer, cardiovascular, or cerebrovascular and inflammatory diseases. Antioxidants found in some herbs and vitamins decrease free-radical formation and oxidation of molecules.

Patient History

When presenting for surgery or invasive procedures, patients need to be questioned concerning their over-the-counter medications and herbal medication intake. Further laboratory tests, such as coagulation studies, may be indicated preoperatively.

Potential Drug Interactions

Vitamin E may increase the blood-thinning effects of anticoagulant medications. The anticoagulant effects of other herbal medications and other blood-thinning medications (e.g., aspirin, NSAIDs) taken on a routine basis may also be enhanced.

Patients taking iron supplements should be aware that these supplements destroy vitamin E. The absorption of vitamin E may be decreased by large doses of vitamin A. Alcohol and mineral oil should be avoided in vitamin E–deficient individuals because these agents also reduce vitamin E absorption.

Patient Education

Patients should be educated about the anticoagulant effects of vitamin E. In addition, patients with low platelet counts (thrombocytopenia) and other clotting disorders should be warned about the use of herbal medications that have anticoagulation effects. Patients should discontinue taking vitamin E 10 to 14 days before invasive procedures or surgery and inform their surgeon that they have a history of vitamin E use. Patients with vitamin K problems or retinitis pigmentosa should not take vitamin E. Very low doses (3 IU) of vitamin E do not seem to worsen retinitis pigmentosa.

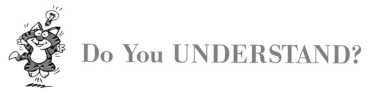

Do You UNDERSTAND?

See page 253 for Learning Activities related to this topic.

http://www.usda.gov/cnpp/
http://www.nutrition.org/
nutinfo/
http://web.indstate.edu/thcme/
mwking/vitamins.html

Key Word

Free radicals Reactive molecules with unpaired electrons that may destroy or damage other molecules to accept an electron. Free radicals may interfere with oxidative metabolism of nutrients and cause an increased incidence of cancer and cardiovascular, cerebrovascular, and inflammatory diseases. Antioxidants found in some herbs and vitamins decrease free-radical formation and oxidation of molecules.

PART II

Nonpharmacologic Therapies

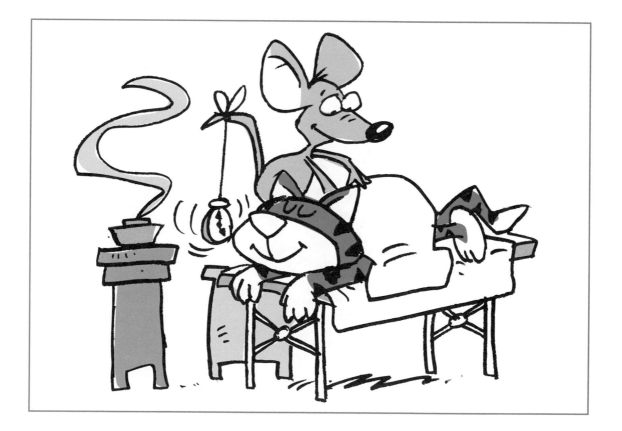

Healing with Physical Power

CHIROPRACTIC THERAPY

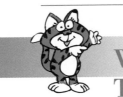

What IS Chiropractic Therapy?

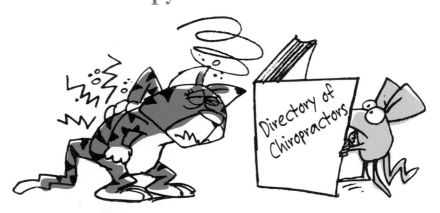

Chiropractic therapy uses spinal manipulation and adjustments to bring about healing. Chiropractic therapy views improper alignment of the vertebral column as the basis of disease. Improper alignment of the vertebrae causes impingement on the spinal nerves where they exit from the spinal column. Spinal nerves carry important messages from the brain to the body for the purpose of maintaining bodily functions. Impingement of these nerves disrupts the flow of messages from the brain to the body, resulting in malfunction, pain, and disease.

What You NEED TO KNOW

Benefits and Uses

Chiropractic therapy can be used to treat the following conditions:

- Arthritis
- Acute pain syndromes
- Carpel tunnel syndrome
- Chronic pain syndromes
- Headaches
- Hyperactivity
- Muscle pain
- Neuritis
- Sprains

Risks and Precautions

Worsening of the pain a day or two after spinal adjustment is not uncommon. Spinal manipulation may result in spinal injury, vascular injury in the cervical or spinal areas, nerve injury, neuralgias, or paresthesias. Rarely, overzealous manipulation may cause cerebral vascular hemorrhage, paraplegia, or quadriplegia.

More than one treatment is usually needed to treat the condition adequately. Patients with chronic conditions may be overexposed to x-ray photography as a part of diagnosis and treatment. Caution should be exercised in the number of x-rays taken annually.

Chiropractic therapy should not be used for emergency or life-threatening situations, and it is not recommended as the first-line treatment for cervical neck rotation.

What You DO

Patient Education

Patients should understand that research into the uses and benefits of chiropractic therapy is limited. Chiropractic therapy has been approved for low back pain and is reimbursable by many insurance companies for this indication.

TAKE HOME POINTS

1. Some chiropractors also use physical therapy, nutritional therapy, herbals, and diet supplements during treatment to aid healing.
2. Massage and acupuncture may be used with spinal manipulation during treatment.

Practitioners

In the United States, college training and a certifying examination is required for practice. The 4-year college degree includes a 1-year residency requirement. Chiropractic therapy is also taught to practitioners of naturopathy and osteopathy. The American Chiropractic Association and the International Chiropractors Association are representative associations for chiropractic practitioners.

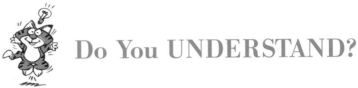

Do You UNDERSTAND?

www.aacp.net
www.chirobase.org/
  07strategy/goodchiro.html   See page 254 for Learning Activities related to this topic.

MASSAGE THERAPY

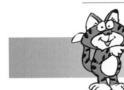

What IS Massage Therapy?

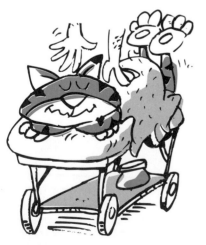

Massage therapy uses various hands-on techniques to carefully manipulate the skin, muscle, and connective tissue (soft tissue) to positively affect well being and health. The effects derived from massage depend on the type and speed of the movements, the area being treated, and the degree of pressure exerted by the therapist's hand, fingers, or thumbs.

Massage and touch have been an important part of healing for many cultures and civilizations throughout time. Massage was used as a therapy modality by the ancient cultures of the Greeks, Hindus, Chinese, Egyptians, and Persians. Nurses have used effleurage, kneading, and percussion as forms of massage. Florence Nightingale used back rubs to enhance skin integrity, soothe patients, and promote relaxation and sleep.

Massage is a nonpharmacologic and holistic nursing intervention that promotes a mind-body connection and relieves discomfort and pain. With shortened hospital stays, high-tech units, increased use of technology and machines, and decreased staffing, massage is a comfort measure that has all but disappeared. In many instances, nurses touch patients only when performing intrusive and painful procedures. Massage is a way to communicate caring and compassion for patients who respond to the unfamiliar hospital environment and procedures with isolation, passivity, and defensiveness. Massage invites the patient to participate in her or his healing process, and it contributes to a balance between dependency and autonomy.

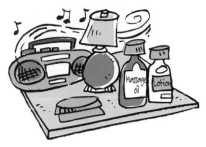

 # What You NEED TO KNOW

Benefits and Uses

Benefits

The purpose or goal of massage is to increase health and well being and—in the case of illness—to help the body heal itself. The skin is the largest organ in the body, containing over 5 million touch receptors that send messages to the brain. Research has shown that the rhythmic stroking and pressure of massage lowers blood pressure and heart rate, improves blood circulation, carries oxygen and other nutrients to cells, and removes waste products (such as lactic acid) from muscles. Massage also promotes the flow of lymphatic fluid, lowers stress hormone levels, and increases production of endorphins, thereby enhancing the immune system. The physiologic, psychosocial, and spiritual benefits derived from massage are many, including:

- Tension relief and relaxation
- Deeper breathing
- Decreased blood pressure and heart rate
- Improved quality of sleep and relief from insomnia
- Increased endorphins and decreased need for pain medication
- Decreased pain
- Greater energy
- Enhanced mobility and improved range of motion
- Decreased stress and anxiety
- Decreased sense of isolation resulting from unconditional one-on-one attention

Many cultures and families share a great deal of physical contact. Other cultures exhibit minimal tactile contact between members of the family. Be aware of cultural and individual differences related to touch and massage.

1. Massage therapy has helped preterm infants gain weight, increase responsiveness, and get discharged earlier compared with those who did not receive massages.

2. Compared with those who did not receive therapeutic massage, term babies who received regular massage were more content, laid down myelin more rapidly, exhibited less irritability, had fewer episodes of colic, and developed strong attachment bonds with parents or siblings as a result of the physical contact between them.

3. In children with asthma, massage therapy resulted in increased peak air flow, improved pulmonary function, and decreased stress hormone levels.

- Mental and tactile stimulation
- Improved sense of well being
- Increased feeling of calm
- Improved immune response
- Speedier recovery from illness
- Softening of contracted muscles
- Prevention of muscle atrophy
- Diversion

Uses

Massage therapy has been used effectively with almost all patient populations, including:

- Children and adults with cancer
- Children with posttraumatic stress disorder
- Children with asthma
- Infants with cerebral palsy
- Hospitalized depressed children
- Term and preterm infants
- Cocaine-exposed and human immunodeficiency virus (HIV)—exposed infants
- Pre- and postoperative patients
- Athletes
- Pregnant women and laboring women
- Terminally ill patients
- Homebound patients
- Nursing home residents
- Patients with myofascial pain, headaches, or temporomandibular joint (TMJ) pain
- Patients with neuromuscular disorders
- Sexually and physically abused children
- Nursing students

Risks and Precautions

It is important for the nurse to know the patient's medical history and current state of health to determine whether a patient is a candidate for massage. Massage is not recommended for patients with the following:

- Fever; massage may further increase surface temperature, leading to discomfort
- Skin rashes, contagious or infectious disease, bumps, lumps, or broken skin
- Acute, undiagnosed back pain

- Phlebitis or deep vein thrombosis; light hand massage may be performed to reduce anxiety, but do not massage feet, legs, or trunk
- Varicose veins
- Low platelet counts (leukemia, purpura, or taking anticoagulants); massage should be performed *very gently*
- Lymphoma
- Certain cardiac problems
- Pregnant women in the first trimester (do not massage over abdomen, legs, or feet)
- Psychosis
- Osteoporosis; use caution when massaging these patients
  Areas of the body that you should NOT massage include:
- On or near malignant tumors and bone metastasis
- Over bruises (until after the fourth day)
- Open wounds
- On or near recent fracture sites
- Overinflamed joints
- Abdomen of patients with mononucleosis or peptic ulcers

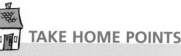

TAKE HOME POINTS

1. For patients with HIV, massage therapy increased the natural killer cells and significantly reduced stress, anxiety, and cortisol levels.
2. Hospice patients reported massage as comforting, luxurious, and beneficial.
3. Massage has been therapeutic for women with pelvic and low back pain associated with endometriosis; it also improves premenstrual syndrome (PMS) symptoms.
4. For women in labor, massage promotes relaxation and pain control.
5. Massage provides relief for patients with chronic back pain.
6. Shiatsu massage has been used to successfully treat constipation.

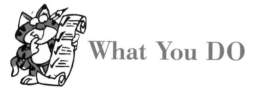

What You DO

Patient Education

Although the effectiveness of massage may be temporary in nature, benefits are reported to last from hours to a week. Massage is a therapeutic intervention that nurses can teach family members to perform at home. The potential of massage for reducing the need for pain medications, sleep medications, and anxiety medications makes massage cost-effective. Massage is often done in a private, comfortable environment; dimmed lighting, relaxing music, and essential oils may be used.

Practitioners

The American Massage Therapy Association (AMTA) requires a training minimum of 500 hours of classroom instruction from a school accredited by the Commission on Massage Therapy Accreditation (COMTA) or from a school that is a member of AMTA. Within the 500-hour training, at least 300 hours of massage therapy theory and technique, and a minimum of 120 hours of anatomy, physiology, and pathology is included in the curriculum.

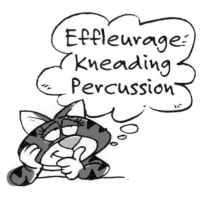

Effleurage
Kneading
Percussion

Currently, no national standard or requirement exists to be a massage therapist; qualification is determined at the state level. Certification by the National Certification Board for Therapeutic Massage and Bodywork is an indication that a massage therapist has the required hours of education, has passed a comprehensive written examination, and is qualified to practice.

The Professional Organizations for Massage Therapists offers certification programs and continuing education and set the standards for practice. These organizations include the AMTA, Associated Bodywork and Massage Professionals, and the National Association for Nurse Massage Therapists.

For more information on massage, a recommended book is Montague's *Touching: The Human Significance of the Skin.*

Do You UNDERSTAND?

See pages 254 and 255 for Learning Activities related to this topic.

Key Word

Endorphins Naturally occurring substances in the body that help provide pain relief.

www.amtamassage.org
www.abmp.com
www.imagroup.com

QIGONG AND TAI CHI

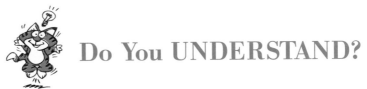

What IS Qigong and Tai Chi?

Either standing or sitting tai chi is appropriate for geriatric and frail older adults with chronic illnesses.

Qigong is considered part of traditional Chinese medicine (TCM), along with herbs and acupuncture. Qi refers to life force, and gong means practice; together, these terms are the practice of working with qi to improve health and well being through movements, abdominal breathing exercises, and concentration or meditation. Qigong promotes the flow of qi through the body's meridians, which enhances health and healing. Tai chi was derived from qigong. Tai chi translates into "grand ultimate fist." Originally used as a martial art, tai chi also has therapeutic uses.

What You NEED TO KNOW

Qigong and tai chi are several thousand years old, and many styles exist. The different styles are associated with specific individuals, family names, animals, or specific religions. Just as there are variations in styles and forms, there are slight variations in spelling found in literature on qigong and tai chi. As part of TCM, the principles of yin and yang are very important, as is the concept of balance of our internal and external influences. Balance, cultivation, and flow of qi are associated with health, which are basic reasons to practice qigong and tai chi.

Qigong works with qi through active or passive techniques. In addition, internal healing or external healing is possible. Active qigong involves slow movements, which moves qi throughout the meridians and organs, whereas passive qigong is meditative and cultivates qi for storage in the dan tien. Both techniques improve the mind and body. Internal qigong promotes self-healing while external qigong requires a qigong master to transfer the healing energy to a patient. The qigong master can treat organ systems or body areas either with contact (in the form of acupressure or massage) or without contact.

Tai chi involves almost weightless, fluid movements, with a focus on breathing, balance, and the concept of empty and full. Several forms and styles exist, which mimic the movements of animals and have martial arts applications. Practicing tai chi is equivalent to walking 6 kilometers per hour. Tai chi chih style is frequently used in research involving patients with decreased exercise tolerance or chronic disease. Participants perform tai chi chih either sitting or standing at a slow to moderate pace. The exercise consists of 20 movements with an ending pose, requiring 8 to 10 lessons to learn and taking about 30 minutes to perform.

1. **Headache is possible if qigong is performed in a strong wind.**
2. **Asthma may prevent deep breathing (as may a full stomach) during practice.**
3. **Some movements put strain on knees of already arthritic or injured joints.**
4. **Avoid strenuous or low positions during pregnancy or menstruation.**

Benefits and Uses

Benefits

Benefits of qigong include:

- Increased blood flow to brain, hands, and feet
- Increased bone density
- Increased strength, appetite, and weight gain in patients with cancer
- Decreased blood pressure
- Decreased stroke and stroke mortality
- Increased testosterone levels
- Increased estrogen levels

Benefits of tai chi include:

- Improved balance
- Improved postural stability
- Increased range of motion
- Increased flexibility
- Increased muscle strength
- Increased cardiorespiratory functioning
- Increased bone density
- Increased effectiveness of cancer therapy
- Decreased falls
- Decreased blood pressure
- Decreased pain
- Decreased stress
- Decreased stroke and stroke mortality
- Increased well being
- Slowed aging

Many of the benefits of qigong and tai chi practice are related to decreased sympathetic response and hormonal alterations. Numerous studies have been conducted on tai chi effectiveness in the United States related to balance improvement and fall reduction in older adults. However, extensive research on the effectiveness of qigong is limited to China and is published in Chinese. Furthermore, nursing research is sparse on the effective use of qigong and tai chi as a nursing intervention.

Uses

Qigong and tai chi are beneficial for many patient populations and require no special equipment. Ideally, for best results, the session is practiced outdoors, near nature, and sat about 6:00 AM, either individually or as part of a group.

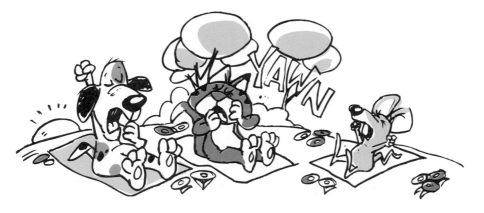

Uses for qigong include:
- Arrhythmias
- Coronary heart disease
- Fibromyalgia
- Heart failure

- Hypertension
- Rheumatic heart disease
- Stroke

Uses for tai chi include:
- Cardiac rehabilitation
- Heart failure
- Hypertension
- Low back pain
- Multiple sclerosis

- Nightmares
- Osteoarthritis
- Pain
- Rheumatoid arthritis
- Stress reduction

Risks and Precautions

As with any exercise program, a medical evaluation before starting is important, especially in the presence of low exercise tolerance or cardiac history. Performing tai chi chih expends metabolic equivalents similar to those of the "Sit and Be Fit" exercise program used for patient with heart failure and people with low exercise tolerance.

Side effects are variable, with most avoidable by not overworking the body and doing what feels comfortable. Instructors can point out ways to modify movements if needed. Limitations of tai chi practice are related to patients with angina and ventricular dysrhythmias.

1. Li family qigong and Chen xi-yi qigong are examples of styles named after a family or an individual.
2. Examples of styles named after animals include crane, snake, dragon, bear, and tiger.
3. Some early qigong practices come from Buddhist, Daoist, or Confucius philosophy.
4. Qigong is sometimes spelled as chi kung, while tai chi is written as t'ai chi or taijiquan.

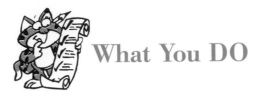

What You DO

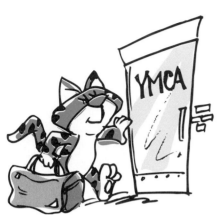

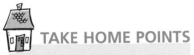

TAKE HOME POINTS

1. Yin refers to female, light, internal, and passive.

2. Yang refers to male, dark, external, and expressive.

3. The five-element system of TCM involves fire, earth, metal, water, and wood.

4. Six external influences affecting health are cold, heat, dampness, dryness, summer heat, and wind.

5. The seven emotions that can cause organ disharmony are joy, grief, sadness, fear, fright, anger, and worry.

6. The dan tien is a center of qi energy storage located three fingers below the umbilicus, mid-abdominal line.

7. Tai chi chuan is the most recognized style and is the original martial art form.

8. Yang is the most popular style of tai chi.

9. Chen is the oldest style of tai chi.

Patient Education

Qigong and tai chi classes and seminars are frequently taught at community centers, martial arts studios, hospitals, colleges, health clubs, YMCAs, and YWCAs. An effective way to learn qigong or tai chi is to find an instructor who teaches a style or form you like and makes you feel comfortable during class. Many instructors have advanced students who assist with their classes. Remember that these skills take years to develop; many qigong masters say they still learn each day.

To develop as an effective qigong or tai chi student or practitioner involves being receptive to the teachings. Much of the practice focuses on listening to your breathing and listening to your heart beat. Often you center your awareness on the dan tien and become aware of your flow of qi. Movements originate from the dan tien, for active qigong and tai chi, and are consistent, smooth, and effortless. Standing meditation is a frequently practiced qigong exercise, which balances the flow of qi.

Standing meditation:

1. Stand with feet shoulder-width apart, weight evenly balanced.

2. Whole body relaxed, knees slightly bent.

3. Shoulders and neck relaxed.

4. Spine straight and erect with head evenly balanced.

5. Sacral area tucked to decrease lumbar curve.

6. Tongue touching roof of mouth.

7. Eyes open but not focused on any object.

8. Arms rounded as if around a tree or holding a beach ball with hands at height of dan tien, chest, or face.

9. Keep hands above elbows.

10. Use relaxed, diaphragmatic breathing, which sinks qi to the dan tien with inhalation.

11. Concentrate on your breathing and feelings.

12. Gradually increase standing meditation time to a minimum of 20 minutes and a maximum of 40 minutes.

Practitioners

Certification ranges from level one to ten, with level seven as instructor status and level ten as sifu, or master. Several professional organizations may be found in the United States, including the National Qigong Association of USA, Qigong Association of America, International Yang Style Tai Chi Chuan Association, and Chinese Tai Chi Chuan Association of Southern California, to name a few. Each association has its own teacher registries or member pages that can be found on its web site. The Qigong Institute promotes research into the effectiveness of qigong and publishes the *Qigong Database*, which highlights research and scientific papers involving qigong.

www.acupuncture.com
www.geocities.com/ctcca_home/
www.nqa.org
www.qi.org
www.qi-journal.com
www.qigonginstitute.org
www.tai-chi.com
www.yangfamilytaichi.com

Do You UNDERSTAND?

See pages 255 and 256 for Learning Activities related to this topic.

REFLEXOLOGY

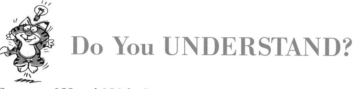

What IS Reflexology?

Reflexology is a touch modality (some people say a science) built around the principle that reflexes exist in each foot and hand that correspond to the glands, organs, and parts of the body (Figure 1). Reflexology is not new and was practiced by Egyptians as early as 2330 BC. Today, reflexology is practiced worldwide. Eunice Ingham, a pioneer of this field, brought reflexology to the United States, first publishing on the topic in 1938. Her nephew, Dwight Byers, is director of the International Institute of Reflexology and has continued her work around the world.

1. **Reflexology should not be used on women who are in their first trimester of pregnancy.**
2. **Wide variability exists among individuals in the tolerance of pressure and the amount of sensitivity that they have in their feet and ankles.**

Examples of Reflex Points

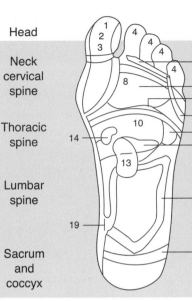

Head

Neck cervical spine

Thoracic spine

Lumbar spine

Sacrum and coccyx

1. Head and brain
2. Pituitary and pineal glands
3. Throat and thyroid gland
4. Sinus
5. Eyes and ears
6. Shoulder
7. Heart
8. Lungs and thymus gland
9. Diaphragm and solar plexus
10. Stomach
11. Liver
12. Gallbladder
13. Kidney
14. Adrenal gland
15. Spleen
16. Pancreas
17. Small intestine
18. Large intestine
19. Bladder
20. Sacrum and sciatic nerve

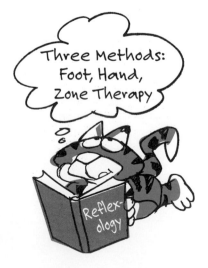

Three Methods: Foot, Hand, Zone Therapy

Reflexology is considered by many researchers to be a valuable therapeutic nursing skill that may potentially show cost savings in both preventative health care and disease management. Although three different methods (foot, hand, and zone therapy) are practiced, emphasis in this section is given to reflexology involving the foot.

What You NEED TO KNOW

Reflexology uses the thumb and fingers to apply pressures to specific reflex points for the purpose of relaxing the patient and enhancing the functions of various body organs (see illustration). Although the mechanism of action remains unclear, one theory is that lactic acid gathers in the feet as microcrystals. Reflexology crushes these crystals, permitting the free flow of energy. Another theory suggests that nerve endings in the feet connect with different areas of the body and that the finger pressure applied to the feet stimulates the corresponding area of the body. This process, in turn, produces relaxation, relieving tension and stress. This exercises affects the autonomic nervous system and eventually the endocrine, immune, and neuropeptide systems. Finally, the simple psychologic explanation holds that reflexology, similar to other forms of human touch, is an outward show of care and concern for the person and which are responsible for the changes seen in the recipient.

Generally, 10 minutes is required to provide pressure to points on each foot for a total of 20 minutes to achieve desired results. Application of pressure to the points can be repeated as needed.

Benefits and Uses

Although reflexology is increasing in the United States, little research has been done that tests its effects in controlled studies. Research studies have shown the following: (a) alterations in baroreceptor reflex sensitivity, which may produce the positive benefits of reflexology; (b) psychologic benefits; (c) improved respiratory rates in cardiac surgery patients; (d) significant decreases in pain and anxiety seen in patients with cancer; and (e) significant decreases in premenstrual symptoms.

Uses of reflexology include the following:
- Anxiety reduction
- Facilitator to sleep onset
- Stress and tension reduction

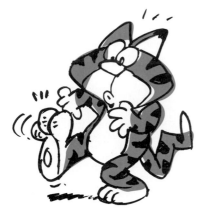

Risks and Precautions

Reflexology does not have risks when used by trained practitioners. The purpose of reflexology is not to diagnose or treat specific diseases, but rather, to stimulate specific points to improve whole-body functioning or healing in specific body areas.

Reflexology should not be used on an inflamed (reddened and swollen) foot or on a foot in which an intravenous needle or cannula is inserted.

Other general considerations that may be a contraindication include the following:

- First trimester pregnancy
- Altered skin integrity on the foot or ankle
- Phlebitis in the foot or lower leg
- Broken bones in the foot or ankle
- Unexplained swelling in the foot or ankle

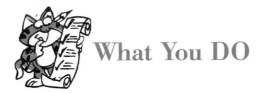

What You DO

Patient Education

Patients should be questioned concerning the use of reflexology to determine their knowledge level and whether any contraindication exists as to the use of reflexology.

Some patients may have misconceptions about touch modalities in general, fears about being touched by another person, or high sensitivity to touch to the feet and ankles that can foster resistance to using this modality. Thus accurate information should be provided about reflexology before using this modality. Important, too, is that the person hold an appropriate level of expectation about what can be achieved using this modality.

Practitioners

Training facilities are available across the United States, Canada, Europe, Japan, and China. Many professional organizations for reflexology exist, including the International Council of Reflexologists (in California) and the Reflexology Association of America. The American Reflexology

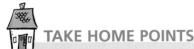

TAKE HOME POINTS

1. Reflexology is a simple, safe technique that does not require special equipment (only the practitioner's hands) and can be taught to family member caregivers as well.

2. Reflexology is used worldwide, with increasing use and research in the United States.

Certification Board offers a certification examination. Continuing educational opportunities are available through several schools and training institutions. Some states require licensure for practice. Eligibility for licensure varies by state and may include a minimum educational hour requirements, national certification, or written and practical examinations administered by state or city of licensure or practice.

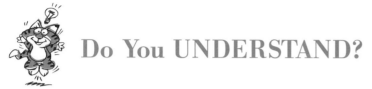

Do You UNDERSTAND?

See page 256 for Learning Activities related to this topic.

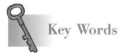

Key Words

Reflexology A touch modality (some people say a science and art) built around the principle that reflexes are present in each foot and hand that correspond to the glands, organs, and parts of the body that, when stimulated, improve the function of the whole body or specific body areas away from the area being stimulated.

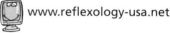

www.reflexology-usa.net

ROLFING

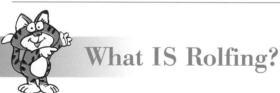

What IS Rolfing?

Rolfing is a form of deep-tissue manipulation that strives to return the patient to proper alignment. Rolfing therapists believe that the body's problems are a result of gravity's influence. This constant fight against gravity affects the body's ability to stay in alignment. Rolfing therapists believe that misalignment leads to muscle and neural problems. Rolfing therapy attempts to strengthen the body's connective tissue, thus strengthening the whole system.

Dr. Ida Rolf, a biochemist, discovered in the 1930s that fascia covers the body's muscles and bones. She also determined that fascia may be manipulated and reshaped. Dr. Rolf concluded that gravity affects the body, and,

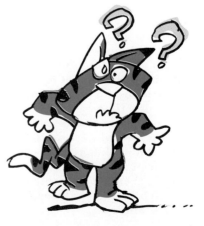

over time, the fascia becomes misshapen and out of alignment. As the basic support structure of the body becomes out of alignment, the effects of gravity become more apparent and problematic.

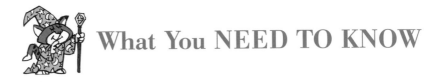

What You NEED TO KNOW

Benefits and Uses

Rolfing is not meant to be a cure, but rather, a means to restore the body to balance. Benefits of rolfing include the following:

- Decrease in headaches
- Ease of chronic stress symptoms
- Improved body definition
- Improved circulation
- Increased breathing capacity
- Increased confidence
- Increased immune function
- Increased range of motion
- Pain relief
- Relaxation

Almost all age groups may benefit from rolfing; however, it is primarily used with adult patients. Rolfing is used for the following conditions and reasons:

- Asthma
- Better sports performance
- Chronic stress
- Constipation
- Headaches
- Menstrual disorders
- Poor flexibility
- Poor posture
- Whiplash

When used as adjunct to other health promotion and therapeutic modalities, rolfing can facilitate tension release. Many people, when they are sick—especially with a chronic illness—will have many years of tension built up. According to rolfing practitioners, some of the chronic health problems that affect patients are worse because the body is out of alignment.

Rolfing is similar somewhat to regular massage, but because the focus is on the deep connective tissue, some patients may find rolfing uncomfortable. Rolfing is usually done in a series of 10 sessions. Each session lasts about 1 1/2 hours and can take place 1 week to 3 weeks apart. Each session has its own focus, with the end result being all 10 sessions building on each other. The effects of rolfing are cumulative and long lasting.

Risks and Precautions

Because deep-tissue manipulation is involved, some patients may experience discomfort, while others may experience warmth to the area. Rolfing is not

1. **People who do not like to be touched should avoid Rolfing therapy.**
2. **Rolfing should not be considered a cure for any specific illness.**
3. **A rolfing series will run over several weeks, with at least a week between sessions. Patients benefit the most from all 10 sessions, which requires a strong commitment.**

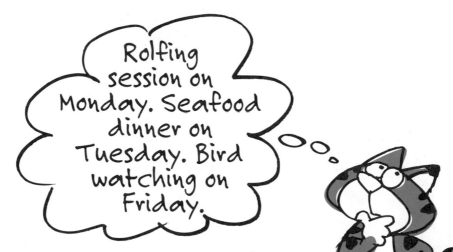

a cure for any specific disease and should not be considered as such. Patients who try to avoid close contact may find rolfing uncomfortable. Rolfing may be very uncomfortable for individuals with arthritis. A modified form of rolfing is needed for the pregnant patient.

What You DO

Professional nurses see many patients that may benefit from certain types of complimentary therapy as they return to wellness. Although rolfing may not be routinely administered or recommended in the hospital setting, nurses who work in offices and clinics may find rolfing being prescribed.

Practitioners

Training in rolf therapy is usually a 4-year college degree. The first 2 years of education is dedicated to science courses, and the final 2 years involve rolf therapy studies and clinical activities. Some states require certification or licensure (or both) for practitioners of rolfing therapy. The Rolf Institute is the only certifying agency for rolf therapists.

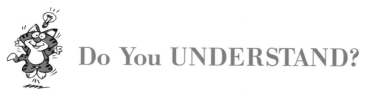

Do You UNDERSTAND?

See page 257 for Learning Activities related to this topic.

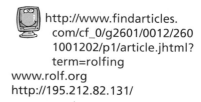

http://www.findarticles.com/cf_0/g2601/0012/260
1001202/p1/article.jhtml?
term=rolfing
www.rolf.org
http://195.212.82.131/

YOGA

What IS Yoga?

Yoga is an ancient science and philosophy of the mind, body, and soul. Practiced for approximately 5000 years, yoga describes the nature of human consciousness and outlines four paths that individuals can follow to achieve enlightenment. These paths include **Karma yoga, Bhakti yoga, Jnana yoga,** and **Raja yoga.** "Yoga" is a Sanskrit word that means to unite or join. The aim of all yogic paths is to unite the mind, body, and soul to go beyond the self, liberate the soul, and join with the supreme consciousness.

Raja yoga is the path with which most people are familiar. Raja yoga includes the physical postures and breathing exercises most often associated with yoga. Raja yoga, however, is more than postures and breathing. Raja yoga involves the way in which an individual approaches others and self, as well mental techniques that allow the person to quiet distracting thoughts and experience a higher consciousness. Around 300 BC, the sage Patanjali described the three disciplines of yoga: (1) ethical practices and principles, (2) emotional and mental discipline, and (3) the successful quest of the soul. Patanjali also identified steps within each discipline that outline a path towards enlightenment (Table 1).

What You NEED TO KNOW

Benefits and Uses

Yoga is among the oldest health practices. Yoga philosophy proposes that health is not just a physical phenomenon, but also, one that includes the mind and the spirit. A central belief of yoga is that a person cannot be healthy unless the mind, body, and spirit are healthy. Thus yoga encourages physical and mental practices that strengthen and join together the mind, body, and spirit. Benefits of practicing yoga include improved mental clari-

Table 1 Disciplines and Steps of Raja Yoga

DISCIPLINE	STEP	SANSKRIT WORD	DEFINITION
Ethical practices and principles (Bahiranga-sadhana)	1	Yama	Nonviolence, freedom from avarice, truthfulness, chastity, and freedom from desire
	2	Niyama	Cleanliness, contentment, austerity, study of self, and devotion
	3	Asanas	Physical postures
Emotional and mental discipline (Antaranga-sadhana)	4	Pranayama	Breathing techniques
	5	Pratyahara	Detachment from the senses
Successful quest of the soul (Antaratma-sadhana)	6	Dharana	Concentration
	7	Dhyana	Meditation
	8	Samadhi	Fusion of the knower, the knowable, and the known; unity with the supreme consciousness

ty, an enhanced sense of well being, increased physical strength and flexibility, a sense of connection, and a feeling of balance.

Yoga can also help individuals who suffer from chronic conditions and disease. Using yoga to alleviate specific physical and psychologic conditions is referred to as yoga therapy. Yoga therapy uses specific postures and sequences of postures to stretch or block areas of the body. In doing so, blood and energy are redirected and allowed to flow more evenly through the body. The selection and sequence of the postures are determined according to the individual's health concerns. It is important to note that, although it appears physically focused, yoga therapy also emphasizes the mental and spiritual aspects of health.

Yoga therapy is said to help many conditions, including diabetes, epilepsy, obesity, asthma, irritable bowel syndrome, depression, and PMS. Unfortunately, limited research exists supporting the effectiveness of yoga therapy. A recent study showed that individuals with carpal tunnel syndrome who received yoga therapy had better outcomes than did either controls or those who wore a wrist splint. Other studies showed that yoga helps patients with osteoarthritis and cardiovascular disease. However, further research on the therapeutic benefits of yoga is needed to demonstrate its positive effects.

Contraindications and Precautions

Many styles of yoga are practiced. Differences between styles concern the level of emphasis given to the physical, mental, and spiritual aspects of yoga. Some styles of yoga are extremely physically demanding. Other styles emphasize relaxation through meditation and chanting or the ethical aspects of yoga, such as selfless service and proper diet. It is important to understand the differences between various styles before attending classes or referring a patient to a yoga class. Almost anyone of any age can practice some type of yoga, and everyone is welcome. Although spiritual, yoga is not a religious practice. People of all faiths practice yoga. A description of some of the more common styles of yoga is presented in Table 2.

Some types of yoga are too physically demanding for people with chronic health conditions. These types also may not be suitable for beginners.

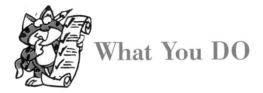 # What You DO

Patient Education

Although an increasing number of people are becoming aware of and practicing yoga, a need to educate patients about the potential benefits of yoga still exists. A person can practice yoga at any age with virtually any condition. Nurses must emphasize that yoga is not a cure, but it can help a person manage physical pain and mental stress and promote spiritual growth. If a nurse recommends yoga, it is important that he or she considers the patient's individual challenges and needs.

Practitioners

Nurses need to be informed about the yoga schools and instructors in their area. Although some yoga instructors are certified, no formal, required certification process exists. Thus the level of education and expertise among yoga instructors varies. Before referring a patient, the nurse should research

Table 2 Popular Styles of Yoga

STYLE	DESCRIPTION
Ananda	Emphasizes preparing the student for meditation. Postures used to expand self-awareness. Also includes techniques that help a student learn to direct energy to specific parts of the body. Unique features include using affirmations and deeply relaxing in poses.
Asthanga	Physically demanding, flowing sequence of postures. Includes 240 postures performed in six successive series. Postures are linked by breath. A unique feature is the continual flow of action.
Bikram	Two-part series with 26 postures. Postures are held for approximately 10 seconds and repeated twice. The same postures and sequences are performed each time. Also includes some breathing exercises. A unique feature is that Bikram yoga is practiced in a room that is at or above 80° F. Students often bring water.
Kripalu	Emphasizes the mental and emotional states that students experience in each pose. Has three stages: willful practice, will and surrender, and surrendering to the body's wisdom. Practice is inner-directed, and students are encouraged to spontaneously assume poses following the body's wisdom. Postures are held for a long time.
Kundalini	Specifically designed to bring forth kundalini. Kundalini is an energy reservoir stored in the base of the spine. Students are taught to use breath, chanting, posture, and meditation to stimulate the Kundalini and bring it up the spine.
Lyengar	Rigorous, scientific, and therapeutic approach. Emphasis on the details of each pose and correcting structural imbalances. A unique feature is the extensive use of props that allow individuals of all abilities to experience postures.

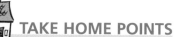

TAKE HOME POINTS

1. Yoga is an ancient science and philosophy of the mind, body, and soul.
2. Yoga offers different paths; however, all paths lead to the same goal: uniting the mind, body, and soul and connecting the self to the supreme consciousness.
3. Yoga benefits people who are healthy, as well as those with physical or mental challenges.
4. Almost anyone can practice some type of yoga; however, individual needs must be considered when selecting a style.
5. If nurses are going to recommend yoga, they must be knowledgeable about the different styles of yoga and informed about the instructors in the community.

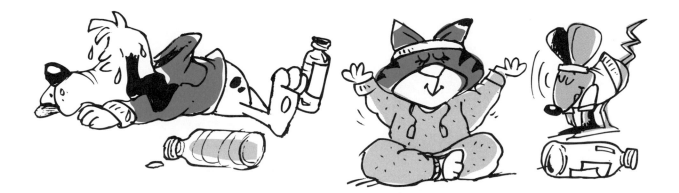

the instructors in the area. Personal interviews with instructors or their students (or both) are good ways to evaluate yoga teachers. Some questions to ask include: how many years they have studied and taught yoga, how often they attend workshops, what type of personal practice they maintain, how they integrate yoga philosophy with practice, and how they work with persons with physical or mental challenges. Also recommended is that the nurse attend an instructor's class before referring a patient. Attending class allows the nurse to experience the pace of the class, its level of difficulty, and the way in which the instructor integrates the physical, mental, and spiritual aspects of yoga. Finding a skilled and knowledgeable instructor is extremely important. Improperly practiced, yoga can aggravate or create more problems for a patient.

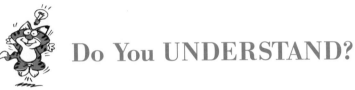

Do You UNDERSTAND?

See pages 257 and 258 for Learning Activities related to this topic.

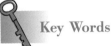

Key Words

www.yogatherapy.com
www.yogasite.com
www.bikramyoga.com
www.iyengar-yoga.com
www.yogajournal.com

Karma yoga Path of selfless action.
Bhakti yoga: Path of prayer and devotion.
Jnana yoga: Path seeking knowledge and wisdom.
Raja yoga: Path to achieving mental and physical control.

4 Healing with the Mind

BIOFEEDBACK

What IS Biofeedback?

Biofeedback is a noninvasive, therapeutic intervention in which biologic information is measured and "fed back" to an individual. Having access to this information allows a person to change physiologic processes that are normally beyond awareness. Biofeedback is based on the principles of learning theory and the field of **cybernetics.** The basic principle of cybernetics is that having information about a variable allows the individual to learn to control the variable. The information that is presented to the individual is referred to as "feedback."

Perhaps the simplest feedback device is a mirror. Using visual cues from a mirror, a person can make adjustments to appearance, posture, or expression. Biofeedback instruments behave much as does a mirror; however, they are designed to measure and provide information about physiologic phenomena. These physiologic phenomena include heart rate, skin conductance, muscle tension, temperature, and brain-wave activity. The phenomena are measured by attaching sensors to a person, which are connected to a biofeedback instrument. The biofeedback instrument measures the phenomenon so individuals will know how close they are to the desired value for the particular phenomenon. The "desired" value level is determined by the therapist according to the individual's needs. The goal of biofeedback therapy is for clients to self-regulate. In other words, individuals become aware of their own internal cues and control physiologic phenomena without using a biofeedback instrument.

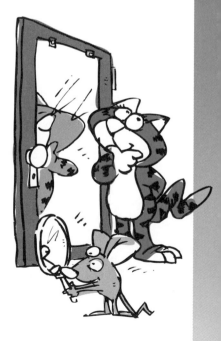

What You NEED TO KNOW

Benefits and Uses

Biofeedback has many uses and has been used to help people manage conditions without medications. Biofeedback is used in adults and children and can be used to treat the following conditions:

- Anxiety disorders
- Asthma
- Attention-deficit hyperactivity disorder
- Cerebral palsy
- Disorders of intestinal motility
- Enuresis
- Epilepsy
- Essential hypertension
- Headache
- Incontinence
- Insomnia
- Motion sickness
- Neuromuscular disorders
- Pain
- Raynaud's disease
- Stroke

Risks and Precautions

Biofeedback is a remarkably safe intervention, and virtually no risks are associated with biofeedback therapy. However, reports of negative reactions to biofeedback therapy have surfaced. These reactions are related to the opposite effect that relaxation can have on an individual. This reaction is referred to as relaxation-induced anxiety. Relaxation-induced anxiety may occur with any relaxation procedure and results from an increase in physiologic and psychologic phenomena associated with anxiety. For example, individuals undergoing relaxation training may experience an increase in heart rate and muscle tension; they may also experience feelings of a loss of control. Other potential adverse effects include unwanted changes in muscle activity (e.g., tics, cramps), disturbing sensory experiences, increased sympathetic nervous system activity, intrusive thoughts, and uncomfortable feelings. Reports of negative reactions are infrequent; however, the actual incidence of adverse reactions is unknown.

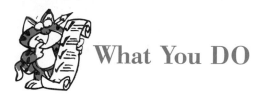

What You DO

Patient Education

Nurses are in an ideal position to identify clients who may benefit from biofeedback therapy. Nurses often assist with the care for people with chronic conditions, many of whom can be helped by biofeedback therapy. This approach is particularly relevant to older adult populations with chronic conditions such as diabetes, hypertension, and incontinence. Many older adults are on multiple medications to regulate these conditions and are unaware of nonpharmacologic therapies such as biofeedback therapy. Nurses can educate these people about biofeedback therapy as an alternative or adjunct to drug therapy.

Patient education should include information about the potential benefits and risks associated with biofeedback therapy. The benefits include symptom relief and an improved sense of well being. The most common risk is increased anxiety. Importantly, nurses must emphasize that if an individual is taking medications for a condition, these should not be discontinued when beginning biofeedback therapy. If one of the goals of biofeedback is to reduce or eliminate the need for medication, this must be done under the supervision of a physician. Discontinuing or reducing a medication is a complicated process that can cause serious problems if done improperly.

Practitioners

Biofeedback therapy began in the United States in the 1950s. Many fields contributed to the development of biofeedback, including medicine, psychology, biomedical engineering, and cybernetics. Biofeedback continues to be an interdisciplinary field, and practitioners come from many different disciplines. Physicians, counselors, psychologists, and nurses are among the professionals who provide biofeedback therapy. Certification is not required to practice biofeedback therapy; however, an organization has been formed to certify practitioners. This organization, known as the Biofeedback Certification Institute of America (BCIA) offers certification to individuals who meet rigorous educational criteria and pass both a written and practical examination. Once certified, a biofeedback practitioner must participate in continuing education courses to remain certified. People who are certified

TAKE HOME POINTS

1. Biofeedback therapy is a non-pharmacologic intervention through which a person becomes aware of and learns to regulate physiologic processes.

2. Biofeedback has been shown to be an effective treatment for many conditions. In particular, biofeedback has been successfully used to help manage chronic conditions across all age ranges.

3. If the goal of biofeedback therapy is to manage a chronic disease, the therapist should consult with the client's physician.

4. With their unique knowledge of physiology, disease, and holistic caring, nurses are among the best professionals to become biofeedback therapists.

www.aapb.org
www.bcia.org
www.bfe.org
www.snr-jnt.org

are eligible to join the Association for Applied Physiology and Biofeedback (AAPB). This professional organization maintains a list of certified practitioners and provides information to the public and to the association's members.

Do You UNDERSTAND?

See pages 259 and 260 for Learning Activities related to this topic.

Key Word

Cybernetics A field that studies information processing.

HUMOR THERAPY

What IS Humor Therapy?

Humor therapy uses the ability of an individual to laugh as a means of effecting changes in physiologic and psychologic states. The terms *humor, laughter,* and *jocularity* are often used interchangeability to describe this whole process of finding fun or funniness in a given situation. Laughter can diminish pain, cause relaxation, decrease anxiety, and strengthen self-esteem.

What You NEED TO KNOW

Benefits and Uses

Humor is useful for a diverse patient population—primarily any patient who has the cognitive abilities to laugh at the humorous incident. Humor can be used with any patient who is mentally intact and is not comatose or heavily sedated. Humor lends itself to any size group, large or small, but is often better with smaller groups or even just one.

Older adult patients with depression have experienced increased self-worth and less depression with humor therapy.

As an adjunct to other health promotion and therapeutic modalities, humor can affect both the ill and healthy person by enhancing relaxation and decreasing stress. Humor and laughter has been shown to strengthen the respiratory system, with increased rate and depth of breathing. Laughter increases the heart rate, causing the circulation to speed, increasing oxygen delivery to the tissues. After laughter, relaxation often occurs with reduced muscle tension, lowered heart rate, and decreased blood pressure. Humor has been shown to cause a release of the body's own natural pain-killing substances (endorphins) assisting in pain control, as well as providing a feeling of well being.

Humor has positive psychologic effects as well. Some evidence suggests that humor can help cure disease by creating a more relaxed atmosphere. Tension, anxiety, and fears can all be released in an appropriate manner with humor. In summary, the benefits of humor include:

- Decreased heart rate
- Increased endorphins
- Increased feeling of well being
- Increased immune system functioning
- Increased oxygen delivery
- Muscle relaxation

- Protection from chest infections
- Pain reduction
- Reduced depression
- Reduced self-destructiveness
- Relief of anxiety
- Stress management

> ⚠️ **Patients with heart problems will need to be monitored during humor therapy.**

Risks and Precautions

Although humor is safe in almost all circumstances, the continued use of extreme jocularity might affect patients with a respiratory disorder if they laugh so much it affects their breathing. Heart patients may need to be observed so that they do not overdo laughter, causing the heart to increase workload too much.

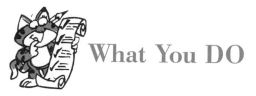 ## What You DO

Patient Education

Nurses should encourage the use of humor with their patients. Humor is not costly, can be done almost anywhere, and needs no formal education. Humor is whatever the person finds as funny. In many stressful situations in the hospital, the nurse can encourage patients and families to look at the experience with laughter, thereby breaking the tension and relaxing all involved.

www.aath.org
www.phoenix5.org/
    humor/HumorTherapyACS.
    html
www.holistic-online.com/
    Humor_Therapy/humor_
    therapy.htm

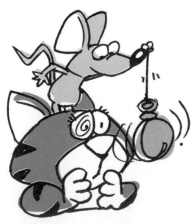

Humor is individualized; everybody has his or her own perspective. What one person finds as humorous may not be to the next. The health care provider may need to work to find what strikes the funny bone of the patient. Humor should be appropriate to the patient, time, and circumstances. If the patient does not find something humorous and the professional keeps pushing that item, the patient will not get the benefits that humor can supply.

Practitioners

Anybody who can laugh or see the funny side of things is a practitioner of humor therapy. No formal training is required unless the individual wants to attend Clown College or the College of Buffoonery.

Do You UNDERSTAND?

See pages 260 through 262 for Learning Activities related to this topic.

HYPNOSIS

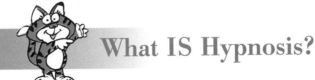

What IS Hypnosis?

Hypnosis is an alternate state of consciousness in which the patient's attention is focused away from current reality and toward particular images, thoughts, perceptions, feelings, motivations, sensations, behaviors, or any combination that the clinician suggests. Patients often experience hypnosis as a condition of intense focal concentration, with decreased peripheral awareness, increased visual imagery, increased suggestibility, and feelings of automaticity. Behavioral changes following hypnotic suggestions are associated with changes in cerebral activation and functional neuroanatomy.

What You NEED TO KNOW

Hypnosis is initiated by the clinician using a hypnotic induction. The induction is a set of verbal and nonverbal instructions and cues that establishes the context as hypnotic, captures the patient's attention, and prepares him or her for therapeutic change.

Although an induction may be used with virtually any patient, only those patients possessing at least moderate hypnotic ability, or hypnotizability, are capable of experiencing a hypnotic state. Hypnotizability approximates a normal distribution among the general population. However, certain clinical groups, including those with posttraumatic stress disorder, phobias, bulimia, and chronic pain, are thought to be higher in hypnotizability.

Following the induction, verbal instructions and suggestions are used to reframe or alter patient behaviors, emotions, sensations, physiologic responses, cognitions, or any combination. A hypnotic induction is thought to augment the effects of any verbal instructions. Hypnotic suggestions may be aimed at producing immediate effects within the hypnotic session or posthypnotic responses. The particular suggestions used may depend on the patient's hypnotizability, age, level of maturity, and presenting problem, as well as the treatment goals.

Benefits and Uses

Hypnosis is not therapy itself, and, in the strictest sense, it is not accurate to use the term "hypnotherapy." Therapists use hypnotic techniques, including hypnotic inductions and suggestions, to enhance an established psychosocial or medical treatment. Thus a clinician using hypnosis to treat a patient for any condition should have received adequate conventional training in the use of hypnosis. In the hands of a trained professional, hypnosis can help alleviate a wide array of psychologic and medical problems in children and adults.

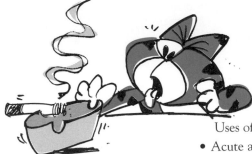

Contrary to popular belief, hypnotic effects are not simply the result of relaxation, expectancies, a placebo response, or compliance with the clinician's suggestions. Indeed, hypnotized individuals can produce dramatic changes in perceptual processing and physiologic activity that may not be attainable without using hypnosis.

Uses of hypnosis include the following:

- Acute and procedural pain
- Asthma
- Athletic performance enhancement
- Burn pain and treatment
- Cancer pain and chemotherapy side effects
- Childbirth
- Chronic pain management (except headaches)
- Eating disorders

- Enhancement of normal memory
- Forensic investigation
- Headaches
- Irritable bowel syndrome
- Past life regression
- Smoking cessation
- Stress management and relaxation
- Trauma resolution
- Warts

Risks and Precautions

The most common aftereffects of hypnosis are temporary relaxation and drowsiness, although a small fraction of patients experience headaches or nausea. The large majority of individuals describe hypnotic procedures as pleasant, and when negative experiences do occur, these are usually mild and transient.

The only contraindications to hypnosis are poor clinical training and poor therapeutic boundaries on the part of the clinician. The patient's motives when hypnosis is requested are also important to consider. For instance, is the patient hoping for a miracle cure in which he or she does not have to be an active participant? Last, individuals predisposed to psychologic instability or with weak boundaries, as well as certain diagnostic categories (e.g., borderline personality, dissociative disorders, posttraumatic stress disorder), require greater clinical skill when working with hypnosis.

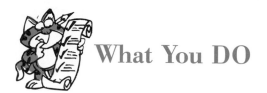

What You DO

Patient Education

Many patients, as is the case with the public at large, have misconceptions or fears about hypnosis that can foster treatment resistance. Patients may be afraid of the label "hypnosis" but not the procedures used in hypnosis interventions. Therefore the nurse should assess each patient's beliefs and provide accurate information about hypnosis before treatment. Patients must also have appropriate expectations for hypnosis. Excessively high expectations may result in disappointment.

The following are some common myths that may need to be addressed:

1. *Myth:* Hypnosis is similar to sleep. *Fact:* Hypnosis is a state of mental activity and focused awareness, not sleep.
2. *Myth:* In hypnosis, the person is under the control of the hypnotist. *Fact:* Hypnosis involves the mobilization of the patient's existing psychophysiologic resources, not the control of the hypnotist.
3. *Myth:* Only gullible people can be hypnotized. *Fact:* The ability to be hypnotized is not a sign of weak-mindedness.

The nurse should also address common patient fears such as fear of losing control or fear of embarrassment.

Practitioners

Workshop training and materials on hypnosis are available through the International Society of Clinical and Experimental Hypnosis, the American Society of Clinical Hypnosis, and the American Psychological Association. The American Society of Clinical Hypnosis is a certifying body for clinical hypnosis practitioners.

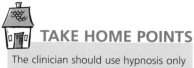

TAKE HOME POINTS

The clinician should use hypnosis only for conditions that are within the scope of her or his clinical training and practice.

www.asch.net
http://.www.apa.org/
divisions/div30.html

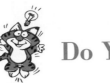

Do You UNDERSTAND?

See page 262 for Learning Activities related to this topic.

Key Words

Hypnotic induction A set of verbal and nonverbal instructions and cues that establishes the context as hypnotic, captures the patient's attention, and prepares the person for therapeutic change.

Hypnotizability The measured ability to respond to standardized hypnotic suggestions. A variety of standardized measurement scales have been developed for the clinical and experimental assessment of hypnotizability.

MEDITATION

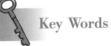

What IS Meditation?

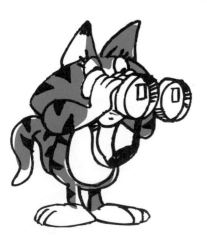

Meditation is cultivation of the mind through quieting and observing inner thoughts, emotions, and bodily sensations that continually rise up and fall away with each passing moment of time and space. The process and practice of meditation involves deeply observing one's inner state. Meditation is learning to slow down and examine passing sensations in minute detail. The technique involves concentrated attention and regular practice on focusing the participant's attention with passive, nonjudgmental observation. Meditation comes from spiritual traditions but is widely used now as a practice to promote health, as well as a form of spiritual development and awakening.

Meditative practices, traditions, and techniques are various. Common, modern forms of meditation include transcendental meditation, mindfulness-insight meditation, mantra-oriented meditation, relaxation-response meditation, Zen meditation, and breath-focusing techniques. Other forms of meditation include "moving meditation." Yoga, stress-relaxation-visualiza-

tion approaches, qigong, chi kung, and tai chi are examples of moving meditation. Generally, however, all of the different traditions use similar underlying principles. Principles of *Vipassana*, a universal form of meditation, tend
to go beyond all the various approaches and are not dependent on any spiritual and religious tradition. Common principles include, for example, concepts such as mindfulness, impermanence, and cultivation of loving-kind-
ness (equanimity).

Mindfulness is being attentive, actively conscious, and acutely aware of
mind-body reactions. Mindfulness allows a person to observe and detect
while being nonjudgmental. Mindfulness helps the individual become
extraordinarily attentive to ordinary experiences. Impermanence is a flowing of perception and mindful attention to the smallest sensation through
which we sense all aspects of our experiences. All meditative approaches
share a love of silence, stillness, and attentiveness or mindfulness. Each
approach leads the participant out of destructive emotions, thoughts, wor-
ries, and internal chatter, which can absorb the human psyche. The cultivation of equanimity refers to a mindfulness of observing and experiencing the
sensation without interfering with it. By focusing on harmful emotions or
sensations, discomfort and suffering may be created. Instead, emotions such
as envy, resentment, jealousy, hatred, or emotional responses to pain and
disease, can be translated through meditative practices of equanimity and
loving kindness. This technique allows clearer thinking and insight in to the
emotions, revealing deeper emotions, which will lead to further processes of
change and impermanence of all of life. The cultivated practice of mindfulness meditation gives rise to feelings and thoughts of forgiveness, gratitude,
equanimity, and loving kindness.

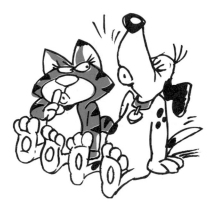

Through the practice of meditation, the individual can allow the pain,
emotions, and bodily sensations to move through as a natural process of life
energy. Individuals are then able to witness and experience impermanence,
which is the foundation of all human suffering. The deep experience of meditation offers quiet, peace, and calmness. Positive emotions and thoughts
evoke higher thinking beyond the material world of daily events, disease,
marital-family-work relationship problems, finances, ego concerns, or com-
petition. Meditation and contemplative views help us pause from placing all
our life energy on those external concerns, which are often driven by money,
fear, and ingratitude. Once we enter into a regular practice of meditation,
the deep insights and discoveries are such that we realize our true nature is
more than identification with body or mind. Indeed, we discover we cannot
restrict our views of our humanity to the mind and body, which is always
changing.

What You NEED TO KNOW

Benefits and Uses

Research has found meditation to be helpful for relaxation. A clinical intervention program of meditation for patients with chronic pain and diseases brought about a deep relaxation response, which is opposite to the fight-or-flight response. Changes took place in the autonomic, endocrine, immune, and nervous systems. For example, deep relaxation was found to increase peripheral blood flow and the electrical resistance of skin, slow electroencephalogram (EEG) alpha waves, and improve immune function. Deep relaxation (through meditation and other means) decreases oxygen consumption, respiratory rate and volume, and heart rate. Skeletal muscle tension, epinephrine level, gastric acidity and motility, and sweat gland activity were also decreased. The blood pressure, especially in hypertensive patients, was decreased as well.

Meditation has also been helpful in treating the following conditions:
- Anxiety
- Insomnia
- Pain syndromes
- Phobias
- Posttraumatic stress disorder

Risks and Precautions

Meditation should not be used to treat conditions in their acute or emergency state. Practitioners are cautioned to slowly rise from the sitting position to avoid **orthostatic hypotension.**

The important aspect of meditation is the discipline required. The discipline comes from serving as a loving, kind self-guide. This kind discipline increases as the practice grows and continues. The essential aspect of meditation, especially in the beginning, is that it be practiced daily. If the individual skips meditation, the mind begins to race away, and the hurried pace continues throughout the day, without awareness. Yet, although daily practice is most desired for its benefits, perhaps it is more important that practice is sustained on a regular basis. However, the daily and regular practice of meditation, best practiced in the early morning, results in a quieting of the mind. This technique best helps our efforts to slow down at work and in our daily life. Similarly, we become more attentive to the ebb and flow of our emotions and senses that are often our driving forces at work and other aspects of living.

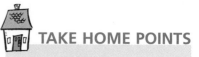

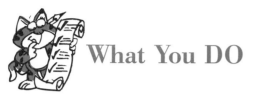

What You DO

Patient Education

Basic principles that guide the practice of meditation include having a regular daily time to meditate, usually best in the early morning. The participant needs to create a quiet, pleasant, calm room. A comfortable but upright posture, usually crossed-leg on a pillow, or upright in a chair, is helpful. Disciplined concentration with **mantra** use or another approach, such as being extraordinarily attentive and mindful of all of the person's inner experiences with focused concentration, should be practiced. When the mind strays, it should be brought back to the process of concentrating. The individual enters into this meditative experience and inner process only through practice.

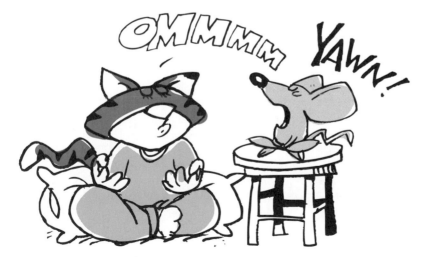

Practitioners

Meditation techniques can be taught by trained instructors or self-taught.

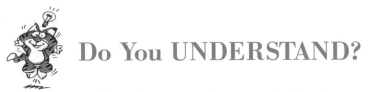

Do You UNDERSTAND?

See pages 263 and 264 for Learning Activities related to this topic.

Key Words

Mindfulness Being acutely attentive to ordinary experiences; cultivation of one-pointed concentration; disciplined awareness without judgment; learning to be present to the *now*.

Impermanence The realization that all life events, both external and internal, including the person's body, mind, and emotions, are all constantly rising up and falling away, expanding and contracting. Experiencing and being present to flux and change as a universal law of life.

Cultivation of loving kindness (equanimity) Cultivation of *mindfulness* reveals life's *impermanence*, which gives rise to universal connections with that which is greater than self, giving rise to feelings and thoughts of forgiveness, gratitude, loving kindness, compassion, and equanimity toward self and others.

Orthostatic hypotension Drop in blood pressure on standing up.

Mantra An object of concentration or inner, silent word chant that has special meaning.

www.shinzen.org
www.minet.org

MUSIC THERAPY

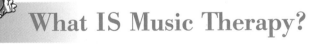

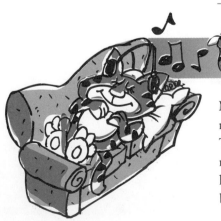

What IS Music Therapy?

Music therapy, a sphere within complementary medicine, uses harmonic melody to affect changes in behaviors, emotions, and physiologic responses. To diminish stress, pain, anxiety, and isolation, music therapy enhances relaxation, learning, creativity, self-awareness, and coping. As an allied health service, such as occupational or physical therapy, music therapy is a behavioral science integrating mind-body healing.

What You NEED TO KNOW

Benefits and Uses

Benefits of music therapy include:

- Decreased analgesic requirements
- Decreased muscle tension
- Decreased release of stress hormones
- Enhanced immune function
- Enhanced memory and recall
- Enhanced sensory stimulation
- Exercise
- Improved language and speech skills
- Improved motor functioning and skill
- Increased attention span
- Increased endorphin release
- Increased mental acuity
- Increased reality orientation
- Increased social interaction
- Learning reinforcement
- Pain distraction and focus
- Positive mood changes
- Reduced blood pressure
- Relaxation and sedation

Target populations for music therapy include the following:

- Bone marrow transplant
- Burn patients
- Children
- Emergency departments
- Hospital employees
- Hospice care
- Intensive care
- Nursing homes
- Obstetrics
- Older adults
- Premature infants
- Psychiatric care
- Neonatal intensive care
- Surgical patients

1. Older adults often have several conditions (CVA, mobility dysfunction, anxiety, depression, Parkinson's or Alzheimer's disease, or chronic pain) that are amenable to treatment with music therapy.

2. Autism, developmental delays, and speech or language dysfunction are special problems of childhood that may be assisted by music therapy.

Preoperatively, music may decrease anxiety. Surgical patients exposed to perioperative sedative music may have diminished analgesic and hypnotic medication requirements during conscious sedation. Postoperatively, music may improve satisfaction, diminish pain and the need for analgesics, increase mobilization, and decrease fatigue on hospital discharge.

Music therapy is useful for diverse patient populations and easily transportable to implement in a variety of clinical situations. Music lends itself to large social gatherings, or it can be enjoyed by one individual.

As an adjunct to health promotion and exercise, music is therapeutic for both the healthy and ill by enhancing relaxation and reducing stress. Music has physiologic effects as well. Heart rate, blood pressure, and respirations vary directly with the pace and volume of the music. Thus music with slow rhythms tends to have calming effects, while music that is quickly paced tends to energize a person. When selecting music for therapeutic effects, the

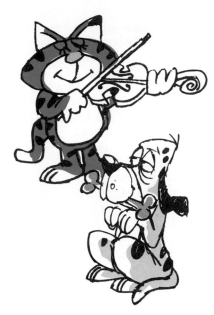

nurse must remember that making generalizations about types of music and their effects is difficult. The effects of music are related to harmony and pace rather than category. For instance, classical music can elicit many types of emotions. *Flight of the Bumble Bee* by Rimskij-Korsakov is energetic. However, Bach's *Sheep May Safely Graze* is soothing. Last, music (similar to art) is highly individualized in its appeal, as well as its effect.

Music has many positive psychologic and intellectual effects. Music production provides an avenue for creativity, improving mental acuity, memory, recall, and attention span. Creating, playing, and listening to music is a positive approach to releasing many types of emotions. Self-esteem is promoted and enhanced as emotions are dealt with and released. Music will also allow individuals with speech difficulties (neuromuscular impairments, diminished intellectual ability) to communicate without using words.

Music is also useful in developing and maintaining neuromuscular system functioning. Learning how to play an instrument promotes fine muscle control and hand-eye coordination. Music promotes bodily movement, promoting the use of arthritic or spastic extremities, enhancing joint functioning, and encouraging range of motion.

In summary, music therapy can be used to treat the following conditions:

- Acquired immunodeficiency syndrome (AIDS)
- Alzheimer's disease
- Anorexia nervosa
- Anxiety disorders
- Asthma
- Autism
- Brain damage
- Cerebrovascular accidents (CVA)
- Chronic pain syndromes
- Depression
- Developmental disability
- Neuromuscular dysfunction
- Parkinson's disease
- Psychosis
- Personality disorder
- Posttraumatic stress disorder
- Schizophrenia
- Substance abuse

Risks and Precautions

Although music is a safe, inexpensive, and effective therapy for many conditions, raucous music may agitate with discordant messages, chords, counts, rhythms, or beats. Any type of music may elicit distressing memories or experiences. Optimally, trained practitioners should implement music as a therapeutic modality.

1. **Patients with Alzheimer's disease may have increased agitation when exposed to bagpipe music.**
2. **Waltz music may trigger holocaust survivors to relive concentration camp experiences.**

www.musictherapy.org
http://home.att.net/ ~preludetherapy
www.warchild.org/projects/ centre/centre.html
www.caregiver.on.ca/ cgcihidmmt.html

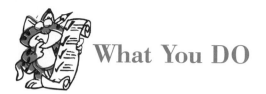

What You DO

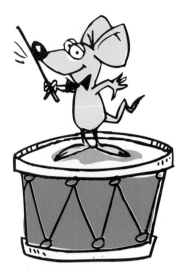

Patient Education

Professional nurses should inform patients of the many positive uses of music therapy. The safety of music therapy, its inexpensive ease of administration and mobility, make it applicable in many settings, such as hospital operating or procedure rooms, elder care facilities, rehabilitation units, mental health clinics, hospices, and psychiatric care facilities, as well as patient residences.

Conversely, nurses should also be keenly attuned to the adverse effects of noxious auditory stimuli in the patient's environment. For instance, the normal frenzy of operating room activity accompanied by clanging and moving of equipment, instruments, and loud talkative personnel will only heighten the surgical patient's anxiety. Preoperative anxiety may aggravate the surgical stress response by increasing the release of stress hormones such as epinephrine and cortisol. Excessive stress may be counterproductive to healing by interfering with sedation, anesthesia, blood-sugar control, wound healing, and postoperative energy levels.

Practitioners

Organized professionally in the United States since 1950, music therapists also practice in many countries, such as Great Britain, Canada, France, and Sweden. Professional therapists hold undergraduate or graduate degrees (or both) in music therapy; the American Music Therapy Association approves training programs. After successfully completing a national examination, board certification is provided through the Certification Board for Music Therapists. Recertification is maintained by continuing education or retesting.

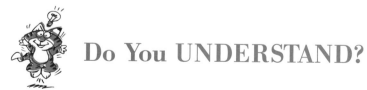

Do You UNDERSTAND?

See pages 265 and 266 for Learning Activities related to this topic.

TAKE HOME POINTS

1. Calming music promotes slower, deeper respirations.
2. Heart rate may increase with the volume or pace of the music.
3. Loud, fast noises may increase blood pressure.
4. Depending on style and sound, music can enhance alertness or promote sedation.
5. During times of stress, levels of epinephrine and cortisol are increased. As a result, the liver releases glycogen, resulting in increased blood-glucose levels.
6. Elevated glucose levels inhibit white blood cell function and may precipitate decreased immune system function and impaired wound healing.
7. The fight-or-flight stress response may cause fatigue resulting from the energy expended in constant readiness and the state of wakefulness needed in preparation for conflict or escape.

PET THERAPY

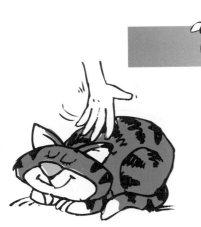

What IS Pet Therapy?

Pet therapy, also known as animal-assisted activities and animal-assisted therapy (AAA/T) involves the use of animals to help individuals attain or improve physical and psychologic wellness and quality of life. Although the benefits of AAA/T have long been acknowledged, it has only been recently that Western health care professionals are increasingly implementing this complementary modality of health care for a wide variety of health care concerns.

What You NEED TO KNOW

Benefits and Uses

Many benefits have been attributed to AAA/T. Human respond to physical, psychologic, emotional, and spiritual distress. The fight-or-flight response to stress triggers the sympathetic response and increases catecholamines, such as epinephrine and norepinephrine, in the body. AAA/T helps decrease stress and the stress response.

For many individuals, the animals arouse feelings of affection, friendship, and nurturing. The animal acts as a human counterpart that accepts its owner unconditionally. The unconditional acceptance and love that the animal offers to humans results in feelings of relaxation, empowerment, and confidence. In addition, watching an animal's behaviors can provide relaxation and diversion. Activities such as stroking fur, talking to animals, and watching bird activities stimulate the production of endorphins, thereby promoting relaxation.

Benefits of AAA/T include:
- Companionship
- Decreased incidence of partner abuse and child battering
- Decreased loneliness and isolation
- Decreased medication use

- Decreased need for physician visits
- Decreased need for cardiovascular disease medication
- Improvement of the individual's sense of well being
- Increased ability to cope with stress and life changes
- Increased ability to adjust to disease or condition
- Improved body image
- Increased independence and security (with trained dogs)
- Increased physical activity
- Increased physical and psychologic health
- Increased reality orientation
- Increased sense of responsibility
- Increased socialization
- Increased trust and self-esteem
- Increased verbal interactions
- Longer survival rate following myocardial infarctions
- Lower plasma triglyceride levels
- Motivate patients to have a positive attitude
- Promote postoperative activity
- Reduction of anxiety
- Reduction of blood pressure and heart rate
- Reduction of cholesterol
- Reduction of pain medication
- Reduction of preoperative stress

AAA/T has been shown to help many diverse patient populations in different ways. Pet ownership provides physical, psychologic, and emotional benefits to most family members. Animal visitation programs involve the animals and their handlers visiting a facility and visiting with the patients. This approach is a short-term intervention intended to increase morale and provide socialization, although other benefits have been frequently documented. Animal-assisted therapy uses animals to help in the healing and rehabilitation of patients with acute or chronic diseases. Target populations for AAA/T include the following:

- Nursing home residents
- Children
- Psychiatric patients
- Rehabilitative patients
- Perioperative patients and families
- Older adults
- Patients in intensive care and critical care units

- Prisoners and inmates
- Patients in acute care settings
- Individuals living alone
- Families of patients undergoing surgery or invasive procedures
- Staff members
- Oncology patients

Some agencies, such as nursing homes, dentist offices, and rehabilitation centers may choose to have animals that live on the premises. Usually, low-maintenance animals such as fish or birds are used, but increasingly, dogs and cats are used. Benefits for the residents include many of the benefits of animal visitation therapy. In addition, long-term residents of health care facilities may assume many of the care activities for the animals, which assist in increased physical activities, increased self-esteem, and increased socialization and decreased levels of depression, loneliness, and despair.

Service animals have been used extensively in AAA/T. Service animals have changed the lives of their owners who are blind, deaf, paralyzed, immobile, or sensory impaired. These animals are trained to open doors and drawers, pick up objects as small as a dime from the floor, indicate when the phone or door bell is ringing, carry packages, pull a wheelchair, and provide a multitude of other services. Service animals may even help their handlers become employed, obtain advanced education, and lead a full and satisfying life.

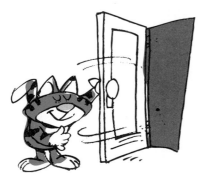

AAA/T can be used to treat the following conditions:

- Anxiety and stress
- Autism
- Cancer
- Cardiovascular disease
- Depression
- Epilepsy
- Motor and neurologic problems
- Paralysis
- Sensory-impaired (blind/deaf)
- Social isolation

Risks and Precautions

Do not use AAA/T with the following individuals:
- Allergic to animals
- Have a fear of animals
- May be immunosuppressed

Infection control personnel should be involved to ensure that transmission of diseases between the patient and animal will be minimized. At this time, no cases of zoonosis have been documented.

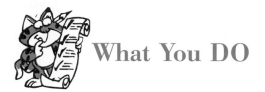

What You DO

Patient Education

Because of the intensive involvement of the nurse in the patient's daily activities, the nurse may be the most appropriate member of the health care team to identify patient concerns that may be relieved by AAA/T. Involvement can take the following forms:

- Become involved in an AAA/T program, including a handler of an AAA/T animal.
- Organize an AAA/T program in the health care facility in which you are working.
- Coordinate AAA/T goals and objectives with the AAA/T team for your patients.
- Update your knowledge concerning the research outcomes and benefits of AAA/T, and communicate these with colleagues and members of the health care team.
- Be open to modalities, such as AAA/T, that may be outside the realm of your current nursing practice.
- Become involved in current AAA/T research. Current areas under investigation include:
  - Patients' retention of discharge instruction in the presence of a therapy animal
  - The reduction of pain medication need when AAA/T is used
  - Stress reduction in waiting areas for family members using AAA/T animals
  - Improvement in postoperative and poststroke functioning with AAA/T
  - Investigating the relationship between the presence of a pet and immune functioning during a stressful life change event
- Work collaboratively with veterinary health care workers in research studies that promote the use of animals in helping with human problems.

Practitioners

At this time, no uniform standards or credentialing criteria exist that apply to all service animal or service dog trainers and animal therapists. Many training organizations offer certification of their animals, indicating that the

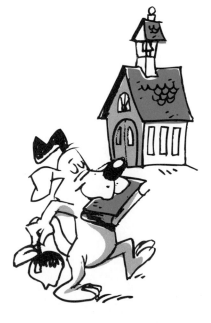

animal has completed the appropriate training dictated by that organization. Without standards for all trainers, the certification criteria vary from agency to agency and are not a guarantee of quality of the trained animal. Organizations such as Therapet and the Delta Society have developed specific criteria to credential animals and volunteers completing their training programs.

Hundreds of AAA/T organizations have been formed, many of them involved at the local or state level. Some organizations working at a national or international level and providing information for consumers for all aspects of AAA/T include the following:

- International Association of Assistance Dog Partners (IAADP)
- American Council of the Blind (ACB) (a complete listing of guide dog schools in the United States)
- Assistance Dogs International (ADI)
- Delta Society
- Paws with a Cause
- Therapet
- Pets As Therapy (PAT)
- Society for Companion Animal Studies (SCAS)
- Children in Hospital Animal Therapy Association (CHATA)
- The United States Guide Dog Council; Seeing Eye, Inc.
- Therapy Dogs International
- Bright & Beautiful Therapy Dogs, Inc.
- The National Association for Search and Rescue

For more information, the following are some recommended books on AAA/T:

- Beck AM, Katcher A: *Between pets and people: the importance of animal companionship,* Ashland, Ohio, 1996, Purdue University Press.
- Burch MR: *Volunteering with your pet: how to get involved in animal assisted therapy with any kind of pet,* Hoboken, NJ, 1996, John Wiley & Sons.
- Davis KD: *Training your dog to reach others,* Hoboken, NJ, 1992, John Wiley & Sons.
- King BL: *Girl on a leash: the healing power of dogs: a memoir,* 1999, Sanctuary Press.
- Levinson BM, Mallon GP: *Pet-oriented child psychotherapy,* Springfield, Ill, 1996, Charles C Thomas Publisher.

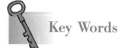

Do You UNDERSTAND?

See pages 266 and 267 for Learning Activities related to this topic.

www.deltasociety.org
www.pawswithacause.org
www.superdog.com/therapy.htm
www.therapet.com

Key Words

Endorphins Neurochemicals with analgesic properties naturally produced by the body.

Zoonosis Infections shared by humans and animals.

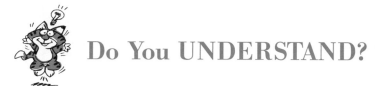

RELAXATION THERAPY

What IS Relaxation Therapy?

Relaxation techniques are probably the least controversial and most widely studied of all complementary and alternative medicine (CAM) therapies. These techniques include a wide range of behavioral (self-regulation) methods used frequently in the treatment of syndromes marked by excessive arousal or stress reactivity.

The most commonly practiced methods of relaxation techniques or therapies include diaphragmatic breathing, progressive muscle relaxation, meditation, visualization, yoga, guided imagery, autogenics, and biofeedback.

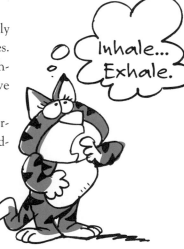

What You NEED TO KNOW

In practice, all relaxation therapies can be used as sole interventions, in combination with other relaxation therapies, or in combination with conventional therapies, such as medication. For instance, breathing retraining is often combined with muscular relaxation exercises. Most cognitive-behavioral interventions and stress-management programs for mental health problems (such as anxiety) include some type of relaxation training as an important component. Moreover, relaxation training is used frequently in interdisciplinary pain management programs. Relaxation therapy is currently one of the few widely practiced alternatives to pain medication and surgery.

The type of relaxation achieved by these techniques is different than simply unwinding with a book or in front of the television. Rather, CAM relaxation therapies are thought to bring about a *relaxation response*. A relaxation response consists of reduced muscle tension, slowed respiration, reduced oxygen consumption, decreased heart rate, decreased blood pressure, and increased slow brain wave (EEG) activity. As might be expected, muscle-oriented methods (such as progressive muscle relaxation) appear to have a pronounced effect on the musculoskeletal system, while breathing techniques appear to have an impact on the autonomic nervous system.

At least 20 different types of relaxation have been studied. These relaxation techniques are *deep methods*, including autogenic training, meditation, and progressive muscle relaxation, and *brief methods*, including paced respiration and deep breathing. Despite differences in rationale and technique, nearly all methods of relaxation training include instructions for focusing attention and altering respiration patterns, which may be the key elements in producing the relaxation response. Interestingly, symptom reduction after relaxation training does not always follow the physiologic changes. Thus the effects of relaxation training may to be related, in part, to increased feelings of control (self-efficacy) and better use of coping behaviors.

Benefits and Uses

Benefits of relaxation therapy include the following:

- Decreased anxiety
- Decreased stress
- Increased coping mechanisms
- Increased mental awareness

- Postoperative pain
- Reduced muscle tension and spasm

Relaxation therapy has the following uses:

- Acute (postoperative) pain
- Anger and aggressive behavior
- Anxiety
- Asthma
- Cancer treatment side effects (nausea and vomiting, pain)
- Childbirth
- Chronic musculoskeletal pain

- Depression
- Headache
- Hypertension
- Insomnia
- Irritable bowel syndrome
- Smoking cessation
- Stress management and muscular relaxation

Risks and Precautions

Relaxation training is considered very safe, and almost no side effects have been reported. Some individuals with chronic pain report increased pain after relaxation training, but these instances are usually the result of improper technique or posture during relaxation sessions. Some patients, however, experience increased anxiety (and related symptoms) during and following breathing exercises. These symptoms will often stabilize over time as patients get accustomed to new breathing patterns. However, in other instance, relaxation training must be terminated. The reasons for this inconsistent response are not fully understood but may be related to hyperventilation.

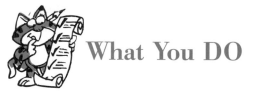 **What You DO**

Patient Education

Relaxation training is usually provided to patients by a trained clinician in weekly sessions over a period of several months. Typical session are 30 to 60 minutes in length, and patients are expected to practice techniques at home to keep anxiety reduced and become more skillful in achieving the relaxation response. Although more abbreviated interventions can often be beneficial, longer training periods have been more effective. Studies comparing different relaxation techniques have not found any one approach to be more effective than is another; however, one approach may be more effective than is another for an individual patient. Therefore patients may benefit from training in more than one relaxation technique.

General information for patients includes the following:

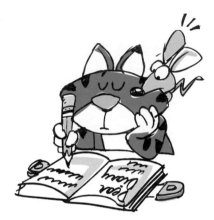

- Relaxation is a skill that requires consistent practice to achieve mastery and hence optimal benefit.
- It is recommended that patients practice a selected relaxation technique for 20 to 30 minutes daily (two 15-minute sessions are optimal). Taped scripts can be useful to assist patients in learning a particular technique, but dependence on audio-taped instructions is best avoided.
- Six to eight weeks of regular practice may be required before clinically significant benefits are achieved, although many patients report immediate benefits.
- Compliance with practice can be improved through the use of a self-monitoring diary. This type of diary also gives patients a method to track their progress.

Practitioners

Relaxation techniques are used in a variety of fields—including psychotherapy, physical therapy, sports medicine, homeopathy, and osteopathy, as well as nursing—to help with stress reduction and improved physiologic functioning. Relaxation should be provided by trained practitioners. Training is usually related to a specific relaxation technique. Relaxation training may also be obtained for self-care.

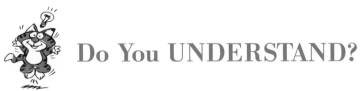

Do You UNDERSTAND?

See page 267 for Learning Activities related to this topic.

http://adultpain.nursing.
uiowa.edu//Nonpharm/
Relaxant.htm

STORYTELLING

What IS Storytelling?

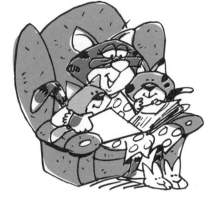

Storytelling is an oral narrative or account of fact or fiction. The use of storytelling as a healing modality has increased in the last few years. This increase is likely a reflection of the rise in divorce, excessive peer group pressure, human immunodeficiency virus (HIV) infection and AIDS, alcohol and drug abuse, homelessness, violence, sexual abuse, suicide, prejudice, and other societal and familial problems in our communities.

Storytelling is simple, inexpensive, noninvasive, and nonintrusive. Storytelling is an independent nursing intervention that contributes to children, adults, and families' healing and well being. Every patient has a life story to tell. Knowing and understanding whom the patient is and what he or she most values is the essence of holistic nursing practice. In our fast-paced, technocratic world, storytelling can be a nurturing way for nurses to connect with patients and to convey comfort.

All of us are a life story waiting to be told. The shared humanity that exists between the patient and the nurse when stories are shared is a therapeutic technique that promotes healing and conveys caring. Studies have found storytelling to be an effective method for transmitting knowledge and instilling hope. When adults shared a story with a child, they both experienced reduced stress levels. When older adults in a retirement community or nursing home participated in group storytelling, they experienced a reduction in depressive symptoms and social isolation. Group storytelling is also known as reminiscence or life review.

What You NEED TO KNOW

Benefits and Uses

Benefits

The benefit of storytelling is found in the theory that the right cerebral hemisphere is the part of the brain that usually interprets imagistic and emotional processes. Listening to stories stimulates imagery and visualizations, allowing release of emotional energy. This release can be therapeutic. As is common with many complementary and alternative therapies, little quantitative research about the use of storytelling as an independent healing modality has been conducted. Nurses often combine storytelling with other interventions. This combination makes it hard to show which benefits were derived from which interventions. However, qualitative studies have assessed storytelling's value and meaning in healing.

Some of the many therapeutic benefits of storytelling include:

- Healing by releasing emotions and feelings
- Coping more positively with illnesses
- Helping dying children and adults become less afraid by lending structure to events that may seem meaningless
- Helping sick children learn how to handle discomfort, confinement, and fear
- Learning how to empathize with others who have different experiences, values, and beliefs
- Stretching our capacity to feel many emotions
- Stimulating language development
- Promoting creativity
- Teaching concentration
- Enhancing interpersonal skills
- Helping develop a keen listening ability
- Providing emotional distance for those unable to deal with direct confrontation of problems or issues via the third-person nature of stories; perceived as less threatening by the patient

Uses

The main purpose of storytelling is to share. Storytelling is an ageless tradition used by humankind to transmit important cultural, religious, moral, and social information. Storytelling passes down values from one generation to the next. Storytelling is a way of making sense of the world. Storytelling helps provide facts, concepts, and information that help us understand people. Storytelling also promotes release of tension and emotions.

Storytelling also is used to state ideas and help the person learn effective ways of solving problems and making decisions. Stories can help the patient see the situation from a different perspective. Stories can heal, educate, inspire, build relationships, empower, motivate, entertain, and transform. Stories encourage people to develop their imagination and consider new and inventive ideas, which builds self-confidence and instills personal motivation. Stories can challenge, raise consciousness, create discomfort, change behavior, and give meaning to life situations. Stories feed our spirit.

The nurse's therapeutic use of storytelling conveys sympathy and understanding. Nurses can use storytelling to comfort the sick and dying, to promote healing, and to create a nurturing and safe environment in which patients can deal with the trials of pain, grief, and suffering.

Risks and Precautions

Storytelling is *not* a cure-all for deep-rooted psychologic problems. These problems need intensive therapeutic interventions under the guidance of an experienced nurse therapist or mental health professional.

Some stories can excite and disturb; create anger, fear, and chaos; upset; and sadden some patients. Nurses must be prepared for these feelings and behaviors. Not all storytelling will be therapeutic. Some patients may use stories and books for escape purposes only; others may rationalize rather than face their problems or may not be able to transfer insights into real life.

Simply reading a story may not be therapeutic; you must have follow-up discussion to reinforce the issue at hand and encourage open expression of feelings. Discussions will help the patient better understand what is being said in the story and how to apply this theme to her or his situation.

Being familiar with the book before you use it is always important. Do not expect immediate healing to occur. In some resistant children, for example, storytelling may not work right away. Time is an important factor to consider as children deal with stressful issues similar to their own terminal illness or the death of a loved one or a pet.

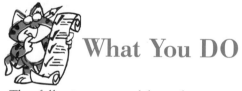 # What You DO

The following are guidelines for incorporating storytelling into clinical practice:

- Match the individual with an appropriate book. Whatever the issue with which the person is dealing (e.g., divorce, a death in the family, a birth in the family, drug or alcohol use), find a book with a theme that matches the crisis. For young children, find books or stories that impart the message through fantasy characters or personified animals. Older children respond well to values-clarification or consciousness-raising stories. Adolescents respond well to comic books or comic strips.
- Those who cannot read can have the story read to her or him.
- Give the person time to digest the story and to think about it.

• Have follow-up activities to use after the reading and digesting. These activities can include writing, drawing, discussing, and dramatizing or retelling the story by using puppets. With very young children, you may want to observe them in play or family interactions to assess any changes in their behavior following the story intervention.

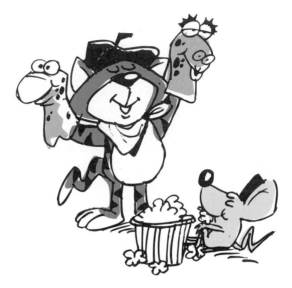

• Let the person talk about the relationship the story has to her or his life.
• Help the person achieve closure by discussing and listening to possible solutions.

Suggested books for storytelling for the pediatric patient include the following:

• *Where Do Babies Come From?* by Margaret Sheffield (New York, 1972, Alfred A. Knopf). This book answers the questions young children have about birth in a gentle, loving, direct way. Nurses, parents, or teachers can use this information to educate children who are curious about the beginnings of life.

• *Saint George and the Dragon* by Margaret Hodges (Boston, 1984, Little, Brown and Company). This book is a story about empowerment and a battle between "good" and "evil," with "good" prevailing. The book is full of beautiful metaphors and is about George, a poor young man who ends up marrying a princess and becomes ruler of the kingdom after fighting and killing a dragon.

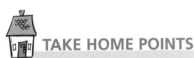

TAKE HOME POINTS

1. You do not have to be a professional storyteller. You can use books that are already in print.

2. Storytelling can be used with individuals or in groups.

3. The storyteller can be the patient or the nurse, or both can create the story together.

4. Stories can be combined with music and dance.

5. Stories can come from books, movies, or the patient's life.

6. The story must be short enough to complete in one sitting and rich enough in detail to capture and maintain the listener's interest.

- *The Blind Men and the Elephant* by Karen Backstein (New York, 1992, Scholastic, Inc.). This children's book is about six blind men who each had a limited understanding of what an elephant was because each touched only one part of the elephant's body. Not until these blind men put all their stories together did they finally understand what an elephant was really like. The book is a good story to bring up similar events in a child's life and teaches how important it is to have the "whole" picture so as to make correct judgments.

Storytelling props that are readily available in the hospital include masks, booties, caps, supply boxes, and syringes. Tools that can be used for storytelling include:

- Brown paper lunch bags
- Construction paper
- Dolls
- Glue
- Gloves
- Markers

- Puppets
- Scissors
- Tongue depressors
- Video camera
- Your index finger

www.storytellingfoundation.com/
artsedge.kennedy-center.org/aoi/opps/spin/storyart3.html
www.maginationpress.com/
falcon.jmu.edu/~ramseyil/bibliotherapy.htm
www.clevelandclinic.org/childrensrehab/programs/bibliotherapy/

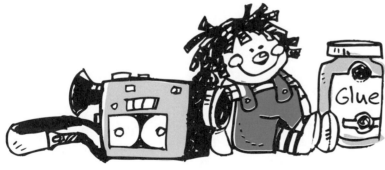

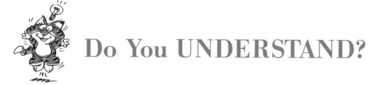

Do You UNDERSTAND?

See page 268 for Learning Activities related to this topic.

SECTION 5
Healing with Subtle Energy

ACUPRESSURE

What IS Acupressure?

Acupressure is an ancient Oriental therapy that applies finger pressure on **pressure points** to relieve pain and discomfort and promote healing. The Chinese and Japanese have used acupressure for over 5000 years. Similar to acupuncture, acupressure releases blockages of energy, also called **chi** or qi. Chi circulates through the body in patterns called yin or yang energies. The energy pathways or **meridian** channels are associated with organs. The balance of chi is constantly changing, and disturbances in the flow of chi may lead to health problems. Trigger point areas that are painful may have blocks to the natural flow of chi. Health is promoted by balancing yin and yang energies of the body, mind, and spirit. Acupressure treatments target specific points in the meridian channels that may need blockages in energy flow removed.

The precise way that acupressure works has not been determined. Stimulating acupressure points may release neurotransmitters in the brain and cause the release of **endorphins.** Another theory is that pain or nausea signals transmitted by small nerve pain fibers may be blocked by signals from acupressure. These signals are carried by the large nerve fibers in the same segment of the spinal chord. Acupressure therapy may stimulate circulation, promote blood flow, release tension and **lactic acid** and thereby promote muscle relaxation.

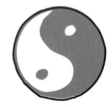

Yin and yang symbol

179

What You NEED TO KNOW

An individual or therapist can administer acupressure. Self-care may use meditative, breathing techniques or massage while applying acupressure to pressure points. Brisk, rhythmic, firm pressure is applied with fingers and hands, or sometimes with elbows or knees, by circular rubbing of points for 30 seconds to 3 minutes or longer. *Acu-yoga* uses stretching and yoga exercises with stimulation of the acupoints. *Jin shin jyutsu* acupressure uses self-care with gentle pressure and touch. *Do-in* self-care acupressure uses massage of muscles, acupoints, and meridian pathways with deep breathing and exercise. *Shiastu*, a term derived from the Japanese word *shi* (finger) and *atsu* (pressure), applies vigorous, firm, finger pressure to points.

Benefits and Uses

Benefits

Acupressure can be given by finger pressure or with "Seabands." Seabands is a wrist bracelet that applies pressure to an antiemetic acupuncture point. This point is located on the each side of the front forearm about three finger's widths up from the first wrist crease between the tendons. Acupressure with wrist pressure bands was as effective as antiemetic medication was in preventing nausea and vomiting during spinal anesthesia for cesarean section. However, acupressure was not effective in children undergoing outpatient strabismus surgery.

Acupressure also works for other causes of nausea and vomiting. Acupressure helps women undergoing chemotherapy for breast cancer experience less nausea and nausea intensity than do women receiving the usual care. In addition, acupressure wristbands help in the treatment of nausea and vomiting for the first trimester of pregnancy.

Resistance to colds or influenza may be increased by acupressure. Stimulation of pressure points between the spine and top of the scapula, back, abdomen, elbow, anterior foot, kneecap, wrist, or hand may increase immune system function. Stimulation of acupressure points on the face is used to relieve nasal congestion. Other acupressure points on the neck and shoulders or chest can be pressed to relieve coughing or respiratory distress. Acupressure treatment helps patients with severe chronic obstructive pulmonary disease experience significantly less dyspnea.

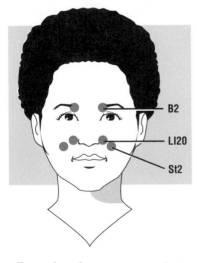

Examples of acupressure points

Uses

Acupressure can be used to relieve stress on organ and meridian pathways that may be fatigued by physical activities. By correcting energy imbalances, acupressure may be useful in relieving muscle pain, headaches, chest or nasal congestion, or dyspnea. Acupressure can also be used to treat or prevent nausea and vomiting during pregnancy, labor, and delivery or postoperatively. Acupressure may minimize symptoms of respiratory illnesses.

Acupressure can be used to treat the following conditions:

- Allergies
- Anxiety
- Back pain
- Chronic fatigue
- Digestive disorders
- Fibromyalgia
- Headache
- Labor
- Insomnia
- Menstrual pain
- Nausea
- Neck pain
- Pregnancy
- Stress
- Tennis elbow
- Vomiting

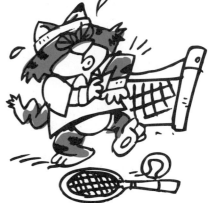

Risks and Precautions

Acupressure should not be applied just after eating a full meal. Acupressure therapy may increase a patient's susceptibility to cold because the body temperature is lowered during treatment. Acupressure should not be used on body parts that are infected, burned, scarred, or ulcerated. Pressure should not be applied to abdominal points in seriously ill patients, especially those with gastrointestinal cancer. Acupressure stimulation of abdominal points may cause premature labor in pregnant women. Acupressure should be carefully applied to sensitive or painful areas of the body.

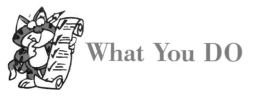

What You DO

Patient Education

Patients should be educated about acupressure before receiving treatment. Applying firm pressure on acupoints may cause soreness or aching pain on

1. **Acupressure should not be applied to the neck of patients with carotid artery disease.**
2. **Patients with cancer, tuberculosis, or cardiac disease should not have abdominal acupressure.**
3. **Pregnant patients should not have acupressure on the abdomen.**

www.acupressure.com
www.dishant.com/
acupressure/

the point. This type of pressure may also cause pain in a related part of the body as energy blocks are released. After obtaining a medical history and finding painful body areas, the therapist may have the patient lie unclothed on a massage table covered by a sheet, exposing only the body part that is being treated. Acupressure should not replace appropriate medical care.

Practitioners

The American Oriental Bodywork Therapy Association accredits practitioners and creates standards for treatments. License in massage therapy does not ensure that a practitioner has been trained in acupressure therapy.

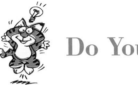

Do You UNDERSTAND?

See pages 269 and 270 for Learning Activities related to this topic.

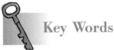

Key Words

Pressure points Numerous symmetrically paired specific points on the body that may conduct electrical energy through meridian pathways.

Chi Subtle energy that circulates through the body.

Meridians Pathways in the body that conduct energy and connect acupressure or acupuncture points with the organs.

Endorphins Neurochemicals with analgesic properties naturally produced by the body.

Lactic acid A toxic by-product of metabolism that may accumulate and cause acidosis when inadequate oxygen supply is delivered to the cells.

ACUPUNCTURE

What IS Acupuncture?

Although many nurses consider acupuncture as a new alternative or complimentary approach, it has been a fundamental part of Chinese health care for at least 2500 years. Acupuncture involves the insertion of thin-gauged needles into the body over strategic points to modify physiologic function. Acupuncture may be used in conjunction with electrical stimulation, applied heat, and or herbs. The National Institutes of Health (NIH) estimates that over 1 million Americans receive acupuncture treatments each year.

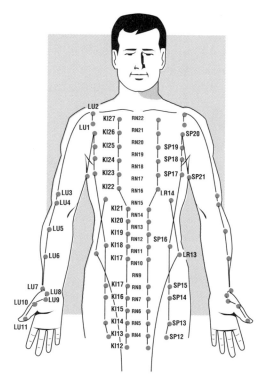

Examples of acupressure points

What You NEED TO KNOW

Theories suggest that patterns of energy flow (denote as qi, pronounced "chee") are present through the body that are responsible for homeostasis; when disrupted or imbalanced in some way, health consequences occur in the form of pathophysiologic responses. A body of literature examining mechanisms and efficacy of the approach has been presented. The literature has been favorable enough to cause the U.S. Food and Drug Administration to remove acupuncture needles from the category of "experimental medical devices."

In the traditional model, qi seems to reflect the spiritual, emotional, mental, and physical aspects of a person's life. Qi has two key components as defined by their attributes: yin (passive, dark, cold, moist, moving medially) and yang (light, active, warm dry, moving laterally). Qi flows through the body along pathways termed "meridians" or "channels," occurring symmetrically on each side of the body. Twelve organ meridians are present in each half of the body and two unpaired, midline meridians. The primary acupuncture points are located where the meridians run close to the skin. Disruptions in qi, or imbalances in yin and yang, are thought to undermine homeostasis.

Researchers and traditional practitioners cite a number of possible, and at this time not clearly defined, explanations for the way acupuncture might work. Among these explanations are the following:

1. Select neurotransmitters are released (e.g., serotonin) that change brain biochemistry.
2. Opioid systems such as endorphins are stimulated.
3. Circulatory modification occurs in which blood vessels may dilate or constrict as a result of release of substances such as histamine.
4. Augmentation of immune function is generated by the release of immune system mediators.
5. "Processing alteration" involves the "gate control" theory; here, connections in the nervous system receive too many impulses, become overwhelmed, and "close" or "open" as a gate.
6. Conduction and simulation of electromagnetic signals take place.

Nine types of acupuncture needles are used, though most practitioners use only six. Needles vary in length, gauge, and shape. Ideally, the needles

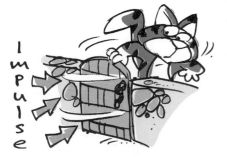

Impulse

should be disposable, otherwise standard sterilization procedures should be followed. Nonpainful sensations (termed "deqi," pronounced "dah-chee") are elicited. Once placed, the needle may be twisted, moved up and down, or vibrated.

Electro-acupuncture uses small electrical impulses in conjunction with needle placement. Sound waves, lasers, and heat may also be used. *Auriculotherapy* is based on the belief that the ear is rich in nerve and blood supply and has connections to many other parts of the body; strategically stimulating the ear is thought to generate certain phenomena in distant parts of the body. *Moxibustion* involves the application of heat to the acupuncture sites, while *cupping* is the stimulation of acupuncture points by the application of suction. *Acupressure* can be considered as acupuncture without needles.

Benefits and Uses

The World Health Organization has noted that acupuncture *may* be effective in carefully selected patients suffering from the following conditions in their respective illness domains:

- Musculoskeletal: arthritis, back and muscle pain, sciatica
- Emotional: anxiety, depression, insomnia
- Respiratory: asthma, bronchitis, common cold, smoking cessation
- Eye-ear-nose-throat: tinnitus, headache, toothache
- Digestive: cramping, diarrhea, constipation
- Gynecologic: menopausal symptoms, premenstrual syndrome
- Other: acute and chronic pain, chronic fatigue syndrome, addiction

Risks and Precautions

No matter what the application and the mechanism, considerable variation exists in patient response. This disparity may be a function of the acupuncturist, the improper application of acupuncture to a specific condition, and patient specific factors, as well as other factors (e.g., patient "belief," concomitant traditional therapy, power of suggestion, and so forth). Limitations such as these have plagued controlled trials studying efficacy and safety. It must be cautioned that the research is extremely uneven and plagued by many problems, making interpretation complicated. Consensus opinions are hard to achieve, and the arguments often seem fueled as much by emotion as it is by science and clinical observation.

Side effects of the therapy are rare, although case reports have surfaced of inadvertent pneumothorax when chest needles were inserted too deeply.

Bleeding and infection can occur in the event of improper insertion technique or poor decontamination procedures.

The practitioner must keep in mind that the use of acupuncture, as with many other complimentary therapies, has resulted in a tremendous amount of anecdotal evidence. Some points to keep in mind are include the following:

- Lifestyle, age, physiology, and mindset combine in predictable and unpredictable ways that facilitate or antagonize the effects of acupuncture.
- Do not rely on a diagnosis of a disease by an acupuncturist who does not have substantial conventional medical or nursing training.
- Health care providers should acquaint themselves with expert, licensed acupuncturists. A good place to obtain a referral is with the American Academy of Medical Acupuncture.
- An essential component is to protect the patient from disease transmission by strictly following universal blood and fluid precautions in technique applications.
- Your attitude and understanding go a long way in establishing a positive atmosphere for acupuncture or any medical or nursing intervention.
- It is important to support and educate consumers and practitioners about the need to be completely aware of all treatments in use (prescription, herbal, over-the-counter, and complementary and alternative therapies) because of the potential for desired and undesired interactive effects.

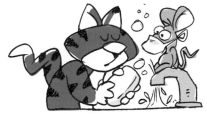

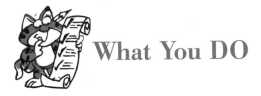

What You DO

Patient Education

Maintaining a positive frame of mind is important when educating the patient about acupuncture. Important teaching points that should be mentioned include the following:

- Maintain a positive, optimistic perspective.
- Selecting an experienced, licensed acupuncturist is important.
- Appreciate the multidimensional way that acupuncture works.
- Third-party payment for acupuncture varies considerably; currently, about 75% of insurers have covered some acupuncture treatments. Generally, physician acupuncturists charge more than do nonphysician acupuncturists.
- Discuss ways that alternative therapies (e.g., acupuncture) and conventional therapies (e.g., traditional medications and interventions) may work in concert.

Practitioners

Acupuncture therapy is allowed throughout the United States. States vary according to practice restrictions and privileges, licensing requirements, training, and certification. In some states, only physicians such as medical doctors, doctors of osteopathy, or chiropractors can administer acupuncture. Other states allow nurses, physician assistants, and trained acupuncture therapists to administer acupuncture. Most states require acupuncture therapists to obtain licensure. The National Certification Commission for Acupuncture and Oriental Medicine administers the national certification examination for acupuncture therapists. Many states require successful completion of this examination to obtain licensure. Acupuncture training is often given at the graduate level, and the Accreditation Commission for Acupuncture and Oriental Medicine (ACAOM) is the accrediting body for schools of acupuncture therapy.

nccam.nih.gov/health/
    acupuncture
nccam.nih.gov/research/concepts/
    consider/acupuncture.htm
http://www.acupuncture.com

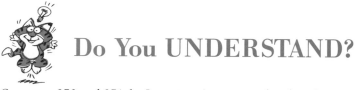

Do You UNDERSTAND?

See pages 270 and 271 for Learning Activities related to this topic.

AROMATHERAPY

What IS Aromatherapy?

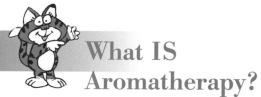

Aromatherapy is the external use of essential oils of plants or herbs for therapeutic medicinal purposes. The pure essential oils of plant flowers, roots, seeds, berries, or leaves are obtained by water or steam distillation or by carbon dioxide or solvent extraction. Essential oils may also be extracted by cold pressing, as is used to extract orange oil from the peel. Aromatherapy with essential oil was used in ancient Egypt in 3000 BC. In the 1800s, a French nurse developed aromatherapy massage.

What you NEED TO KNOW

Benefits and Uses

Benefits

Essential oils may have sedative, stimulatory, analgesic, antispasmodic, or antibacterial effects. Aromatherapy may be helpful for many conditions, such as relief of anxiety or nausea. The essential oil of lavender has been found to have sedative and relaxant effects and is a soothing antiflatulent. Dental patients who were exposed to the aroma of the essential oil orange (*Citrus sinensis*) in waiting rooms reported less anxiety, a more positive mood, and improved calmness than did those exposed to no odor. Reduced anxiety may also be the result of masking of unpleasant odors, such as dental cements containing eugenol. The smell of peppermint may decrease postoperative nausea and vomiting in surgical patients. Peppermint has been also used to relieve irritable bowel syndrome. Peppermint and menthol may relax smooth muscles by inhibiting calcium channels.

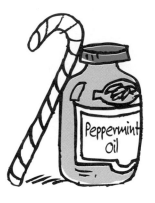

Uses

Essential oils are separated into minuscule droplets to administer by inhalation using heated lamps or burners or electric nebulizing diffusers. The olfactory stimulation of smelled oils may trigger memories or emotional responses that affect neurotransmitters in the limbic system of the brain for a therapeutic effect. The epithelial cells of the mucus membranes or respiratory tract may absorb aerosolized molecules of the essential oils for therapeutic effects. For instance, the smell of eucalyptus oil may cause bronchodilation. Inhalation of menthol vapor may decrease airway resistance in patients with asthma.

Oils may be applied the body to during massage. Essential oils may also be used in baths or lotions or applied in compresses. Combined with massage, aromatherapy can decrease the stress response and improve immune function and tissue oxygenation. Aromatherapy foot massage was found to psychologically benefit postoperative cardiac surgery patients.

Essential oils may also be used as perfumes to mask unpleasant odors. A drop of peppermint oil on a nurse's surgical mask may decrease the offensive odors of fecal incontinence or a ruptured bowel obstruction. Anesthesia circuit masks may be scented with essential oils to diminish children's anxiety during inhalational induction of general anesthesia.

Aromatherapy can be used to treat the following conditions:

- Anxiety
- Arthritis
- Asthma
- Colds
- Depression
- Digestive problems
- Hypertension
- Insomnia

- Migraines
- Muscular pain
- Nausea
- Premenstrual syndrome
- Skin conditions
- Stress relief
- Wound healing

1. **Essential oils should be kept out of the reach of children.**
2. **Pregnant patients and individuals with hypertension, epilepsy, or allergies should not use aromatherapy.**
3. **Allergic reactions from aromatherapy may cause skin inflammation or irritation.**

Risks and Precautions

Essential oils should be used cautiously during pregnancy or by patients with epilepsy, high blood pressure, or allergies. Just as with ingested herbs, vaporized essential oils may interact with medications. Some essential oils may have toxicities. Vaporized essential oils may cause allergic skin reactions. Topical application of essential oils such as dill, lime, orange, or rue may cause photosensitivity and sunburn with prolonged exposure to ultraviolet light. Excessive external use may also result in toxicity. Ingestion of spearmint, birch, or wintergreen may cause renal damage; pennyroyal has been associated with miscarriage. Camphor, sassafras, and calamus oils may be carcinogenic. Certain oils such as sage may be neurotoxic. Topical application of mustard or horseradish oil may cause skin irritation. With all essential oils, avoid contact with eyes or mucous membranes, and keep away from children.

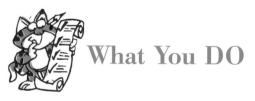

What You DO

Patient Education

Patients should understand that only small doses of vaporized essential oils should be used. Prolonged exposure may increase the toxicity of essential oils. Nebulizing diffusers should be used with one to three drops of essential oil for 15-minute intervals and no more than three times daily. Although the oil may not be smelled after a time, the medicinal effects may continue. Refrigeration of essential oils may prevent chemical breakdown.

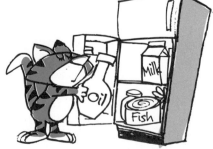

www.naha.org/
www.nature-helps.com/
agora/agora.htm

Practitioners

In the United States, the National Association for Holistic Aromatherapists or the American Alliance of Aromatherapy may recommend practitioners, although many aromatherapists may have no formal training or credentialing. Currently, the Natural Association of Holistic Aromatherapists is promoting curriculum and licensing standards for the practice of aromatherapy.

Aromatherapy is most popular in Great Britain. England, France, Switzerland, and New Zealand have licensing requirements for aromatherapists. In England, the Aromatherapy Organizations Council was formed to recognize standards of training for aromatherapists. Massage therapists may receive education and training about essential oils during their education.

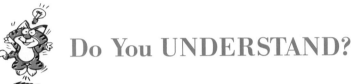

Do You UNDERSTAND?

See page 272 for Learning Activities related to this topic.

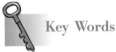

Key Words

Essential oils Aromatic plant oils isolated by steam distillation often used for perfumes, aromatherapy, or medicinal effects. Many essential oils have antispasmodic, expectorant, sedative, analgesic, or antimicrobial activity.
Carcinogenic Capable of producing cancer.

COLOR THERAPY

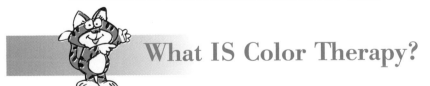

What IS Color Therapy?

Color therapy uses the seven colors of the rainbow to bring about balance, health, healing, relaxation, inspiration, and protection of the body and mind. Color therapy is also known as chromatherapy, light therapy, or colourology. Color therapy uses the healing powers within colors to achieve its goals.

What You NEED TO KNOW

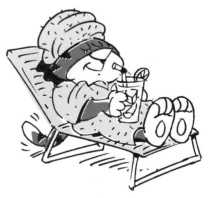

Color therapy comes from Ayurveda, an ancient medical practice developed in India. Ayurveda states that there are five basic elements to the universe: earth, air, water, fire, and space. These elements are also present in humans. The relationship and amounts of each element will determine individual personality traits and characteristics. Illness results from an imbalance of the elements. Color is composed of differing frequencies and wavelengths (vibrations) of light energy. Light energy is the form of energy seen by humans. Microwaves, radio waves, x-rays, and ultraviolet rays are types of energy that are invisible to the human eye. Ayurveda uses color and its energy transmitted through vibrations to restore an individual's elements to the proper level. When the elements are balanced, wellness occurs. The level needed for each element varies among individuals. The seven colors of light energy correspond to specific body regions, or chakras. Treatment colors are chosen depending on the affected body region:

CHAKRA	COLOR	BODY REGION
First	Red	Root or base of spine
Second	Orange	Sacral or pelvis-groin area
Third	Yellow	Solar plexus
Fourth	Green	Heart
Fifth	Blue	Throat
Sixth	Indigo	Brow
Seventh	Violet	Crown

Color therapy is given in a variety of ways. Patients can be wrapped in colored cloth or bathed in colored light. Patients may receive color-treated water to drink. Water is color treated by wrapping water containers in clear, colored paper or plastic wrap and then placing the container in direct sunlight. The water soaks up the color energy and would then contain restorative properties. Room coloring, window treatments, and even individual clothing can be used for their specific healing properties.

COLOR	NOTE
Red	G
Yellow	A sharp
Blue	D
Violet	E
Orange	A
Green	C
Indigo	D Sharp

Color therapy is often combined with hydrotherapy and aromatherapy in spa-type settings. When used in this manner, warm or hot water treatments with essential oils and color energy are combined to restore and relax. Through mathematical manipulations, other therapists have associated colors with musical notes. Sounds and music are composed to enhance the therapeutic effects.

Benefits and Uses

Each color is useful for healing specific conditions and restoring certain body areas:

COLOR	ACTION	HEALTH CARE USE
Red	Energy, empowerment, stimulation; awakens physical energies	Enhances circulation; increases red blood cell production to treat cancer and analgesia; promotes wound healing
Orange	Pleasure, enthusiasm, sexual stimulation	Antibacterial; used to treat digestive system distress; increases immunity; increases sexual function; used to treat chest and kidney ailments
Yellow	Sensory stimulant, wisdom, clarity, uplifting	Decongestant; antibacterial; gastrointestinal stimulant; enhances lymphatic system; used to treat skin problems
Green	Balance, calming, stability, security	Antiseptic; germicidal; antibacterial; used to repair ulcers, used to treat broken bones; regenerates tissue
Blue	Enhances communication and knowledge; calming, comforting	Purges toxins; used to treat liver disorders, jaundice; reduces fever, bleeding
Indigo	Sedative, calming, promotes intuition	Used to treat bleeding, abscesses, congestion, conditions of ears, nose, eyes, sinuses
Violet	Spiritual awakening, enlightenment, balance physical and spiritual energies	Muscle relaxant; soothes nervous system; used to treat rheumatism, epilepsy, analgesia; repairs deep tissue

Risks and Precautions

Color therapists recommend using a variety of colors because using one color (monochromic) can cause imbalances. Prolonged exposure can lead to overstimulation and complications, related to the effects of each color:

- Red: agitation and aggression
- Orange: nervousness and agitation
- Yellow: exhaustion and depression
- Green: negativity
- Blue: depression
- Indigo: headache, drowsiness
- Violet: loss of reality base

Color therapy research is minimal. Therefore color therapy should be viewed as an enhancement to conventional medical therapy and not as a replacement.

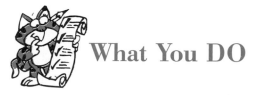

What You DO

Patient Education

Patients should understand that, although color therapy is a useful tool for promoting relaxation, it should not become the mainstay of treatment for patients with serious mental or physical ailments. Patients should seek health care management of their condition by qualified health care practitioners.

Practitioners

Color therapists do not undergo certification or licensure. Training usually involves modern applications of color therapy, as well as study of the historical development and use of color therapy. Color therapists usually received instruction in using color therapy as an adjunct to other alternative therapies, such as aromatherapy and reflexology. Color therapy is practiced throughout the United States, United Kingdom, Europe, Hong Kong, and South Africa. The International Association of Colour and Colour Therapy Association represents color therapists.

Do You UNDERSTAND?

See page 273 for Learning Activities related to this topic.

FENG SHUI

What IS Feng Shui?

Feng shui (pronounced "fung-shway") is translated as "wind and water" from Mandarin Chinese. Feng shui is a picture word for the flow of life force that animates all of creation. Our vitality is dependent on fresh air and pure water; it also depends on the change of seasons, time of day, structure of buildings, color of surroundings, and symbolism contained in works of art. All of these elements contribute to the science of feng shui, which was developed in China more than 3000 years ago. The principles of feng shui are universal. Indeed, similar systems have been developed in India, Japan, and ancient Europe. Feng shui can be seen as a bridge between medicine and environmental design.

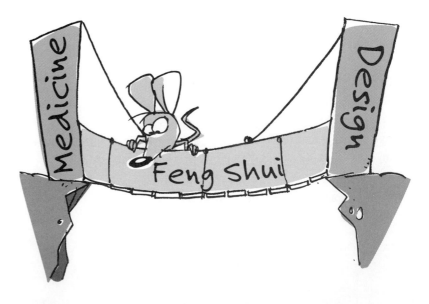

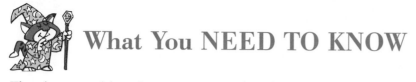

What You NEED TO KNOW

The objective of feng shui is to improve lives by improving the environment. A qualified practitioner, specific to a client or patient, chooses the methods of improving the environment.

Chi (pronounced "chee") is the Chinese word for breath or life force essence. Chi can be cultivated, directed, or dissipated; however, individuals cannot live without it. Chi can be affected by interventions directed inside or outside of the body. Acupuncture, exercise, and nutrition develop chi in the body. Feng shui deals with chi outside the body in our buildings, environment, and landscapes.

The yin-yang symbol is an ancient emblem of the balance of life. The white side is yang, which symbolizes all things masculine, expansive, exterior, hot, and heavenly. The black side is yin, which symbolizes all things feminine, contracted, interior, cool, and earthy. Yin and yang exist only in relationship to each other. All life is made of their constant cycle. This concept is referred to as tai chi, which means "embracing unity." Tai chi is at the center of feng shui's most common tool, the bagua. Sometimes spelled pakua, bagua means eight trigrams. Eight trigrams are made of three lines representing yin (broken lines) and yang (solid lines). Each gua, or side of the octagon, has many attributes and qualities. Sometimes called the eight life aspirations, the guas are:

- Jen
  - Associated with family and ancestors
  - Symbolized by green, wood, feet, thunder, spring
- Shun
  - Associated with wealth and abundance
  - Symbolized by purple, red and green, wood and wind, hip, and bones
- Li
  - Associated with reputation and fame
  - Symbolized by red, fire, eyes, and summer
- Kun
  - Associated with marriage and partnership
  - Symbolized by pink, organs, earth, and women
- Dui
  - Associated with children and creativity
  - Symbolized by white, metal, mouth, autumn, and lakes

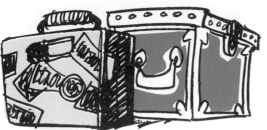

- Chyan
  - Associated with travel and helpful people
  - Symbolized by metal, gray, head, father, and sky
- Kan
  - Associated with career and ability
  - Symbolized by black or deep blue, ears, winter
- Ken
  - Associated with knowledge and education
  - Symbolized by green and black, hands, earth
- Tai chi
  - Associated with mental and physical well being

Benefits and Uses

Physical health, better careers, and more harmonious relationships are just some of the benefits of creating a better environment that supports the circulation of chi.

Risks and Precautions

Feng shui is a safe, effective therapy with no known side effects or risks.

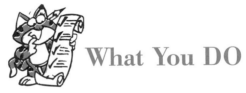

What You DO

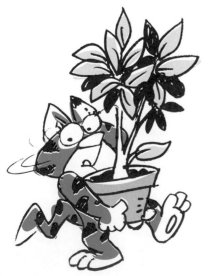

Feng shui has many exciting applications that can be used in the hospital and home environment. Feng shui can be used to complement a patient's health needs. Specific guas can be increased or decreased depending on the patient's signs and symptoms. Color, placement of objects, plants, and water structures are used to direct the flow of chi. At home or in a patient's hospital room, the movement of chi should be smooth, not too fast or too slow. In the workplace, faster-directed chi for traffic areas would be appropriate. Nurses may use the principles of chi, harmony, and unity in structuring a patient's room.

Practitioners

Many schools for training in feng shui exist in the United States. Feng shui is practiced internationally in Australia, Israel, Mexico, Switzerland, and the United Kingdom, to name a few. National and international societies (see web sites) exist for the purposes of training, continuing education, research, and practitioner databases.

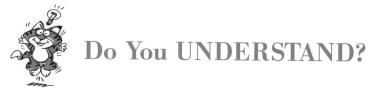

Do You UNDERSTAND?

See pages 273 and 274 for Learning Activities related to this topic.

See pages 273 and 274 for Learning Activities related to this topic.

 www.fengshuiguild.com/
www.fengshuisociety.
org.uk

HOMEOPATHY

What IS Homeopathy?

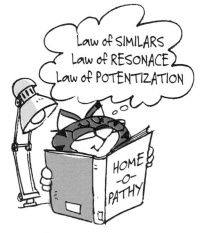

The term *homeopathy* is a word derived from "homeo," meaning similar, and "pathos," meaning suffering. From this definition, homeopathy deals the question of disease and suffering. In so doing, homeopathy uses a few fundamental principles: the Law of Similars, the Law of Resonance, and the Law of Potentization. These principles were developed by Samuel Hahnemann, a German physician, who practiced medicine in the late 1700s, at a time when medicine was in a state of chaos.

What You NEED TO KNOW

Hahnemann was born in a small town in Saxony, Germany in 1755. Hahnemann practiced medicine during a period when popular medical treatment involved purgation, emesis, bloodletting, and administration of belladonna or the poisons mercury, arsenic, and snake venoms. Hahnemann's greatest concern about the use of these "medicines" of his time was that no one knew how the medicines worked or their primary influence on the body. In this environment, Hahnemann practiced medicine, but he could not accept the harm these practices caused on patients already ill and weak. Hahnemann extensively studied chemistry and was fluent in many languages. Because he was unable to agree with current medical practices, he translated medical texts from Latin, English, and Greek into German. During this time, Hahnemann was exposed to many prominent philosophers, chemists, and botanists who later influenced his thinking about health and healing.

While translating *A Treatise on Materia Medica* by the Scottish physician William Cullen, Hahnemann began to discover the foundations he would use for homeopathy. This text was an account of a drug called cinchona or Peruvian bark that Dr. Cullen had used to treat malaria. Dr. Cullen hypothesized that the herb constituted "factors" that affected the malaria. However, Hahnemann observed that, although other substances contained these same factors or ingredients, they did not cure the malaria. He reasoned that another factor must be present in cinchona that cured the malaria, and he set out to prove his theory. To test this idea, Hahnemann took cinchona until he produced a reaction in his body. He experienced symptoms such as cold feet and fingertips, heart palpitations, tremors, thirst, intermittent fevers and perspiration, extreme headache, and drowsiness. Hahnemann called this result the "totality of symptoms." He called the process of demonstrating what a substance in its pure form does to a healthy body a "proving." Through the process of proving, Hahnemann was able to show that the totality of symptoms in malaria were identical to those produced by taking cinchona. Hahnemann then used this herb to treat and cure malaria. This result encouraged Hahnemann to conduct more provings on other chemical and botanical substances. Hahnemann then developed a system to categorize each substance. The collection of categorized provings can be found in the *Homeopathic Materia Medica Pura*. After successfully treating a malaria patient with cinchona, Hahnemann treated other diseases by giving substances to produce the same clinical picture as did the illness. Hahnemann called this treatment process *similia similibus curentur* or "like cures like" (Law of Similars).

The process of provings led to the development of another principle of homeopathy: the Law of Resonance. Hahnemann noted that giving strong medications to sick patients often produced side effects and unwanted damage to other body systems. Hahnemann searched for a method to minimize the negative effects of medicines. Hahnemann believed that humans are a series of magnetic fields and subtle energy bodies or electrodynamic systems. This electrodynamic energy is referred to by the Chinese as "chi." According to the principles of physics, matter and energy interchange in bioenergetic fields that can be measured in waveforms. If the frequencies of the subtle fields of both substances are close enough in frequency, they will resonate. Tuning forks resonate to each other when toned at a distance. By administering substances, the symptom picture of which resonates to the symptom picture of the illness, the body can augment its own curative processes. That is, the body can heal itself. Because the body's own healing processes are increased, decreased amounts of medications are needed to cure the patient.

Using medications in smaller amounts decreases toxicity problems and reduces unwanted side effects in the patient.

The maximal healing potential of a medication is achieved when it is able to release its healing energy and make it more available to the electro-dynamic field of the body. This process is known as the **Law of Potentization** and is done by administering a physical force such as succussion to the diluted substance. By increasing potentization, homeopathic remedies increase the body's defensive immune system to help the body heal.

Homeopathy recognizes that symptoms are the body's efforts to deal with stress. The signs and symptoms produced in an individual are a unique picture of the state of the body's defense mechanisms. Inherent to the practice of homeopathy is the taking of a meticulous case history of symptoms an individual exhibits during the illness, and how factors in the physical, emotional, and mental environment affect the illness. After the case history of the totality of symptoms has been taken, a remedy is chosen. This process is known as "individualizing" the case. For example, during an influenza outbreak, affected individuals may have similar symptoms of nausea and vomiting, cough, irritability, and drowsiness. However, one person's cough may be loose with thick yellow phlegm, and another's cough may be dry and harsh with clear thin nasal drainage. Both patients have coughs, but each cough is different and is influenced by the individual's environment and physiologic defense mechanisms. This difference is what is known by homeopaths as distinguishing the subtle variations of every individual case, thereby treating the individual and not the disease.

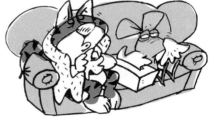

Benefits and Uses

Homeopathy has been used for many conditions, including:

- Allergic reactions
- Asthma
- Attention deficit disorder
- Bed wetting
- Colds
- Colic
- Constipation
- Depression
- Diarrhea
- Ear infections
- Headache
- Hemorrhoids
- Influenza
- Low back pain
- Motion sickness
- Postoperative infections

Risks and Precautions

Homeopathy should not be used for emergency or life-threatening conditions. For example, eminent appendicitis rupture or fractured bones should be treated by conventional surgical techniques.

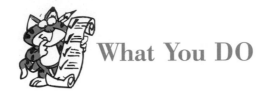

What You DO

Patient Education

Patients should understand that homeopathy is not meant to stabilize emergency or life-threatening conditions. Traditional medical treatment should be sought for these conditions. Homeopathy does offer treatment of less severe problems with the benefits of decreased side effects. Homeopathy also treats the patient as a holistic being and views illness on an individual basis, assessing the physical, mental, and contextual factors that affect the patient.

Practitioners

Homeopathy training involves 3 to 4 years of schooling after high school. Master's and doctorate degrees in homeopathy are also available. Some states require certification for licensure and practice. Some insurance companies also require certification for reimbursement. Certification bodies include the American Institute of Homeopathy, Homeopathic Academy of Naturopathic Physicians, and the National Center for Homeopathy.

Do You UNDERSTAND?

See page 274 for Learning Activities related to this topic.

Key Words

Law of Potentization Diluting substances to minimize the toxicity level while maintaining curative properties.

Law of Resonance When two energy fields vibrate in near unison, they become linked and augment the action of each other.

Law of Similars Substances that cause symptoms in healthy people can be used to heal unhealthy patients who exhibit the same (or similar) symptoms.

www.homeopathic.org/
www.homeopathyusa.org/

INTUITIVE SPIRITUAL HEALING

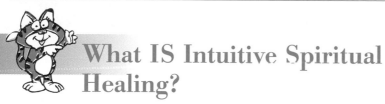

What IS Intuitive Spiritual Healing?

Intuitive spiritual healing (ISH), or the "laying on of hands," is a transfer of energy by a trained spiritual healer. ISH has been practiced for thousands of years by peoples and cultures around the world. ISH can aid patients in healing not only their physical body, but also the emotional, mental, and spiritual aspects of their being. Patients often use ISH as an adjunct to traditional medical treatment.

What You NEED TO KNOW

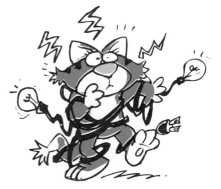

Whether it is to place a hand on a fevered brow or to massage a stiff muscle, touch has always had a place in medicine as a diagnostic or therapeutic tool. Practitioners of ISH work by placing their hands on the patient's body or holding them slightly above the body and connecting with the patient energetically. These therapists use touch and contact with the patient as an assessment tool and a therapeutic device.

The human body is an energy field. The anatomic makeup of the physical body creates an electrical field in and around the body. Traditional medical physicians recognize disturbances in the energy flow of organs in the body as indicative of disease. For example, physicians use recordings of the electrical activity within the body, such as electrocardiograms (ECG), electroencephalograms (EEG), and electromyelograms (EMG), as diagnostic tools to diagnose these disturbances. The healing practitioner assesses the patient by connecting with the subtle energy field that surrounds and penetrates the physical body. This energy field is composed of at least seven layers consisting of the same substance that creates the physical body. The only difference between the solid substance of the physical body and the subtle energy that comprises the energy field surrounding the body is the vibration of the energy. The different vibrations of the physical body and the energy field make it possible for both to exist within the same space.

Each layer of the energy field has a different function and level of reality. The first three energy field layers comprise the physical plane of the body. The fourth layer is the astral plane, which acts as a bridge between the physical and spiritual levels of the body. The last three field layers comprise the spiritual plane. The energy field layers hold our thoughts, emotions, and memories from which our physical reality is created. The creation of a healthy balanced life begins with an idea or belief that is brought down from the higher spiritual levels of our being. When this idea is in alignment with universal law and is able to pass down through the layers of the field without distortion, a healthy part of our life manifests in the physical world. Often, however, our reactions to specific events or memories create distortion in the field layers. Ideas filtering down from our spiritual levels become distorted by distortions present in the field. As this distorted idea enters into the physical world, imbalances are created in the physical body, eventually leading to disease states.

A session with a practitioner of ISH will last anywhere from 30 minutes to 1 hour. The patient remains clothed and is usually lying down for the healing. Initially, the healing practitioner uses a series of hand movements on the patient's body, which create a foundation on which deeper healing work can be done. The patient may experience the healing energy as heat, pulsations, vibrations, or a tingling sensation. Through contact with the patient's subtle energy field, the healing practitioner is able to detect disturbances in the flow of the energy field. Disturbance can be exhibited as blockages, depletion, or oversupply of energy to one part of the body. Practitioners gather information about the condition of the patient's body, as well as the emotional, mental, and spiritual states, which then helps them to move intuitively to where healing is most needed at that moment. The patient may be surprised to learn that the healing practitioner does not necessarily work on the area where the patient is complaining of symptoms.

Intuition can be defined as the act of knowing or sensing without the use of a rational process, such as having a hunch or an impression about something. For example, when the telephone rings, have you known who was calling and it turns out to be that person? Intuition is just one of the tools that an ISH practitioner uses to gather information about a patient.

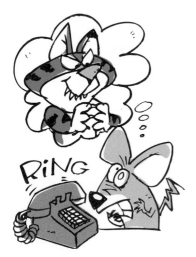

The five senses—sight, hearing, touch, smell, and taste—are also used to gather information. All of us have skills in using our senses to collect information from the world. Often, because our brains deem a lot of the information that we gather as unnecessary, we are unaware of using our senses in these subtle ways. For example, this instance is where we get the expression "you can even smell the fear." Another example is when nurses just "know" that a patient is becoming ill.

Practitioners of spiritual healing have discovered which of their senses they best use to access information from the world. These senses are then expanded with practice over a length of time.

We know these concepts of expanded senses by other terms such as clairvoyance, clairaudience, and clairsentience.

Ideas to help you understand which sense with which you perceive might include the following:

1. Which of these phrases do you use in conversation?
   a. I see what you mean.
   b. I know what you mean.
   c. I hear you.
2. When I _____ a baby _____, my heart opens.

ISH is concerned with treating the patient who just so happens to have a disease, instead of focusing primarily on the patient's disease. ISH is a safe adjunct to traditional medical therapies used in treating medical or emotional disease states. Trained practitioners of ISH can work cooperatively with traditional medical doctors in many ways to assist the patient on the path to wellness. For example, ISH can be used to help the preoperative patient prepare for surgery in bringing relaxation to the patient. ISH can be used postoperatively to facilitate a quicker, smoother recovery from the effects of surgery. ISH can help patients receiving treatment for cancer because the healing work can help remove debris left from radiation and chemotherapy. This action will help decrease debilitating side effects.

Benefits and Uses

ISH allows and encourages the patient to be a full participant in the healing process. Simply fixing the physical problem may not address underlying emotional and spiritual problems that contribute to disease states or develop because of the disease. When underlying emotional and spiritual problems are not addressed, the disease state may likely recur.

ISH works on all levels of the patient's energy field to correct distortions that are present and contribute to the disease state. Healing of this type is not spontaneous, as might occur with "faith" healing. Improvement in a patient's physical condition will occur gradually over time. ISH can lead the patient to deeper understandings of themselves and open themselves to deeper spiritual realities.

Target populations for ISH include:

- Adults
- Children
- Chronic disease patients
- Coronary care patients

- Hospitalized patients
- Infants
- Oncology patients
- Surgical patients

Intuitive spiritual healing can be used to treat the following conditions:

- Acquired immunodeficiency syndrome (AIDS)
- Alcoholism
- Anxiety
- Arthritis
- Asthma
- Back pain
- Cancer
- Depression

- Epilepsy
- Heart disease
- Headache
- Hypertension
- Immunosuppression
- Menstrual pain
- Preoperative relaxation
- Postoperative pain and healing
- Posttraumatic syndrome disorder

Risks and Precautions

ISH has no known risks or precautions.

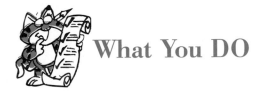 **What You DO**

Patient Education

Many hospitals have a complimentary and alternative medicine department available for patients. This department may employ an intuitive spiritual healer. If this is the case, as a professional nurse, you can inform patients of the positive effects and uses of ISH. If patients are already seeing a healer outside of the hospital, they might ask if their healer might work on them while they are in the hospital. Patients may desire that their healer accompany them into the operating room or join them in the postanesthetic care unit (PACU). The healing practitioner will need the permission of the attending physician to work on the patient in the hospital. The healer may also need to meet with personnel in charge of the units in which the healer would be treating the patient. As a nurse, you may be asked to help facilitate this process by giving the healing practitioner information concerning hospital rules and regulations. It may be necessary to schedule time during the patient's day when the healing practitioner might work with the patient.

After receiving a healing, the patient may experience a sense of deep relaxation, peace, balance, and centeredness. The patient may experience pain relief and enhanced well being. As the professional nurse who takes care of the patient after a healing, you may need to schedule some quiet time so that the patient can integrate the effects of the healing session.

 www.barbarabrennan.com
www.wholistichealing
  research.com
www.ahna.org

Practitioners

Healers in the United States may be taught by apprenticeship or educated through programs such as the Barbara Brennan School of Healing. In the United Kingdom, spiritual healing is a recognized therapy within the British National Health Service. In England, the National Federation of Spiritual Healers (NFSH) and the Confederation of Healing Organizations (CHO) certifies spiritual healers. The NFSH guidelines restrict healers from making medical diagnoses and require healers to advise patients to consult their own physician.

Do You UNDERSTAND?

See page 275 for Learning Activities related to this topic.

Key Words

Clairvoyance The ability to see beyond what others can see.
Clairaudience The ability to hear things beyond what others can hear.
Clairsentience The ability to feel things beyond what others can feel.

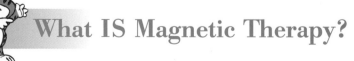

MAGNETIC THERAPY

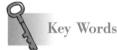

What IS Magnetic Therapy?

Magnetic therapy is the use of magnetic fields to create a static force on the body, often for purposes of relieving pain. The Chinese have used magnets for over 4000 years to reduce pain, promote wound healing, treat epilepsy or diarrhea, and improve eyesight. Acupuncturists may apply magnets to acupuncture points.

Magnets can differ in size, shape, and strength. Strong magnetic fields may pass through bone and tissues. Permanent or static magnets may be unipolar, bipolar, or have alternating poles that contact the body. Pulsating electrical currents may create magnetic fields. Magnets may be placed on or next to the body for therapeutic effects.

The exact way that magnets bring about analgesia and healing is poorly understood. Magnets are thought to possibly stimulate **endorphin** release. Magnets may also block pain transmission by stimulating nerve endings. When magnets stimulate nerve endings, the nerves become "overloaded" and are unable to send pain messages. If pain messages do not reach the brain, pain is not felt. Other theories explain that magnets may dilate blood vessels by creating charged particles in the blood or increase the oxygen-carrying capacity of the blood by action on the iron in hemoglobin. However, hemoglobin is bound to red blood cells and is therefore unable to react to magnetic fields. Some scientists believe that magnets affect cell membranes by affecting calcium binding or ion exchange at the cell wall. Magnets may affect the body's electromagnetic fields to bring about healing or analgesia.

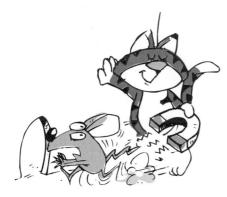

 What you NEED TO KNOW

Benefits and Uses

Magnets are used in many ways. Repetitive transcranial magnetic stimulation (rTMS) with low-frequency magnetic pulses is used for epilepsy, depression, and schizophrenia. Pulsating electromagnetic fields may be used to treat nonhealing fractured bones. The most common therapeutic use of magnets is for pain relief.

Research into the effectiveness of magnetic therapy for analgesia is conflicting. Magnets have been found safe and effective in relieving arthritic knee pain. Applying magnets to the skin for 45 minutes was found to decrease pain in adults who had knee pain resulting from childhood polio. Patients with **diabetic neuropathy** found relief after using magnetic footpads for several months. Another study of patients with fibromyalgia found improved physical functioning in women who slept on magnetic mattress pads every night for 4 months. However, relief of pain and fatigue were not significantly improved. Other studies have found magnets to be ineffective for low back pain or heel pain.

Magnetic therapy can be used to treat the following conditions:

- Arthritis
- Back pain
- Carpal tunnel syndrome
- Chronic pelvic pain
- Depression
- Diabetic peripheral neuropathy
- Edema
- Epilepsy
- Fibromyalgia
- Headaches
- Knee pain
- Low back pain
- Menstrual pain
- Migraine
- Multiple sclerosis
- Muscle spasms
- Neck pain
- Nonhealing fractures
- Obsessive-compulsive disorder
- Osteoarthritis
- Osteoporosis
- Parkinson's disease
- Peripheral neuropathy
- Postpolio syndrome
- Postsurgical wound healing
- Scar tissue
- Schizophrenia
- Stress incontinence
- Tendonitis
- Tennis elbow

1. **Magnets may interfere with pacemaker function.**
2. **Pregnant women should not wear magnetic wraps over the abdomen.**

Risks and Precautions

The magnets used today are generally safe because most magnets generate small electromagnetic fields. Magnets may interfere with electrical medical devices. Cardiac pacemakers can be converted from demand to fixed heart rate firing by putting the magnet over the pacemaker box. Unsupervised small children may swallow magnets, causing gastrointestinal obstruction. Pregnant women should not use magnets because fetal effects have not been determined.

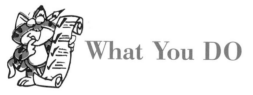

What You DO

Patient Education

Nurses should instruct patients who have pacemakers to not wear magnetic necklaces or wraps that may interfere with the pacemaker. Magnets should not be placed next to electrosurgical cautery grounding pads used in the operating room.

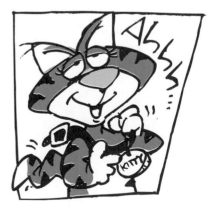

www.umm.edu/cam/
electro.htm
www.sciencedaily.com/releases/
1999/09/990909071842.htm
www.marshfieldclinic.org/
cattails/00/julaug/magnet.asp

Do You UNDERSTAND?

See pages 276 and 277 for Learning Activities related to this topic.

Key words

Endorphins Naturally occurring opioid substances found in the brain and nervous system that bind to neuroreceptors to relieve pain.

Diabetic neuropathy Nerve pain resulting from diabetic disease processes.

PRAYER

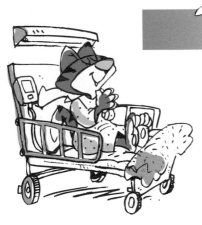

What IS Prayer?

Prayer, a common practice among almost all religions and faiths, uses the faith of the prayer to seek divine intervention in the healing process. This request to God, a divine being, or higher power, can take many forms. Requests for divine intervention might be for a healing, reduction of symptoms, shortened hospital stay, or safety during procedures. These requests are just a beginning list. Ill patients themselves often make these requests. Additionally, other individuals may be praying for patients as well. The people praying have a belief that a higher power hears and answers their prayers.

What You NEED TO KNOW

Benefits and Uses

Prayer is useful for all patient populations and is easy to do. Prayer requires no specific time or place to happen; prayer can be done anytime, day or night, and anywhere. Prayer can be done in large groups, such as in church, or just one person uttering a prayer in a quiet place. This benefit allows prayer to be used anytime a person feels the need to converse with a higher power.

Prayer has many positive effects. The person who is praying often enjoys psychologic benefits such as a feeling of relief of giving control of healing to a higher being. Combined with faith in the works of a higher power, the person now has a reason to feel relaxed because their higher power, who is all mighty, will take control of their illness. Psychologically, many people find it reassuring that a higher power will be assisting the physician, nurse, or therapist in the treatment of the illness and maybe even allowing a miracle to occur. When the patient prays, a time of distraction occurs during the prayer that allows the person to leave their immediate problems behind and focus on their conversation with a higher power. For people praying on behalf of the patient, the time spent in prayer is a time of spiritual renewal and reawakening. In summary, benefits of prayer include:

- Acceptance of what the future may hold
- Church support
- Decreased incidence and severity of depression
- Decreased length of hospital stays
- Decreased morbidity and mortality
- Fewer hospitalizations
- Getting in touch with fellow believers
- Healing
- Improved coping
- Increased relaxation
- Lowered blood pressure
- Miraculous cures
- Peace of mind
- Spiritual awakening

Prayer as a healing therapy is just starting to be studied. Several issues make it difficult to research prayer. Often, prayer and spirituality are considered to be similar and are studied together. Also, it is difficult to maintain a control or "non-prayed-for" group, as the researcher would not deny prayer to a patient requesting such intervention. Last, others would argue that being cured is not an appropriate measure of the power of prayer. To the believer, the success of prayer is in putting the person's trust in a higher power and finding peace to face the future, not solely curing the disease. Many reports about prayer are anecdotal in nature, making it hard for the scientific community to explain or accept. Some people attribute the benefits of prayer to a new medication or a treatment; others find that prayer increases the patient's will to live, which, in turn, assists traditional medical therapies to heal the patient. However, to a person earnestly praying for healing, he or she wholly believes that the healing was a result of prayer.

http://1stholistic.com/
prayer/hol_prayer_home.
htm
http://phoenix.liu.edu/
~dolinsky/pha590/amtherapy/
mindbody/overview/sld067.htm

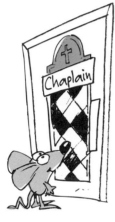

Risks and Precautions

Prayer is a safe, inexpensive, and effective therapy for all conditions. There are no known negative side effects to prayer. In the majority of cases, prayer is an adjunct therapy. Some patients of certain beliefs will use only prayer for healing and may refuse certain medical treatments. This action might cause apprehension to members of the health care team. It should be remembered that this decision, in all but a few instances, belongs to the patient.

Some patients do not believe in prayer or a higher power. This therapy would not be appropriate for these patients.

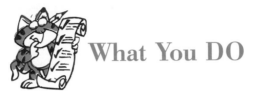

What You DO

Patient Education

Nurses may encourage believers to pray whenever they feel the need. There are no risks. Prayer is totally free, does not require any setup or prior approval, and can be done anywhere by anybody.

If the nurse feels comfortable with prayer, he or she can ask patients if they want the nurse to pray for them. Most believers would find this gesture comforting. Additionally, the hospital chaplain service can provide spiritual and prayer services for patients.

Practitioners

No training is required. Individuals should simply talk to a higher power as they would talk to their closest friend.

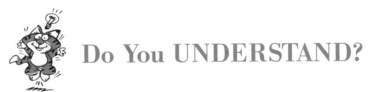

Do You UNDERSTAND?

See pages 277 and 278 for Learning Activities related to this topic.

REIKI

What IS Reiki?

Reiki is a term meaning universal life energy manifested in the physical. Rei and Ki are Japanese characters, where Rei means universal life energy, and Ki (also called chi) is that energy demonstrated through being alive. When this energy is decreased or restricted, a person can become prone to illness. Universal life energy is always present, in and around a person, and can be accessed though conscious intent.

The practice of Reiki is an ancient form of energy work, similar to what was once referred to as "laying on of hands." Reiki is similar to therapeutic touch (TT) in that energies are transferred through the practitioner to the client, but Reiki involves more contact than does TT. Reiki uses the energy of Ki to aid in healing both the practitioner and the recipient by allowing channeling of energy (Ki) to flow easily though the body.

By moving energy through the body, stress can be reduced, and a relaxation response is evoked. Reiki has been used to aid in healing wounds, assisting with pain reduction, and reducing stress.

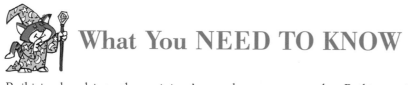

What You NEED TO KNOW

Reiki is placed into the recipient's aura by a master-teacher Reiki practitioner during an attunement. An attunement is when the master-teacher opens certain chakras or energy centers in the recipient's auric field. The symbols that are sacred to Reiki are then placed into these chakras. Once the person has been attuned, the Reiki is permanently embedded into the individual's auric field and is accessible at a thought. Four levels of Reiki are taught: first- through third-degree levels and master-teacher. If a person wishes to use Reiki for himself, herself, or for family members, the first-degree level is sufficient.

Reiki is considered a light-touch application of energetic transfers rather than massage. However, Reiki can be incorporated into massage and other touch therapies to enhance the treatments.

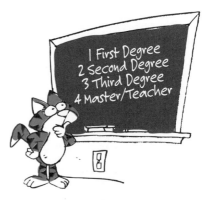

Benefits and Uses

- Stress illnesses
- Chronic illnesses
- Terminal illnesses: assists with achieving acceptance of a person's life
- To aid in psychologic healing (in conjunction with conventional therapies such as psychotherapy)
- Wound healing
- Pain reduction

Risks and Precautions

Reiki has no known risks or precautions.

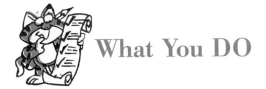 **What You DO**

Patient Education

To receive an attunement, a student contacts a practitioner (Reiki master-teacher). The attunements are given in a series of levels (1 to 3 and master-teacher), and each level involves an empowerment from the master in which sacred symbols are implanted in the auric field. Once the participant has received level-1 Reiki, you may begin using it on yourself and others. This level is the same for patients as well. If a person wishes to go further for the teaching of students, he or she must have the master-teacher level (level 4).

To begin a session, you center yourself, call in the Reiki forces, and direct these forces to what you wish to have done. "Centering" is another term for taking a deep breath, exhaling, and entering into a light meditative state in which external events do not intrude.

The practitioner of Reiki places his or her hands lightly in various positions on the body of the recipient. The process usually begins at the head and works down the front and back of the body. The hands will be left in each position for a few minutes up to 5 minutes per area, and the receiver may feel, warmth, heat, tingling, or coolness. Occasionally, no sensation is felt. The session starts at the front and moves to the back, lasting from 1 to 1½ hours. Most recipients report a very relaxed feeling and fall asleep, while others may have an emotional release, occasionally shedding tears. The giver of Reiki will often feel an energetic flow through herself or himself while administering the session.

 www.atlantic.net/~arma/
www.iarp.org

Practitioners

The International Association of Reiki Professionals (IARP) is the world-wide, representative organization. IARP offers many member benefits, such as liability insurance, publications, programs, and conferences. Currently, no licensing or certification requirements exist for the practice of Reiki.

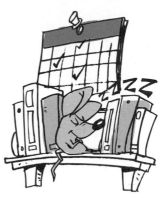

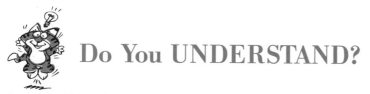

Do You UNDERSTAND?

See pages 278 and 279 for Learning Activities related to this topic.

THERAPEUTIC TOUCH

What IS Therapeutic Touch?

Therapeutic touch (TT) is a holistic method that aims to help or heal using the hands to redirect, focus, and rebalance the body's energy field. Therapeutic touch practitioners assume that the potential to heal naturally resides within the client and energy fields are the basic unit of living beings. Martha Rogers, RN, PhD, describes that we are energetically connected to the universe, theorizing that our bodies are composed of energy fields that affect our state of health. Malinski defines therapeutic touch as "a health patterning modality whereby the nurse and client participate knowingly in the changing human-environmental field process." Dossey, Keegan and Guzzetta describe touch therapies such as TT, which focus on the body's energy meridians to relieve tension, re-establish the flow of energy and restore balance to the human energy system.

First developed in the early 1970s by nursing pioneer Dolores Kreiger, RN, PhD, and psychic Dora Kunz at the University of New York, TT was originally derived from laying-on-of-hands. Although TT practitioners may develop their intuitive capacity, TT practitioners do not use clairvoyant guidance and focus energy exchange from their energy fields.

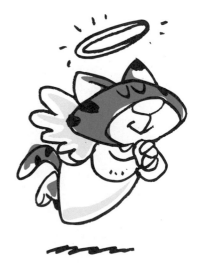

What You NEED TO KNOW

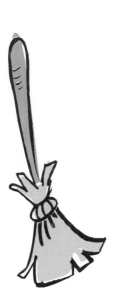

Personal recognition, intention, and acceptance of the role of a healer are necessary for the TT practitioner. Prior to providing therapy, TT practitioners attempt to become mindfully present, centering to reflectively listen, and still the conscious mind to focus their attention upon the intent to heal. The Kreiger-Kunz method of TT utilizes initial assessment of the human energy field, scanning with the hands to detect disruptions in the energy field. The TT practitioner moves his or her hands in non-physical contact or light touch in a sweeping motion above or across the body in a head to foot direction to note differences and asymmetry of energy field disturbance. The TT practitioner "unruffles" or clears the energy field and detects blockages of the flow of energy. The practitioner facilitates the transferred flow of energy from his/her hands to the client's energy field. The TT practitioner may detect energy fields as changes in temperature, vision, color, field disruptions, or sounds.

Benefits and Uses

Although not fully corroborated by research, some reports defend that therapeutic touch may be useful to minimize anxiety, speed wound healing, reduce pain, promote a relaxation response, and stimulate the body's natural healing process. Similar to relaxation therapy, TT was found to significantly decrease self-reported anxiety in patients at a Veteran's Administration psychiatric hospital. Another study of demented Alzheimer's patients who received TT had improved well-being, relaxation, and emotional connection. TT may significantly reduce post-test anxiety scores of hospitalized patients compared to casual touch or no touch.

Therapeutic touch may significantly decrease tension headache pain by 70% but did not affect the postoperative reports of pain or the need for pain medication.

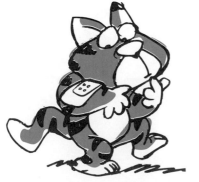

Nevertheless, a double-blind study found that punch biopsies of full thickness dermal wounds had significantly accelerated wound-healing rates with TT compared to placebo. Kreiger's research demonstrated that "laying on-of-hands" significantly increased the post-test hemogloblin levels of ill clients.

TT is used for the following conditions:

- Alzheimer's disease
- Anxiety reduction
- Arthritis
- Autoimmune disorders
- Back pain
- Bone fractures
- Bone marrow harvest
- Breast feeding
- Cancer
- Chronic fatigue syndrome
- Diabetes
- Disease prevention
- General well-being
- Grief
- Headaches
- Heart disease
- HIV or AIDS
- Hypertension
- Multiple sclerosis
- Neck pain
- Pain control
- Premature infants
- Premenstrual syndrome
- Pre- and post-surgical
- Pulmonary disorders
- Rehabilitation
- Skin problems
- Spiritual growth
- Wound healing

1. **Patients with serious or critical illness should not consider TT as a substitute for appropriate medical treatment.**
2. **Increased blood flow from TT treatments may be deleterious for cancer patients.**
3. **Although TT is not a religious practice it may be considered controversial to practice or teach in public institutions.**

Risks and Precautions

TT is not painful and generally regarded as safe. Some patients may become agitated during TT treatments. Those sensitive or adverse to human contact and touching may feel vulnerable and anxious during TT treatments. In contrast, others may become relaxed and too drowsy to ambulate and drive home.

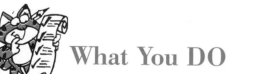 **What You DO**

Patient Education

Patients should understand that there are differing opinions regarding the effectiveness of TT and that TT is not designed to remedy an acute or life-threatening physical condition. TT sessions may last from twenty-thirty minutes, although the length of treatment may vary between practitioners and clients. During treatment, the client remains clothed, either sitting in a chair or lying in a comfortable position.

Practitioners

The Nurse Healers-Professional Associates International is the official organization of therapeutic touch and creates standards for TT practice and education. Therapeutic touch is sometime taught in a 12-hour workshop. However, therapeutic touch practitioners may also undergo a one-year mentorship with an experienced TT provider.

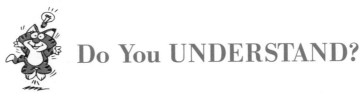

Do You UNDERSTAND?

See pages 279 and 280 for Learning Activities related to this topic.

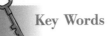

Key Words

Centering Clearing the mind, and relaxing the body to focus on mental stability prior to providing therapeutic touch.

Energy field disturbance A disharmonious disruption of the human energy field surrounding a person that may be disharmonious to the body, mind or spirit.

Intention Motivation and directing attention to healing with therapeutic touch.

Scanning Passing the hands across the human energy field to detect disturbances.

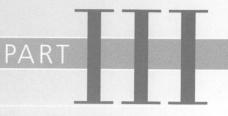

Learning Activities

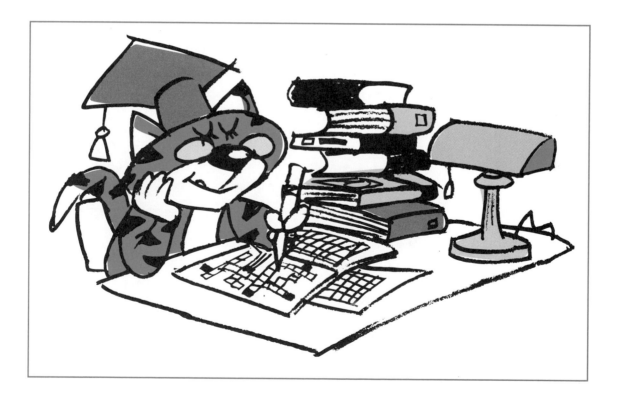

Herbs

ALFALFA

DIRECTIONS: Complete the crossword puzzle related to alfalfa.

Across

1. Bronchoconstriction disease
5. Decrease in all the blood cells
8. How to administer nitro-glycerin (*abbreviation*)
9. Plant chemical that may inhibit coagulation
10. Male child
12. Type 1 or type 2
15. Plant constituents that affect estrogen receptors

18. NPO: nil per _____
19. Alfalfa plant part with hemolytic properties
20. Alfalfa is used for

_____ stones
24. Alfalfa is used for

_____ secondary to plaque (*abbreviation*)
25. Alfalfa is used for

_____ stones

Down

2. Knife, fork, and _____
3. Same as 2 Down
4. A little bit of leftovers or to fight
6. Normal saline (*abbreviation*)
7. Diseases
9. Rope
11. Substance that alters drug metabolism

13. Hot-air _____
14. Entrance
16. Not well
17. Strong _____ an ox
21. Pop
22. Ogle
23. A type of fever

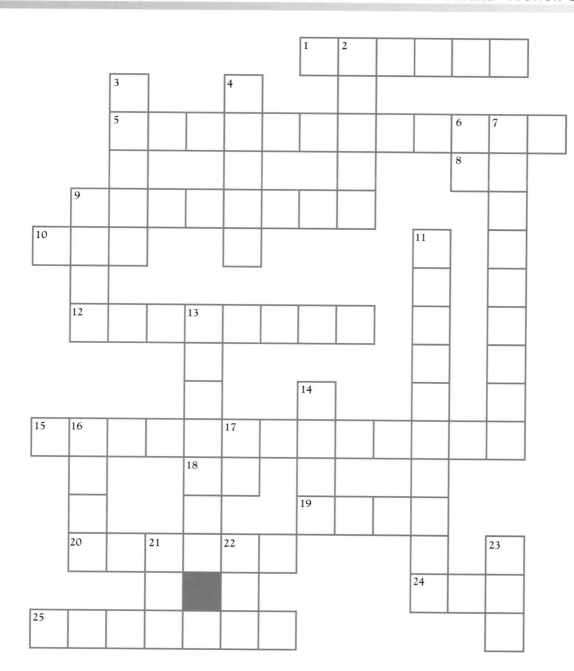

Answers: Across: 1. Asthma; 5. Pancytopenia; 8. SL; 9. Coumarin; 10. Son;
12. Diabetes; 15. Isoflavonoids; 18. Os;
19. Root; 20. Kidney; 24. CVA; 25. Bladder.
Down: 2. Spoon; 3. Spoon; 4. Scrap; 6. NS;
7. Illnesses; 9. Cord; 11. Xenobiotic;
13. Balloon; 14. Door; 16. Sick; 17. As;
21. Dad; 22. Eye; 23. Hay.

Aloe Vera

DIRECTIONS: Complete the crossword puzzle (see the following page) related to the actions, side effects, and uses of aloe vera.

Across

3. An electrolyte imbalance that may occur when using aloe vera
5. Blood in the urine
6. Absence of menstruation
7. A hormone secreted from the adrenal cortex that increases blood glucose levels
9. The form of aloe that causes the most side effects

Down

1. This form of aloe may be used for dermatitis caused by excessive exposure to the sun
2. Taken for constipation
4. Increased amounts of albumin in the urine
8. Aloe may cause potassium to be lost here

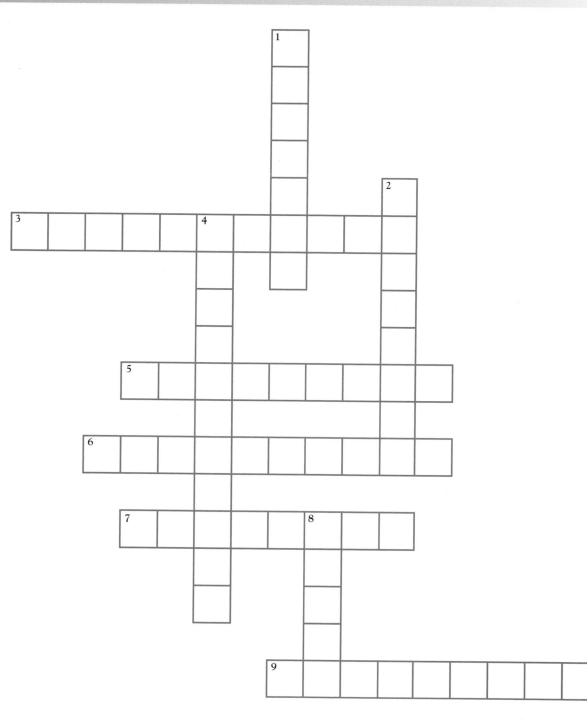

DIRECTIONS: Define the following terms related to aloe vera.

10. Phytochemicals:

_____

_____

_____

11. Anthrones:

_____

_____

12. Bradykinin:

_____

_____

_____

13. Histamine:

_____

_____

_____

DIRECTIONS: Identify the following statements as *true* (T) or *false* (F).

14. _____ The use of aloe may cause hyperkalemia.

15. _____ Aloe stimulates skin cell growth and the production of T cells by the immune system.

16. _____ Aloe contains salicylates that decrease pain and inflammation.

17. _____ Increased peristalsis occurs with ingestion of aloe because it irritates the intestinal mucosa.

18. _____ Aloe gel speeds the formation of thromboxane A, which promotes wound healing.

ASTRAGALUS ROOT

DIRECTIONS: Find and circle the following uses for astragalus root.

AIDS   Chemotherapy   Herpes   Infection
Angina   Diabetes   HF   Influenza
Asthma   Hepatitis   Hypertension   Water retention

Y	B	D	V	X	T	Y	C	E	Q	C	N	N	W	N
Y	P	E	G	N	C	M	Z	S	H	M	O	A	A	V
V	G	A	Z	N	E	U	L	F	N	I	I	B	T	N
J	P	N	R	D	W	H	B	E	S	Q	T	G	E	H
L	D	G	F	E	B	H	M	N	S	K	C	E	R	Q
L	I	I	K	K	H	Y	E	W	D	Q	E	L	R	Q
H	G	N	A	M	H	T	I	P	I	W	F	D	E	Y
Z	E	A	T	B	R	W	O	B	A	S	N	C	T	J
U	H	R	C	E	E	O	P	M	B	T	I	B	E	L
U	W	R	P	Y	Q	T	H	J	E	Y	I	K	N	F
Q	R	Y	I	E	D	T	E	O	T	H	X	T	T	M
Y	H	D	T	V	S	T	V	S	E	Y	C	Y	I	A
L	H	H	T	A	I	V	T	K	S	B	L	C	O	S
V	P	Y	F	A	C	K	E	C	U	B	V	K	N	J

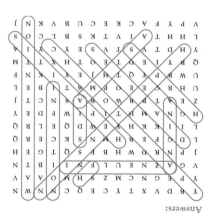

DIRECTIONS: Place a check next to the BEST answer.

1. Astragalus is called an immune system stimulant because it:
   a. _____ Increases the production of hemoglobin.
   b. _____ Causes an acceleration in IgE antibody production.
   c. _____ Accelerates immune cell maturation.
   d. _____ Inhibits free radical production.

2. The positive inotropic effects of astragalus root are demonstrated by:
   a. _____ Increased cardiac output.
   b. _____ Vasoconstriction.
   c. _____ Stroke volume stability.
   d. _____ Capillary refill >3 seconds.

3. Which of the following statements about the side effects of astragalus root is true?

    a. _____ Side effects are mild and rare.

    b. _____ Serious gastrointestinal distress may occur.

    c. _____ Doses above 50 g cause thrombocytopenia.

    d. _____ Fever may be seen when used in children.

4. A potential complication resulting from the use of astragalus in patients undergoing general anesthesia during surgery is:

    a. _____ Thrombocytopenia

    b. _____ Massive fluid shift

    c. _____ Additive hypotensive effects

    d. _____ Prolonged sedation

5. Which of the following laboratory tests will yield the most critical information for preoperative evaluation of a patient using astragalus?

    a. _____ Platelet count and WBC count

    b. _____ Clotting studies

    c. _____ Reticulocyte count

    d. _____ Dimentation rate

Answers: 3. a; 4. c; 5. b.

BLACK COHOSH

DIRECTIONS: Complete the crossword puzzle related to the actions, side effects, and uses of black cohosh.

Across

    1. High blood pressure

    3. Fever reducing

    5. Vomiting

    7. The length of time that black cohosh should be discontinued before surgery

    9. Painful menstruation

Down

    2. Ringing in the ears

    4. "Cohosh" means

    5. An agent that helps clear secretions

    6. A whirling sensation in the head

    8. Black cohosh may _____ the heart rate

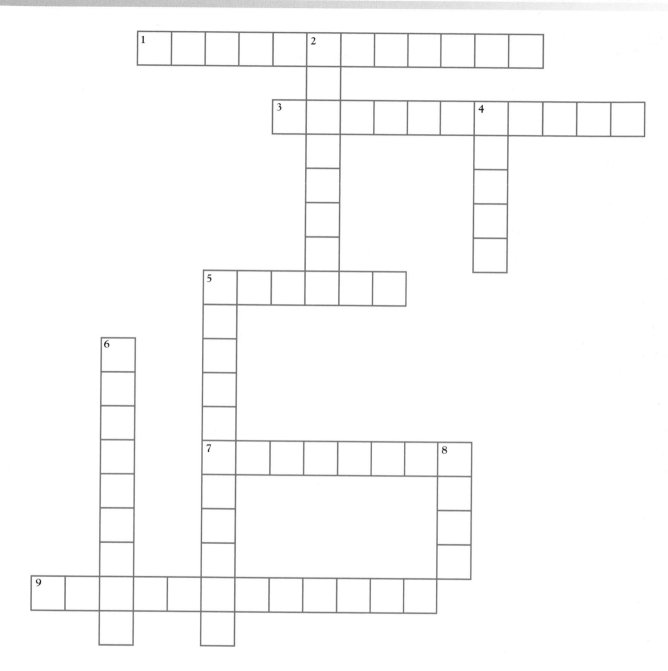

DIRECTIONS: **Select the correct response from the italicized words to make the statement true.**

1. Black cohosh may _____ the hypotensive effects of other prescriptions or herbal medications. (*increase* or *decrease*)
2. Patients _____ take black cohosh during pregnancy. (*should* or *should not*)
3. Undesirable _____ may occur in anesthetized patients who take black cohosh preoperatively. (*hypotension* or *hypertension*)
4. Black cohosh may _____ the vasodilatory and heart rate–slowing actions of clonidine. (*increase* or *decrease*)
5. Black cohosh _____ secretion of LH. (*increases* or *decreases*)

Answers: 1. increase; 2. should not; 3. hypotension; 4. increase; 5. decreases.

DIRECTIONS: **Identify the following statements as *true* (T) or *false* (F).**

1. _____ Administration of black cohosh should be discontinued after 6 months of use.
2. _____ Black cohosh decreases or prevents uterine contractions.
3. _____ Large doses of black cohosh can cause sweating, headache, weight gain, hypotension, or joint pain.
4. _____ Black cohosh is considered a relatively safe herbal agent.
5. _____ Discontinuing black cohosh after achieving hypertension control may result in hypotension.

Answers: 1. T; 2. F; 3. T; 4. T; 5. F.

CAPSICUM

DIRECTIONS: **Define the following terms related to capsicum.**

1. Substance P:

_____

_____

2. Neurotransmitter:

_____

_____

3. Desensitization:

_____

_____

4. Nociceptors:

_____

_____

Answers: 1. A neurotransmitter in pain transmission; located within the spinal cord, brain, and sensory neurons associated with pain; 2. A substance that transmits nerve impulses across a synapse; 3. The process of becoming insensitive or nonreactive to a sensitizing agent; 4. Pain receptors located in the skin.

DIRECTIONS: Complete the crossword puzzle related to the actions, side effects, and uses of capsicum.

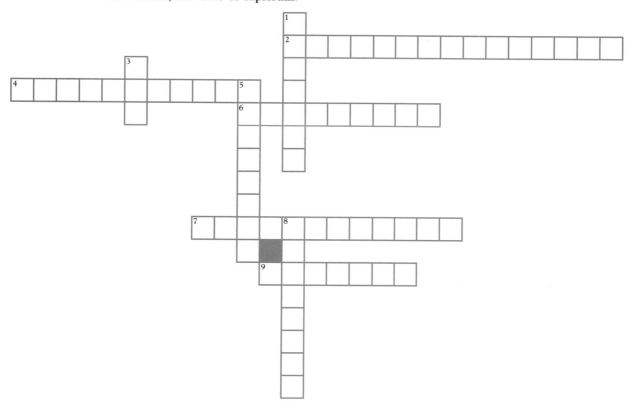

Across

2. Opposite of coagulation
4. Pain neurons in the skin
6. Contact dermatitis
7. Side effects include increased heart rate, nervousness, and upset stomach
9. Sharp odor or taste

Down

1. Another name for capsicum
3. This color of pepper has the highest concentrations of capsaicin
5. Herpes zoster
8. Itching

Answers: Across: 2. Anticoagulation; 4. Nociceptors; 6. Hunan hand; 7. Theophylline;
9. Pungent, Down: 1. Cayenne; 3. Red;
5. Shingles; 8. Pruritus.

CHAMOMILE

DIRECTIONS: **Unscramble the words in parentheses to fill in the blanks.**
1. Chamomile decreases _____ release, which may account for the antiallergy and antiinflammatory actions. (*ehinistma*)
2. Functions of the CNS may be _____ with consumption of chamomile. (*ddeesprse*)
3. Patients with _____ and clotting disorders should avoid chamomile. (*atherniompbotocy*)
4. Although chamomile is recognized as generally safe for human consumption, concentrated tea preparations can cause _____. (*semies*)

Answers: 1. Histamine; 2. Depressed; 3. Thrombocytopenia; 4. Emesis.

CRANBERRY

DIRECTIONS: **Place a check next to the BEST answer.**
1. Prolonged use of large amounts of cranberries or cranberry juice may contribute to:
   a. _____ Bleeding disorders
   b. _____ Kidney stone formation
   c. _____ Dental decay
   d. _____ Urinary tract infections
2. Cranberry juice should not be used by individuals with:
   a. _____ Urinary tract infections
   b. _____ Diabetes
   c. _____ Periodontal disease
   d. _____ Prostatic hypertrophy

Answers: 1. b; 2. d.

DANDELION

DIRECTIONS: **Unscramble the words in parentheses to fill in the blanks.**
1. Dandelion is a natural _____ that does not cause potassium loss as a result of its high potassium content. (*eircitud*)
2. Dandelion may cause _____, thus patients with diabetes need to have blood-glucose levels monitored closely. (*aichpgymloe*)

Answers: 1. Diuretic; 2. Hypoglycemia.

3. The substance _____ within the root of the
dandelion acts as an appetite stimulant. (*nedseslemadiou*)

4. Allergic reactions such as _____

_____ have been known to occur in
people known to be allergic to members of the ragweed, chrysanthemum, marigold, or daisy family. (*tamredsiti*)

DIRECTIONS: **Find and circle the following uses and side effects of
dandelion.**

Antiinflammatory
Diuresis
Diuretic
Eczema

Hepatitis
Hypoglycemia
Hyponatremia
Indigestion

Jaundice
Laxative
Weight loss

V	E	J	G	P	Y	L	X	E	Q	E	Y	H	A	N	I	B	K	H	J	A	S	W	Z	A	I
B	R	A	I	D	O	L	K	A	Q	W	O	S	Q	N	I	E	N	B	M	I	V	P	L	I	U
J	Q	U	H	C	G	X	M	L	C	L	I	P	D	H	L	F	O	E	M	M	E	L	B	M	L
Y	M	N	B	N	E	E	O	I	I	T	J	I	N	C	W	A	V	H	F	E	H	O	S	E	H
R	K	D	A	G	Z	X	T	Q	I	U	G	K	N	U	T	I	Q	Q	H	R	P	V	I	C	O
M	A	I	C	C	R	E	O	T	V	E	H	F	W	H	T	P	A	K	W	T	U	P	S	Y	L
I	Y	C	E	E	R	L	A	Q	S	W	Q	P	S	A	E	E	R	F	P	A	V	U	E	L	Z
A	M	E	L	U	H	P	N	T	O	F	P	K	X	C	B	H	M	M	D	N	V	I	R	G	T
D	X	I	I	P	E	S	I	K	F	R	V	A	O	F	U	R	T	N	A	O	K	K	U	O	Y
C	K	D	C	H	S	O	Z	E	Y	D	L	C	V	I	Y	F	J	C	X	P	S	F	I	P	N
Z	P	N	N	A	N	T	I	I	N	F	L	A	M	M	A	T	O	R	Y	Y	Y	Q	U	D	Y	H
S	G	B	A	W	E	I	G	H	T	L	O	S	S	C	A	I	Z	A	Q	H	R	W	C	H	E

ECHINACEA

DIRECTIONS: **Complete the following statements.**

1. Echinacea _____ the immune system to increase resistance to bacterial, fungal, and viral infections.

2. Some anesthetics, such as _____ or _____, are metabolized by _____ _____ that are inhibited by echinacea, making their actions unpredictable.

3. Echinacea is _____ for systemic diseases such as _____, _____, _____ _____ _____ or autoimmune disorders such as multiple sclerosis.

4. Echinacea may promote _____ of bacteria and phagocytosis.

5. Immunosuppressive drugs such as cyclosporine and corticosteroids might be _____ by taking echinacea.

Answers: 1. stimulates; 2. midazolam (Versed), diazepam (Valium), liver enzymes; 3. contraindicated, AIDS, tuberculosis, collagen connective tissue diseases; 4. encapsulation; 5. counteracted.

DIRECTIONS: **Find and circle the following uses for echinacea.**

Abscesses	Carbuncles	Fatigue	Pharyngitis	Septicemia
Acne	Colds	Flu	Prostatitis	Tonsillitis
Cancer	Eczema	Migraines	Rhinorrhea	Viruses

A	X	K	A	S	A	P	N	K	O	G	P	A	K	W	W	A	U	F	L	E	B	V	I	T	K
D	E	M	S	L	I	L	R	R	C	S	S	M	D	Q	G	B	R	I	E	L	W	A	R	O	S
F	R	H	E	E	C	T	J	O	I	Y	T	E	F	F	Q	A	Q	E	D	S	V	S	D	N	E
U	A	O	R	R	P	K	I	A	S	B	B	Z	S	F	L	S	G	F	C	C	O	D	V	S	L
Q	D	T	C	R	N	T	X	G	X	T	C	C	Q	S	G	L	Y	D	P	N	P	L	I	I	C
P	I	B	I	I	O	U	I	Z	N	W	A	E	P	T	E	X	V	N	K	F	A	O	R	L	N
D	M	Z	M	G	D	N	P	C	D	Y	R	T	D	W	D	C	R	E	B	L	U	C	U	L	U
Q	G	M	Z	V	U	Y	I	L	E	K	R	V	I	L	J	V	S	V	N	L	X	Z	S	I	B
R	P	P	G	A	S	E	Z	H	I	M	R	A	T	T	I	W	T	B	F	C	H	Y	E	T	R
X	F	W	P	N	J	G	E	H	R	U	I	V	H	D	I	O	G	Y	A	M	A	P	S	I	A
M	B	D	Q	U	Q	R	J	Z	I	A	U	A	B	P	A	S	C	H	W	P	K	A	O	S	C
M	Y	E	U	S	Y	E	N	I	A	R	G	I	M	I	G	P	K	P	L	N	O	P	B	W	R

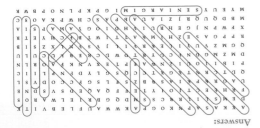

Answers:

EPHEDRA

DIRECTIONS: **Place a check next to the BEST answer.**

1. Ephedra causes weight loss by:

    a. _____ Increasing the body's metabolic rate and increasing appetite

    b. _____ Inhibiting norepinephrine release and increasing appetite

    c. _____ Decreasing appetite and increasing the body's metabolic rate

    d. _____ Promoting norepinephrine release and decreasing metabolic rate

2. The sympathomimetic effects of ephedra are demonstrated by:

    a. _____ Decreased blood pressure, decreased heart rate, and increased cardiac contractility

    b. _____ Decreased blood pressure, decreased heart rate, and decreased cardiac contractility

    c. _____ Increased blood pressure, increased heart rate, decreased cardiac contractility

    d. _____ Increased blood pressure, increased heart rate, and increased cardiac contractility

DIRECTIONS: **Identify the following statements as *true* (T) or *false* (F).**

3. _____ Patients should avoid taking ephedra with coffee, tea, or other caffeinated beverages.

4. _____ Surgical patients should continue taking ephedra until the day before surgery.

5. _____ Use of ephedra can cause cardiac dysrhythmias, myocardial infarction, and cardiac arrest.

6. _____ Ephedra is a bronchoconstrictor, reducing airflow, and is an antitussive.

DIRECTIONS: **Answer the following question.**

7. How does ephedra decrease urinary output in some patients?

_____

_____

_____

_____

Answers: 1. c; 2. d; 3. T; 4. F; 5. T; 6. F; 7. By decreasing renal blood flow, which will decrease urinary output.

EVENING PRIMROSE

DIRECTIONS: Place a check next to the BEST answer.

1. Which of the following laboratory tests may be indicated preoperatively for patients taking primrose?
   a. _____ Platelet count and WBC count
   b. _____ Clotting times
   c. _____ Reticulocyte count
   d. _____ Dimentation rate

2. Evening primrose works as an antiinflammatory agent by:
   a. _____ Reducing environment allergies and blood pressure
   b. _____ Increasing bleeding time by 40% and platelet aggregation by 45%
   c. _____ Decreasing the production of prostaglandins and leukotrienes
   d. _____ Functioning as an antimicrobial and antibacterial agent

3. A potential complication resulting from the use of evening primrose in patients with a history of schizophrenia is:
   a. _____ Increased seizure activity
   b. _____ Prolonged sedation
   c. _____ Increased cardiac output
   d. _____ Gastrointestinal upset

DIRECTIONS: **Unscramble the words in parentheses to fill in the blanks.**

4. Evening primrose decreases the production of _____ and _____. (*spnriosdntaagl*) (*sleenukeiotr*)

5. The use of evening primrose and anesthetic medications simultaneously may result in _____. (*nhyopiostne*)

6. Blood pressure–lowering effects of antihypertensive medications may be _____. (*dinescare*)

FEVERFEW

DIRECTIONS: Label each of the following actions of feverfew as increased (I) or decreased (D) to indicate the appropriate direction of the response.

1. _____ Clotting time
2. _____ Histamine release
3. _____ Uterine contractions
4. _____ Bruising
5. _____ Serotonin release
6. _____ Platelet aggregation

DIRECTIONS: Answer the following questions.

7. Feverfew should not be taken with what other herbal agents? (*List two.*)
   a. _____
   b. _____
8. Identify two NSAIDs that should not be taken with feverfew.
   a. _____
   b. _____
9. List three contraindications for feverfew:
   a. _____
   b. _____
   c. _____

GARLIC

DIRECTIONS: Complete the following statements.

1. Garlic may _____ blood sugar by stimulating the release of insulin from the pancreas.
2. Garlic may irritate the _____ _____ and can cause stomach upset, heartburn, nausea, vomiting, diarrhea, gas, and bloating.
3. Garlic should be _____ before surgery to prevent excessive _____ _____.
4. Patients who take garlic preoperatively should have _____ _____.

DIRECTIONS: **Find and circle the following uses for garlic.**

Allergies   Colds   Otitis media
Arthritis   Diarrhea   Ringworm
Asthma   Hyperlipidemia   Tuberculosis
Candida   Hypertension   Vaginitis

A	I	M	E	D	I	P	I	L	R	E	P	Y	H	O	F	T	A	A	S	C	W	J	Q	B
L	J	Y	S	X	W	N	S	B	I	A	I	Y	C	E	U	K	I	W	Y	N	A	M	V	V
L	M	Z	V	E	W	D	S	W	M	L	P	E	T	B	X	D	C	D	Y	E	B	A	V	A
E	V	Q	D	N	I	D	Z	H	M	E	W	P	E	K	E	H	B	N	I	D	G	X	R	E
R	I	H	K	L	L	J	T	I	R	I	E	R	V	M	W	S	A	W	F	I	O	T	J	H
G	J	H	Q	O	H	S	M	T	S	L	C	N	S	G	Z	C	U	D	N	P	H	C	G	R
I	I	P	C	E	A	I	E	E	W	U	P	I	Y	E	W	Z	S	I	I	R	F	J	F	R
E	W	I	H	B	D	N	I	I	L	L	T	O	Q	H	O	K	T	D	I	D	N	G	X	A
S	I	C	A	K	S	Z	T	O	L	I	N	E	H	R	V	I	V	T	S	V	N	C	F	I
G	Y	Z	I	S	Q	S	B	T	O	A	X	U	Y	S	D	I	Q	W	P	X	A	B	D
E	V	W	O	P	L	I	D	O	R	G	W	H	N	E	N	S	P	N	W	F	B	H	C	P
R	M	N	O	N	S	I	S	J	M	R	O	W	G	N	I	R	M	G	O	V	S	P	U	H

Answers:

GINGER

DIRECTIONS: **Complete the crossword puzzle (see the following page) related to the actions, side effects, and uses of ginger.**

Across

2. Hardening of vessels
6. Active ingredient in ginger
7. Antiplatelet drug
8. Imperfect digestion
9. Vomiting

Down

1. Decreased platelets
3. Disease with painful, stiff joints
4. Headache
5. Pertaining to the contracting ability of the heart

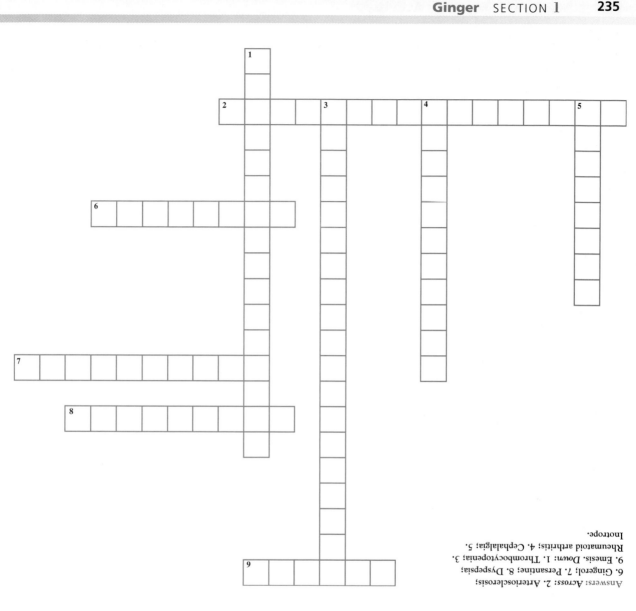

DIRECTIONS: Identify the following statements as *true* (T) or *false* (F).

1. _____ Ginger increases gastrointestinal motility.
2. _____ Heparin or Coumadin may be safely taken simultaneously
with ginger.
3. _____ Coagulation is decreased by the active ingredients in ginger.
4. _____ The use of ginger during pregnancy is advocated.

GINKGO

DIRECTIONS: **Place a check next to the BEST answer.**

1. Ginkgo should not be used in patients with epilepsy because it:
   a. _____ Decreases cerebral perfusion
   b. _____ Lowers seizure threshold
   c. _____ May decrease blood pressure
   d. _____ Causes vasoconstriction of vessels

2. Cross-sensitivity to ginkgo may occur in those who are also allergic to:
   a. _____ Ginger, ephedra, or dandelion
   b. _____ Evening primrose or vitamin C
   c. _____ Echinacea, ragweed, or sunflowers
   d. _____ Poison ivy, poison oak, or poison sumac

3. Garlic, feverfew, ginger, red clover, and passionflower:
   a. _____ Can safely be administered with ginkgo
   b. _____ Add to the anticoagulation effects of ginkgo
   c. _____ Can safely be substituted for ginkgo
   d. _____ Come from the same type of leaves as ginkgo

Answers: 1. b; 2. d; 3. b.

GINSENG

DIRECTIONS: **Unscramble the words in parentheses to fill in the blanks.**

1. Ginseng is composed of numerous active ingredients known as _____ that oppose each other. (*sgiednsiesno*)

2. _____ is the term used to describe the opposing features of ginseng. (*nadegaopt*)

3. Ginseng possesses _____ inotropic and chronotropic effects on the heart. (*engviate*)

4. Large doses of ginseng can lead to excessive estrogen production, which may cause _____. (*amiasglta*)

DIRECTIONS: **Label each of the following actions of ginseng as increased (I) or decreased (D) to indicate the appropriate direction of the response.**

5. _____ Stamina
6. _____ Immune system
7. _____ Anticoagulation
8. _____ Stimulant effects of caffeine
9. _____ Cardiac contractility

Answers: 1. ginsenosides; 2. adaptogen; 3. negative; 4. mastalgia; 5. I; 6. I; 7. I; 8. I; 9. D.

DIRECTIONS: Find and circle the following uses for ginkgo.

Alzheimer's   Headache   PVD (peripheral vascular disease)   Vertigo

Dementia   Macular degeneration   Thrombosis   Tinnitus

Depression   PMS (premenstrual syndrome)

```
R J H Z U P J H K F K N A X Y D J D X R E A O G V V
S I S O B M O R H T S F K G E Y S V J D L S D G E Y
B N D Y T E J W S I L U P P P T M P F Z P N H Z P A
C Q D E P I M Q D I R C R V J S S O H S M J V N S O
I J X E M J N V B I F E N F T D Z E L O S S Y G U P
E N Y R K E U N S O S E W W S M I H G R S D T T X Y
R I X D R B N V I S X C S J E M J I Y K F X G Z M B
C V S O R F I T I T L T A P E U T Y F V U U F V M Q
O M U A N O Q O I U U Y T R X R U W E H A D Q Q S G
C S Y T I P N W V A A S S U E F E S Z U K R Q N E T
H E A D A C H E M I H V N V D Q L H K T R M K M K T
R P P R N O I T A R E N E G E D R A L U C A M B C S
```

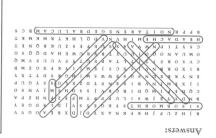

Answers:

GOLDENSEAL

DIRECTIONS: Complete the following statements.

1. An acceptable dose range for oral goldenseal per day is a total dose of

   _____.

2. _____ is the accumulation of bilirubin in
   the brain and spinal cord of a newborn.

3. Goldenseal may _____ the hypotensive
   effects of _____ agents.

4. Goldenseal is a CNS _____ but
   _____ the respiratory center, uterus, and bladder
   in very large doses.

DIRECTIONS: Identify the following statements as *true* (T) or *false* (F).

5. _____ Goldenseal has antibacterial properties.

6. _____ The hypertensive and stimulant effects of goldenseal may be
   increased by anesthetics and narcotics.

7. _____ Goldenseal may demonstrate antioxytocin effects and
   decrease the strength of uterine contractions and prevent
   the progression of labor.

8. _____ When an individual begins taking goldenseal, driving and
   using heavy machinery should be avoided until individual
   susceptibility to the sedative effects can be determined.

Answers: 1. 750 to 1500 mg/day;
2. Kernicterus; 3. increase, antihypertensive;
4. depressant, stimulates; 5. T; 6. F; 7. F;
8. T.

HAWTHORN

DIRECTIONS: Complete the crossword puzzle related to the actions of hawthorn.

Across

1. Prevented by hawthorn's calcium effects
3. Decreased by peripheral vasodilation
4. Blood levels decreased by hawthorn
5. Problem seen in surgical patients using hawthorn
6. Condition in which hawthorn use is contraindicated

Down

1. Agents that help limit tissue damage by free radicals
2. Effect that may increase when hawthorn is used with CNS depressants and anesthetics
7. Increased levels of this increase levels of intracellular calcium in the heart (abbrev.)

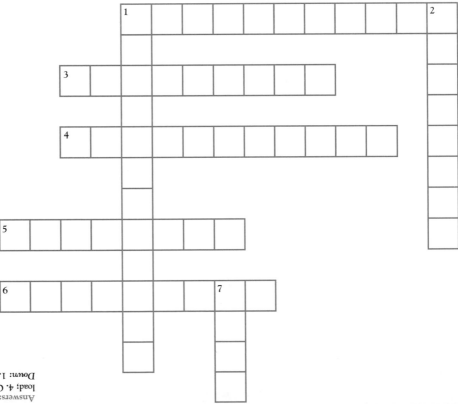

Answers: Across: 1. Arrhythmias; 3. Afterload; 4. Cholesterol; 5. Bleeding; 6. Pregnancy. Down: 1. Antioxidants; 2. Sedative; 7. CAMP.

DIRECTIONS: Unscramble the words in parentheses to fill in the blanks.

1. A positive _____ improves the force of cardiac contraction. (*noroetpi*)

2. When increased _____ enters the heart muscle cells, the force of cardiac contraction is increased. (*miacucl*)

3. When cardiac muscle contraction is improved,

   _____ _____ increases, and blood flow to the tissues is improved. (*ccaaidr ttuuop*)

4. Increasing the cardiac output decreases the amount of blood left in the heart at the end of _____. (*eslyost*)

HOP

DIRECTIONS: Label each of the following actions of hop as increased (I) or decreased (D) to indicate the appropriate direction of the response.

1. _____ Male sex drive
2. _____ Depression
3. _____ Mental acuity
4. _____ Urinary output
5. _____ Male infertility
6. _____ Sedative effects

DIRECTIONS: Place a check next to the BEST answer.

7. Which of the following is the appropriate recommended oral daily dose for hop?

   a. _____ 1 to 3 g three times each day

   b. _____ 0.5 to 1.0 g three times each day

   c. _____ 0.1 to 0.5 g two times each day

   d. _____ 5 to 7 g each day

8. Patients should stop taking hop 2 weeks before surgical procedures. Why?

   a. _____ Severe oversedation may occur when combined with anesthetics.

   b. _____ Anesthetics have decreased effectiveness when combined with hop.

   c. _____ Hop increases pain levels in postsurgical patients.

   d. _____ Hop can cause severe gynecomastia in surgical patients.

9. Hop decreases the male sex drive in some individuals by:

   a. _____ Decreasing testosterone production

   b. _____ Increasing sedation and sleep time

   c. _____ Decreasing mental acuity

   d. _____ Mimicking the effects of estrogen

10. The bitter acid ingredients in hop are responsible for:

   a. _____ Antidysrhythmic actions

   b. _____ Antimicrobial properties

   c. _____ Oxidative actions

   d. _____ Promoting coagulation

11. A known side effect of breathing in hop dust is:

   a. _____ Anaphylaxis

   b. _____ Dysrhythmias

   c. _____ Excitability

   d. _____ Mental confusion

12. Estrogen effects of hop can cause:

   a. _____ Increased growth of sensitive tumors

   b. _____ Increased fertility

   c. _____ Increased secretion of LH

   d. _____ Increased dysmenorrhea

13. Patients presenting for surgical and invasive procedures should be advised to:

   a. _____ Use the minimal dose needed to obtain relief of symptoms.

   b. _____ Discontinue using of hop 2 weeks before the procedure.

   c. _____ Continue using hops until the day of the planned procedure.

   d. _____ Expect a need for increased pain medication while using hops.

Answers: 8. a; 9. d; 10. b; 11. a; 12. a; 13. b.

KAVA KAVA

DIRECTIONS: **Complete the crossword puzzle related to the actions of kava kava.**

Across

2. Skin and nail color resulting from long-term use of high doses of kava
5. Bloody problem reported with kava use
9. Drug property as a result of effect on sodium and calcium channels
10. Kava interferes with the action of this neurotransmitter

Down

1. Condition in which kava use is contraindicated
3. Part of brain that deals with emotions (2 words)
4. Kava's most well known action
6. Throbbing side effect of kava
7. Maximum number of months recommended for kava use
8. Agent that should not be taken together with kava because of sedative effects

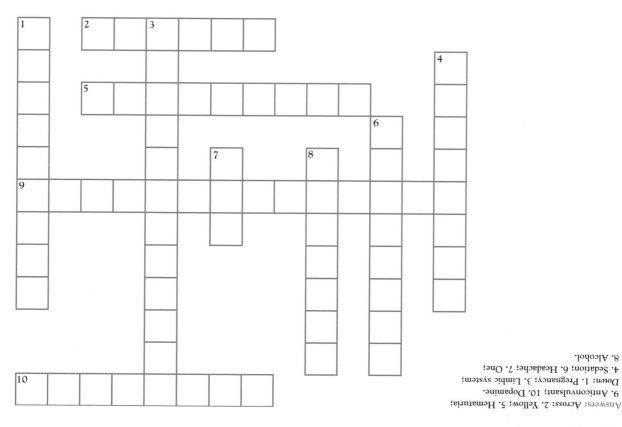

LICORICE

DIRECTIONS: **Complete the crossword puzzle related to the side effects of licorice.**

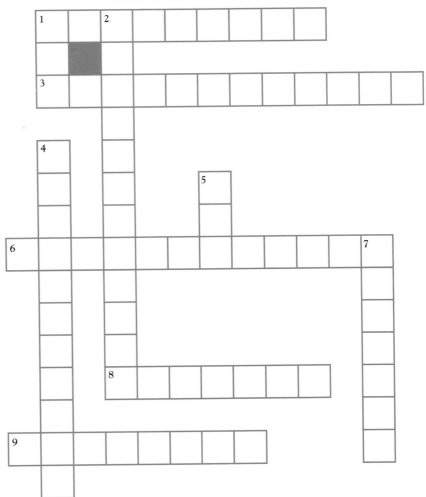

Across

1. Patient population in which licorice safety has not been determined
3. Licorice may cause a decrease of this hormone, leading to sexual dysfunction
6. They occur during labor
8. Co.
9. Disease in which licorice is contraindicated because of its interference with blood glucose control

Down

1. Laboratory test used to assess clotting factor
2. Epinephrine effect increased by hypokalemia
4. Condition resulting from increased renal excretion of potassium in the urine
5. Ventricular tachyarrhythmia caused by licorice-induced hypokalemia (*abbreviation*)
7. Discontinuation of licorice required 2 weeks before this event

DIRECTIONS: **Place a check next to the BEST answer.**

1. An active ingredient found in licorice is:
   a. _____ Glycyrrhizin
   b. _____ Cortisol
   c. _____ Anise oil
   d. _____ Vitamin A

2. A side effect of licorice ingestion that results from decreased metabolism of cortisol is:
   a. _____ Hypocalcemia
   b. _____ Hypertension
   c. _____ Hyperkalemia
   d. _____ Weight loss

3. Licorice is used in cough preparations because it:
   a. _____ Increases production and transport of bronchial mucus
   b. _____ Relaxes smooth muscle in the bronchial tree
   c. _____ Produces increased saliva to soothe throat irritation
   d. _____ Inhibits the cough reflex

4. Coumarins found in the roots of the licorice shrub are responsible for its:
   a. _____ Antiinflammatory action
   b. _____ Antioxidant properties
   c. _____ Blood thinning effects
   d. _____ Effects on platelet adhesion

5. Licorice is used in menopause because it:
   a. _____ Has estrogen-like actions
   b. _____ Has progesterone-receptor binding
   c. _____ Improves sex drive
   d. _____ Induces hot flashes

DIRECTIONS: Match the terms in Column A and phrases related to licorice in Column B.

Column A

1. _____ Addison's disease
2. _____ Pseudoaldosteronism
3. _____ Mineralocorticoid
4. _____ Cortisol
5. _____ Glucosides

Column B

a. Plant metabolites that produce sugars through hydrolysis during metabolism
b. Disease resulting from inadequate secretion of adrenal cortex hormones
c. Glucocorticoid hormone secreted from the adrenal cortex that increases blood glucose levels
d. Hormonal or medicinal activities resulting in sodium and water retention and potassium excretion
e. Condition with alkalosis, sodium retention, and potassium excretion

Answers: 1. b; 2. e; 3. d; 4. c; 5. a.

PASSIONFLOWER

DIRECTIONS: Place a check next to the BEST answer.

1. The primary side effect of passionflower is:
   a. _____ Bleeding
   b. _____ Nausea
   c. _____ Sedation
   d. _____ Tachycardia
2. Which of the following effects may be seen in surgical patients using passionflower?
   a. _____ Increased incidence of anaphylaxis
   b. _____ Decreased incidence of bleeding
   c. _____ Increased time in PACU
   d. _____ Decreased use of pain medication
3. Passionflower is contraindicated in:
   a. _____ Adolescent patients
   b. _____ Older adult patients
   c. _____ Postpartum patients
   d. _____ Pregnant patients

Answers: 1. c; 2. c; 3. d.

DIRECTIONS: Find and circle the following terms related to the actions and uses of passionflower.

Analgesic   Anxiety   Hypnotic   Neuralgia

Antibacterial Burns   Inflammation   Palpitations

Antifungal   Hemorrhoids   Insomnia   Sedative

Antispasmodic

L	A	I	R	E	T	C	A	B	I	T	N	A	B	U
I	I	N	S	O	M	N	I	A	O	O	L	N	A	P
Z	I	F	T	T	B	Y	F	T	B	F	Y	X	V	O
P	A	L	P	I	T	A	T	I	O	N	S	I	P	R
Q	N	A	G	O	S	H	J	N	D	N	F	E	N	O
T	T	M	P	F	B	P	M	X	L	F	P	T	Q	F
X	I	M	U	A	Y	T	A	D	A	M	E	Y	B	L
K	F	A	N	A	L	G	E	S	I	C	I	O	H	K
Y	U	T	V	A	K	W	Z	Z	M	H	S	P	T	J
S	N	I	S	D	I	O	H	R	R	O	M	E	H	L
X	G	O	B	N	N	E	V	I	T	A	D	E	S	E
O	A	N	D	Q	R	C	E	R	G	Y	X	I	A	V
T	L	M	L	F	D	U	N	Y	N	M	R	Y	C	C
U	G	Z	J	I	Q	Q	B	O	D	U	D	R	M	C
C	K	Z	Z	U	E	N	E	U	R	A	L	G	I	A

RED CLOVER

DIRECTIONS: Complete the following statements.

1. Red clover contains active ingredients known as _____ that are responsible for its estrogen-like actions. This results in decreased hot flashes in menopausal women because the secretion of _____ hormone is altered. The production of _____ is increased.

2. Menopausal women using red clover will experience a(n) _____ in arterial compliance, which may assist in reducing the risk of cardiac disease.

3. Red clover may be useful in reducing fractures in older women because it promotes _____ uptake and helps maintain bone _____.

4. Red clover has moderate _____ actions resulting from its salicylates.

5. Side effects from red clover are usually a result of its _____ action and may include _____ enlargement, menstrual changes, and weight _____.

DIRECTIONS: **Find and circle the following terms related to the uses of red clover.**

Acne

Analgesia

Arthritis

Asthma

Bronchitis

Burns

Dermatitis

Eczema

Expectorant

Menopause

Pharngitis

Whooping cough

W	E	X	P	E	C	T	O	R	A	N	T	Q	O	B
H	B	W	I	S	I	T	I	T	A	M	R	E	D	L
O	S	C	M	S	I	T	I	R	H	T	R	A	O	B
O	T	W	E	E	O	T	O	R	S	Z	I	H	B	A
P	H	A	R	Y	N	G	I	T	I	S	G	E	Q	C
I	C	Z	E	L	Y	O	P	H	E	X	N	M	Y	G
N	G	V	O	C	O	Y	P	G	C	C	G	P	H	C
G	S	K	C	Y	X	H	L	A	A	N	X	L	S	P
C	A	M	H	T	S	A	C	L	U	J	O	T	N	X
O	Q	C	I	Y	N	S	B	H	V	S	N	R	U	B
U	G	K	L	A	M	E	Z	C	E	B	E	H	B	F
G	W	Z	E	G	S	E	V	K	P	J	L	V	R	R
H	N	B	H	U	P	I	M	S	R	K	V	Q	N	B

ST. JOHN'S WORT

DIRECTIONS: **Unscramble the words in parentheses to fill in the blanks.**

1. Increased drug _____ can lead to decreased action of theophylline. (*ealimslbtmo*)

2. The risk of _____ is increased in women taking St. John's wort and oral contraceptives together. (*ypcrengna*)

3. The effects of cholesterol-lowering drugs may be
_____ if taken with St. John's wort. *(ddeecur)*

4. Anticonvulsant drugs demonstrate _____
of an effect when combined with St. John's wort. *(sles)*

5. Bronchodilator action is reduced in patients taking St. John's wort,
resulting in increased bronchial _____
and asthmatic episodes. *(noitictrscno)*

DIRECTIONS: **Complete the crossword puzzle (see the following page)
related to St. John's wort.**

Across

1. Class of drugs metabolized by hepatic cytochrome P450.
5. Number of weeks to delay surgery after discontinuing the herb.
7. When drug metabolism is increased, medication action and duration
are _____.
8. Sites stimulated by St. John's wort.
9. Uptake of this potent vasoconstrictor is inhibited by St. John's wort.
12. Eating disorder.
14. Naturally occurring chemical compound that increases heart rate.
15. Best time of day to take St. John's wort.

Down

1. Potent vasoconstrictor.
2. Condition associated with St. John's wort on induction of general
anesthesia.
3. Group of symptoms that may occur when abruptly stopping the herb.
4. Condition commonly treated with St. John's wort.
6. Contraindicated condition for using St. John's wort.
10. Patients with this disease may experience psychotic delirium from St.
John's wort.
11. What may happen to patients with bipolar disease when they use St.
John's wort.
13. Metabolic enzyme system returns to this state when a patient stops
taking St. John's wort.

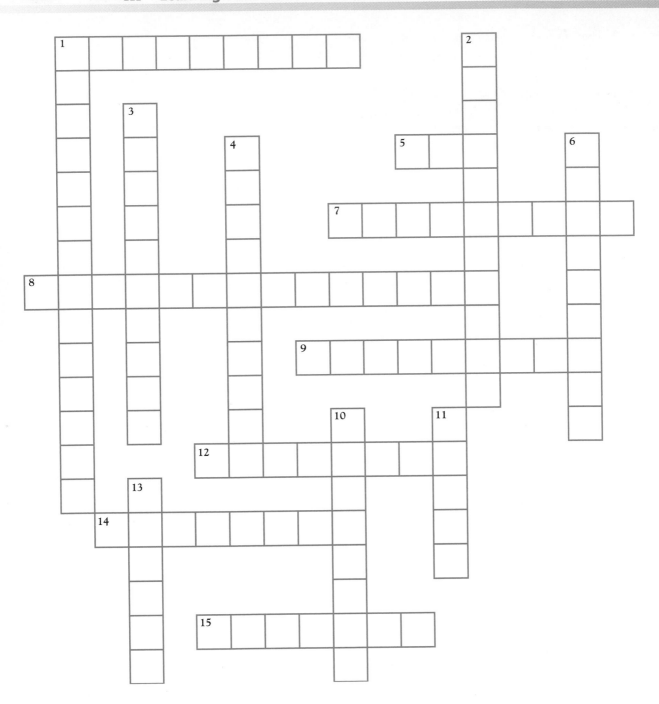

CHONDROITIN

DIRECTIONS: **Complete the following statements.**

1. Only about _____% of chondroitin is available for use after oral intake.
2. A person taking _____ should not take chondroitin.
3. Chondroitin and _____ have similar antiinflammatory actions.
4. Chondroitin is derived from _____ and _____ cartilage.

COENZYME Q10

DIRECTIONS: **Label each of the following actions of coenzyme Q10 as increased (I) or decreased (D) to indicate the appropriate direction of the response.**

1. _____ Cardiac contractility
2. _____ Peripheral resistance
3. _____ Effects of warfarin (Coumadin)
4. _____ Actions of clonidine
5. _____ Cardiac output
6. _____ Stroke volume

DIRECTIONS: Find and circle the following uses for coenzyme Q10.

AIDS	CHF	Mitral valve prolapse
Angina	Dyspnea	Myocardial infarction
Atherosclerosis	HIV	Obesity
Cancer	HTN	Pulmonary edema
Cardiac dysrhythmias	Liver congestion	

```
I  C  B  Z  M  M  Y  O  C  A  R  D  I  A  L  I  N  F  A  R  C  T  I  O  N  E
G  B  V  V  P  Y  M  C  S  U  A  S  D  I  A  G  V  R  Y  S  Q  O  L  H  P  J
S  Z  V  A  E  K  H  Z  C  J  K  B  Z  R  K  S  F  H  T  J  F  K  C  R  I  Q
Z  K  C  P  F  F  J  E  C  N  T  A  N  J  S  G  T  B  I  X  V  B  B  X  L  T
X  D  Y  S  P  N  E  A  N  W  N  F  M  L  S  N  P  G  S  Z  V  T  A  V  Y  T
R  D  T  E  T  D  N  E  G  B  Z  R  G  F  O  C  C  E  Q  Q  T  Y  R  E  A
F  U  N  W  P  C  P  O  I  Y  K  W  F  S  O  I  W  W  B  P  V  C  V  K  J  J
V  P  I  F  E  K  W  N  X  C  N  O  I  T  S  E  G  N  O  C  R  E  V  I  L  S
C  E  O  R  F  T  A  C  C  A  M  E  D  E  Y  R  A  N  O  M  L  U  P  R  H  T
Y  O  C  K  S  T  C  A  R  D  I  A  C  D  Y  S  R  H  Y  T  H  M  I  A  S  K
I  G  G  S  E  S  P  A  L  O  R  P  E  V  L  A  V  L  A  R  T  I  M  A  M  A
X  I  U  S  R  O  S  Z  A  T  H  E  R  O  S  C  L  E  R  O  S  I  S  O  B  A
```

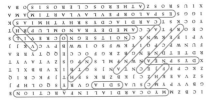

Answers:

FISH OIL

DIRECTIONS: Label each of the following actions of fish oil as increased (I) or decreased (D) to indicate the appropriate direction of the response.

1. _____ Bleeding times
2. _____ Blood pressure
3. _____ Serum glucose levels
4. _____ Vitamin E levels

Answers: 1. I; 2. D; 3. I; 4. D.

DIRECTIONS: **Answer the following questions.**

5. Fish oil should not be taken with what other herbal agents? (*List two*)

a. _____

b. _____

6. Identify three antihypertensives that may enhance blood pressure–lowering effects when used with fish oil:

a. _____

b. _____

c. _____

GLUCOSAMINE

DIRECTIONS: **Identify the following statements as *true* (T) or *false* (F).**

1. _____ It is thought that glucosamine stimulates proteoglycan in the joint cartilage.

2. _____ The antiinflammatory effects of glucosamine are similar to those of NSAIDs.

3. _____ Glucosamine appears to have very mild side effects.

4. _____ Glucosamine should not be taken by people who are allergic to shellfish.

CHONDROITIN AND GLUCOSAMINE

DIRECTIONS: **Label each of the following phrases as applying to chondroitin (C), glucosamine (G), or both (C and G).**

1. _____ Stimulates glucoprotein

2. _____ Derived from bovine cartilage

3. _____ Reduces collagen breakdown

4. _____ 90% absorbed when taken orally

5. _____ Beneficial for joint pain

6. _____ Is slow acting

VITAMIN C

DIRECTIONS: **Complete the following statements.**

1. The recommended daily allowance for vitamin C is

_____.

2. Although rare in adults, side effects of vitamin C may include:

_____, _____,

_____, _____,

and _____.

3. Taking vitamin C with anticoagulants, such as _____

or _____, may decrease the effect of

the anticoagulant.

Answers: 1. 80 to 150 mg daily; 2. Nausea, vomiting, diarrhea, heartburn, intestinal cramping; 3. Heparin, warfarin.

DIRECTIONS: **Match the following terms in Column A and phrases related to vitamin C in Column B.**

Column A

4. _____ Flavonoids
5. _____ Free radicals
6. _____ Antioxidant
7. _____ Pectin

Column B

a. May interfere with oxidative metabolism of nutrients and cause an increased incidence of cancer, cardiovascular, or inflammatory diseases
b. A component of rose hips that has a laxative and diuretic action
c. Plant pigments responsible for the color of fruits and vegetables
d. Responsible for destroying free radicals that can cause cellular damage

Answers: 4. c; 5. a; 6. d; 7. b.

DIRECTIONS: **Find and circle the following uses for vitamin C in the word puzzle on the following page.**

Allergies
Antioxidant
Arthritis
Asthma
Burns
Colds
Collagen development
Depression

Diabetes
Diarrhea
Diuretic
Fever
Gallstones
Gout
Hematuria
Influenza

Laxative
Sciatica
Scurvy
Sore throat
TPN (total parenteral nutrition)
Wound healing

```
H E M A T U R I A C A G A L L S T O N E S D L G T S
A A J N W S B U R N S Z A W A E E D U P O Q T N C T
H J L E O L D N Y D R I M C B X J T U H K R A I X A
A C X L H I T I W V Y E T H I B A Z E J H D C L Q O
Z I N L E D S E A M R S Y I O T J T D B I T B A T R
N T P N F R X S B R J U Y K R S A H I X A Y L E U H
E E D C P E G O E L R N C U D H M I O V U I S H O T
U R Y Q W B F I G R P H B S D S T I C B E P D D G E
L U O P Q U M N E F P N E K P L T R O S U J L N L R
F I I P B A M H T S A E O A Q N V T A F S J O U A O
N D K M Q G H K N T X R D L A A W F E V E R C O O S
I K C O L L A G E N D E V E L O P M E N T S U W Y Y
```

VITAMIN E

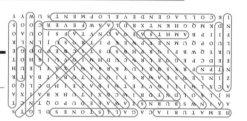

DIRECTIONS: **Identify the following statements as** *true* **(T) or** *false* **(F).**

1. _____ Vitamin E is well tolerated.
2. _____ Patients with retinitis pigmentosa should not take vitamin E.
3. _____ Alcohol may decrease vitamin E absorption.
4. _____ Iron supplements may strengthen the effects of vitamin E.
5. _____ Vitamin E should be held 10 to 14 days before surgery.
6. _____ Men and women can take the same dose of vitamin E.

DIRECTIONS: **Provide answers to the following instructions.**

7. List four foods that contain vitamin E:

_____

_____

_____

_____

8. List four conditions for which vitamin E may be used:

_____

_____

_____

_____

Healing with Physical Power

CHIROPRACTIC THERAPY

DIRECTIONS: **Complete the following statements.**

1. _____ of the pain a day or two after adjustment is not uncommon.
2. More than _____ treatment is usually needed.
3. Caution should be used in the number of _____ taken annually.
4. Chiropractic therapy has been approved for _____ _____.
5. A _____ _____ is required for practice.

Answers: 1. Worsening; 2. one; 3. x-rays; 4. low back pain; 5. certifying examination.

MASSAGE THERAPY

DIRECTIONS: **Complete the following statements.**

1. Massage therapy positively affects _____ _____ and health by using various hands-on techniques.
2. Massage therapy involves careful manipulation of the _____, _____, and _____ tissue.
3. The effects derived from massage depend on the _____ and _____ of the movements, the area being treated, and the degree of _____ exerted by the therapist's hands.

Answers: 1. well being; 2. skin, muscle, connective; 3. type, speed, pressure.

4. As a nonpharmocologic agent, massage therapy relieves discomfort and _____.

5. By inviting the patient to participate in his or her healing process, massage therapy contributes to a balance between _____ and _____.

DIRECTIONS: **Place a check next to the BEST answer.**

1. A physiologic response to rhythmic stroking and pressure of massage is:
   a. _____ Increased mean arterial pressure
   b. _____ Improved oxygen delivery to cells
   c. _____ Increased lactic acid carried to muscles
   d. _____ Increased heart rate

2. Massage therapy enhances immune system functioning by:
   a. _____ Reducing endorphin production
   b. _____ Promoting flow of lymphatic fluid
   c. _____ Enhancing cortisol production
   d. _____ Increasing levels of antibody production

3. Massage is not recommended for patients with:
   a. _____ Lymphedema
   b. _____ AIDS
   c. _____ Phlebitis
   d. _____ Premature birth

DIRECTIONS: **Provide an answer to the following question:**

4. What factors make massage therapy cost-effective?

   _____
   _____
   _____

QIGONG AND TAI CHI

DIRECTIONS: **Define the following terms related to qigong and tai chi.**

1. Qi: _____
2. Gong: _____
3. Tai chi: _____

DIRECTIONS: **Complete the following statements.**

4. Many of the benefits of qigong and tai chi are related to decreased
_____ response and _____
alterations.

5. List two hormones that are increased with qigong.

_____

_____

6. Qigong promotes the flow of _____
through the body's meridians, which enhances health and healing.

7. Qigong is the practice of working with _____
to improve health and well being through _____,
_____, and _____ or meditation.

Answers: 4. sympathetic, hormonal; 5. estrogen, testosterone; 6. qi; 7. qi, movements, abdominal breathing, concentration.

REFLEXOLOGY

DIRECTIONS: **Complete the following statements.**

1. Reflexology is a _____ modality.

2. Reflexology was brought to the United States by _____
_____.

3. It generally takes _____ to provide
pressure points on each foot.

4. Reflexology does not require any _____.

5. People have a wide variety of _____
sensitivity in their feet.

DIRECTIONS: **Identify the following statements as** *true* **(T) or** *false* **(F).**

6. _____ Reflexology is considered to be a valuable nursing skill.

7. _____ Reflexology uses the palm of the hand to apply pressure.

8. _____ Little research with reflexology has been done in controlled
studies.

9. _____ Reflexology has been shown to reduce stress.

Answers: 1. touch; 2. Eunice Ingham; 3. 10 minutes; 4. equipment; 5. touch; 6. T; 7. F; 8. T; 9. T.

ROLFING

DIRECTIONS: **Complete the following statements.**

1. The body's problems are a result of _____.

2. Being out of _____ is what causes most problems, according to rolfing practitioners.

3. _____ is the founder of the rolfing theory.

4. A substance known as _____ covers muscle and connective tissue.

5. _____ _____ can be manipulated to correct deficits.

6. By _____, the rolfing therapist works to create alignment.

DIRECTIONS: **Identify the following statements as** *true* **(T) or** *false* **(F).**

7. _____   Rolfing can be considered a form of massage.

8. _____   Rolfing works to restore alignment.

9. _____   Rolfing is a cumulative process.

10. _____   Rolfing sessions are short.

11. _____   Rolfing needs to be done by a certified practitioner.

YOGA

DIRECTIONS: **Complete the following statements.**

1. Raja yoga includes the physical _____ and _____ exercises most often associated with yoga.

2. Raja yoga philosophy includes the way in which one approaches others and _____, as well as _____ techniques.

3. Yoga philosophy proposes that health is not just a physical phenomenon, but also one that includes the _____ and the _____.

4. Differences between styles of yoga concern primarily the level of emphasis given to the _____, _____, and _____ aspects of yoga.

5. Some styles of yoga are extremely _____ demanding, while others emphasize _____ through meditation.

6. Ethical aspects of yoga can include actions such as _____ service and proper _____.

7. Some types of yoga may be contraindicated for people with chronic _____ _____.

8. Yoga can aggravate or create more problems for a patient when it is _____ practiced.

9. Nurses who recommend yoga should be knowledgeable about the _____ styles of yoga and informed about the _____ in the community.

BIOFEEDBACK

DIRECTIONS: Find and circle the following uses for biofeedback.

ADHD	Epilepsy	Motion sickness
Anxiety	Headaches	Pain
Asthma	Incontinence	Stroke
Enuresis	Insomnia	

M	H	S	Y	Y	S	P	E	L	I	P	E	X
O	W	E	Q	T	I	I	A	K	X	X	Q	H
T	S	H	K	P	E	S	S	R	T	I	Y	M
I	N	C	O	N	T	I	N	E	N	C	E	L
O	X	A	D	H	D	M	X	S	R	H	R	O
N	K	D	M	S	S	S	O	N	M	U	C	S
S	R	A	H	S	S	M	P	K	A	N	N	U
I	T	E	T	N	N	X	Q	B	G	T	D	E
C	K	H	F	I	M	I	B	I	G	G	O	F
K	F	A	A	D	D	Y	A	D	X	C	D	D
N	B	X	K	J	J	E	I	P	E	W	U	K
E	K	O	R	T	S	L	I	C	C	T	H	H
S	D	E	X	U	U	P	B	W	C	F	N	T
S	E	P	F	G	G	N	S	U	W	X	B	J

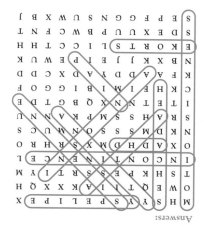

Answers:

259

DIRECTIONS: **Place a check next to the BEST answer.**

1. Biofeedback is based on principles of:
   a. _____ Learning theory
   b. _____ Pathophysiology
   c. _____ Meditation
   d. _____ Biologic control

2. Biofeedback instruments are designed to:
   a. _____ Provide diagnostic data
   b. _____ Measure physiologic phenomenon
   c. _____ Monitor psychologic responses to intervention
   d. _____ Improve compliance with treatment

3. The goal of biofeedback is for clients to:
   a. _____ Decrease dependence on all medications
   b. _____ Self-regulate physiologic phenomena
   c. _____ Control disease progression
   d. _____ Improve muscle strength

4. The most common risk of biofeedback is:
   a. _____ Increased anxiety
   b. _____ Muscle weakness
   c. _____ Depression
   d. _____ Dysrhythmias

Answers: 1. a; 2. b; 3. b; 4. a.

HUMOR THERAPY

DIRECTIONS: **Complete the crossword puzzle related to humor therapy.**

Across

2. Place where formal training in humor therapy can be obtained.
3. State of mind that can be altered by humor.
5. Type of change in body function that can result from humor.
6. Sad state that can be reduced with humor therapy.
7. Type of patient who cannot respond to humor therapy.
8. Word used interchangeably with humor.
9. Natural pain killing substances released when humor is used as therapy.
12. Humor is whatever the person finds as _____.
13. Physiologic parameter that often decreases after laughter and relaxation.

Answers: Across: 2. Clown college; 3. Psychologic; 5. Physiologic; 6. Depression; 7. Comatose; 8. Laughter; 9. Endorphins; 12. Funny; 13. Heart rate. Down: 1. Blood pressure; 4. Jocularity; 10. Heart; 11. Anxiety.

Down

1. Another physiologic measure that may decrease with relaxation.
4. Another word for humor.
10. Type of patient that may need to be observed more closely because of increased workload of this organ.
11. "Uptight" condition that can be relieved with humor.

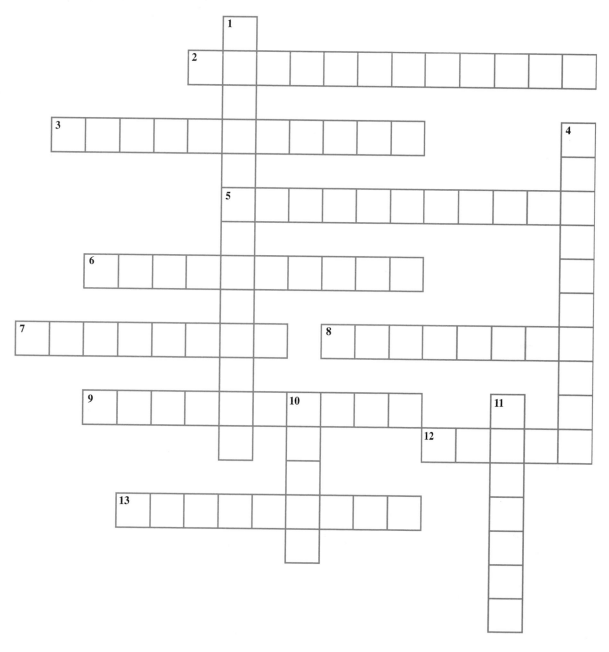

DIRECTIONS: **Identify the following statements as** *true* **(T) or** *false* **(F).**

1. _____ Laughter can diminish pain, cause relaxation, and decrease anxiety.

2. _____ Humor can be safely used with all patients and in all situations.

3. _____ The act of laughing has been shown to cause a release of endorphins, the body's own natural pain killers.

4. _____ Nurses can and should use humor as a means to relieve tension and promote relaxation.

5. _____ Some evidence suggests that humor can cure disease.

6. _____ Laughter increases oxygen delivery to the tissues.

Answers: 1. T; 2. F; 3. T; 4. T; 5. T; 6. T.

HYPNOSIS

DIRECTIONS: **Complete the following statements.**

1. Hypnosis is an alternate _____ of _____.

2. Patients often experience hypnosis as a condition of intense focal _____ with decreased peripheral awareness.

3. Hypnotic _____ is a set of verbal and nonverbal instructions and cues that prepares the patient for _____ change.

4. Particular suggestions used in hypnosis depend on patient's age, level of _____, presenting _____, and treatment _____.

5. Therapists use hypnotic techniques to enhance established _____ or _____ treatment.

6. Hypnotized individuals can produce dramatic changes in perceptual processing and _____ activity that may not be attainable without the use of hypnosis.

7. The most common after effects of hypnosis are temporary _____ and _____.

8. It is important to consider a patient's _____ when hypnosis is requested.

Answers: 1. state, consciousness; 2. concentration; 3. induction, therapeutic; 4. maturity, problem, goals; 5. psychosocial, medical; 6. physiologic; 7. relaxation, drowsiness; 8. motives.

MEDITATION

DIRECTIONS: **Complete the crossword puzzle (see the following page)**
related to meditation.

Across

3. Flowing of perception and mindful attention to all sensations.
6. Object of concentration or inner, silent word chant that has special meaning.
7. Recommended frequency for practicing meditation.
9. Decrease in this physiologic measure is possible with meditation.
10. Example of moving meditation.
12. Number of minutes most desirable for meditation.
13. Research has found meditation to be helpful for _____.
14. Posture recommended for meditation.
15. Leg position usually used in meditation.

Down

1. Being attentive, actively conscious, and acutely aware of mind-body reaction.
2. Common modern form of meditation.
4. Mindfulness of observing and experiencing the sensation without interfering with it.
5. Sleepless condition which may improve with meditation.
8. Type of hypotension that may occur when rising quickly from sitting positions.
11. Best time to practice meditation.

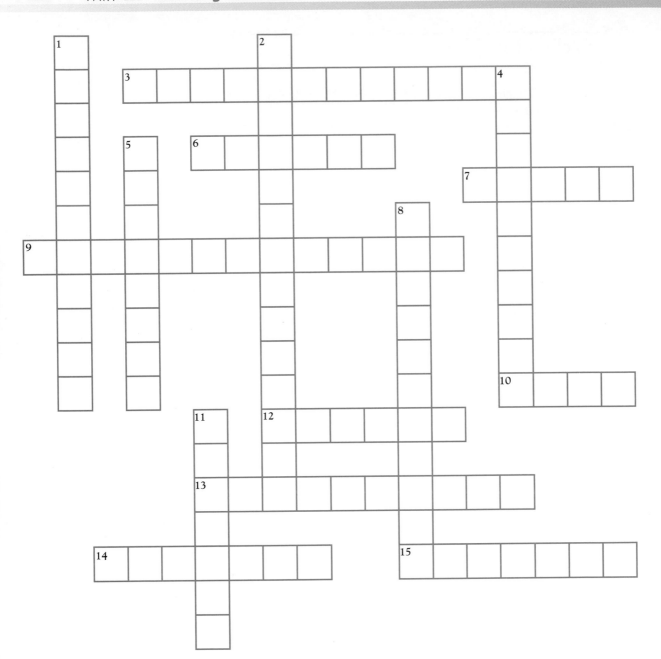

MUSIC THERAPY

DIRECTIONS: **Find and circle the following target populations and conditions treated with music therapy.**

AIDS	Children	Obstetrics
Anorexia	Chronic pain	Psychosis
Asthma	Depression	Schizophrenia
Autism	Elderly	Substance abuse
Brain damage	Hospice care	Surgery
Burn patients	Neonates	

```
S  U  R  G  E  R  Y  X  U  T  X  D  H  N  N
U  T  I  F  B  A  A  S  F  N  C  O  O  U  P
A  I  N  E  R  H  P  O  Z  I  H  C  S  U  D
N  J  T  E  A  A  K  J  L  A  F  H  P  G  X
O  Q  N  O  I  S  S  E  R  P  E  D  I  N  J
R  S  E  B  N  T  Q  N  N  C  Q  F  C  E  R
E  E  R  S  D  H  A  O  E  I  O  Y  E  O  D
X  X  D  T  A  M  U  P  O  N  A  X  C  L  Y
I  I  L  E  M  A  T  K  N  O  Z  B  A  L  S
A  S  I  T  A  O  I  H  A  R  G  I  R  L  Y
R  G  H  R  G  H  S  Z  T  H  U  E  E  A  Y
R  S  C  I  E  K  M  H  E  C  D  B  E  Q  H
P  S  Y  C  H  O  S  I  S  L  J  Q  O  W  K
S  U  B  S  T  A  N  C  E  A  B  U  S  E  O
```

DIRECTIONS: Complete the following statements.

1. Music therapy uses harmonic melody to affect changes in

   _____, _____, and

   _____.

2. Music therapy is used to diminish stress, _____,

   _____, and _____.

3. Music is a behavioral science integrating _____

   healing.

DIRECTIONS: Identify the following statements as *true* (T) or *false* (F).

4. _____   Music with slower rhythms lead to depression.
5. _____   Music allows patients with speech impediments to communicate without the use of words.
6. _____   Joint functioning can be enhanced by music therapy.
7. _____   Heart rate, blood pressure, and respirations vary directly with the pace and volume of music.

Answers: 4, F; 5, T; 6, T; 7, T.

PET THERAPY

DIRECTIONS: Find and circle the following uses for pet therapy.

Anxiety   Cancer   Epilepsy   Paralysis
Autism   Deafness   Heart disease   Stress
Blindness   Depression   Isolation

I	S	O	L	A	T	I	O	N	J	A	N
Q	S	I	Y	T	O	S	X	Q	G	N	O
C	E	N	S	V	S	E	G	K	H	X	I
W	N	P	P	Y	B	S	M	D	C	I	S
Z	D	C	E	Z	L	B	E	E	C	E	S
T	N	U	L	Y	I	A	H	R	I	T	E
A	I	H	I	F	F	H	R	C	T	Y	R
L	L	D	P	N	Y	K	S	A	E	S	P
J	B	H	E	W	I	C	O	N	P	R	E
L	M	S	I	T	U	A	O	C	R	R	D
M	S	W	D	B	D	S	H	E	N	G	K
E	S	A	E	S	I	D	T	R	A	E	H

Answers:

DIRECTIONS: Complete the following statements.

1. A _____ is another term for a pet.
2. _____ are animals that are legally defined through the Americans with Disabilities Act.
3. An animal trained to assist a patient in using arm muscles is known as a _____.
4. A _____ is given to people who have disabilities, but these animals have not completed the service animal training.

Answers: 1. companion animal; 2. Service animals; 3. therapy animal; 4. social animal.

DIRECTIONS: Label each of the following effects of pet therapy as increased (I) or decreased (D) to indicate the appropriate direction of the response.

1. _____ Anxiety
2. _____ Blood pressure
3. _____ Heart rate
4. _____ Cholesterol
5. _____ Socialization
6. _____ Need for cardiovascular medication
7. _____ Preoperative stress
8. _____ Reality orientation
9. _____ Pain medication use
10. _____ Physical activity

Answers: 1. D; 2. D; 3. D; 4. D; 5. I; 6. D; 7. D; 8. I; 9. D; 10. I.

RELAXATION THERAPY

DIRECTIONS: Identify the following statements as a benefit (B) or a use (U) of relaxation therapy.

1. _____ Decrease anxiety
2. _____ Decrease stress
3. _____ Anxiety
4. _____ Chronic pain
5. _____ Acute pain
6. _____ Increased mental awareness
7. _____ Hypertension
8. _____ Reduce muscle tension

DIRECTIONS: Complete the following statements.

9. Relaxation therapy is considered _____ and has almost no _____ _____.
10. There are two basic types of relaxation: _____ and _____.
11. It may take _____ of regular practice to see benefits.
12. Relaxation is a _____ that requires consistent practice to master.

Answers: 1. B; 2. B; 3. U; 4. U; 5. U; 6. B; 7. U; 8. B; 9. safe, side effects; 10. deep, brief; 11. 6 to 8 weeks; 12. skill.

STORYTELLING

DIRECTIONS: **Complete the following statements.**

1. Knowing and understanding whom the patient is and what he or she values is the essence of _____ nursing practice.

2. Storytelling is not a cure-all for deep-rooted _____ problems.

3. Listening to stories stimulates imagery and allows release of _____ energy.

4. Qualitative research studies have documented the _____ and _____ in healing derived from storytelling.

5. Storytelling is an effective method for transmitting _____ and instilling _____.

6. Group storytelling among a group of older adults can result in reduction of _____ symptoms and social _____.

7. The therapeutic use of storytelling by nurses conveys _____ and _____.

8. _____ is an important factor to consider as children deal with stressful issues.

Answers: 1. holistic; 2. psychological; 3. emotional; 4. value, meaning; 5. knowledge, hope; 6. depressive, isolation; 7. sympathy, understanding; 8. Time.

5 Healing with Subtle Energy

ACUPRESSURE

DIRECTIONS: Complete the following statements.

1. Acupressure works by applying finger pressure on
   _____ _____ to relieve
   pain and discomfort and promote _____.

2. Acupressure is similar to acupuncture in that it releases blockages of
   _____ known as chi.

3. Chi circulates through the body in patterns called
   _____ or _____ energies.

4. Disturbances in the flow of chi may lead to _____
   _____.

5. Health is promoted by balancing yin and yang energies of the body,
   _____ and _____.

6. Acupressure targets specific points in the _____
   channels that may need _____ in energy flow
   _____.

7. Stimulating acupressure points may release neurotransmitters in the
   brain and cause the release of _____.

8. Acupressure promotes muscle relaxation by stimulating circulation,
   promoting _____ flow, and releasing
   _____ and _____ acid.

Answers: 1. pressure points, healing;
2. energy; 3. yin, yang; 4. health
problems; 5. mind, spirit; 6. meridian,
blockages, removed; 7. endorphins;
8. blood, tension, lactic.

269

DIRECTIONS: Find and circle the following uses for acupressure.

Allergies	Headache	Postop nausea
Anxiety	Insomnia	Pregnancy
Congestion	Labor	Stress
Dyspnea	Muscle pain	Vomiting

```
P  D  Y  S  P  N  E  A  B  M  K  N
O  A  Y  C  N  A  N  G  E  R  P  O
S  G  I  K  O  X  E  O  L  O  T  I
T  N  E  U  I  H  Z  C  O  B  C  S
O  I  H  Y  T  E  I  X  N  A  D  S
P  T  C  S  S  E  R  T  S  L  G  E
N  I  A  P  E  L  C  S  U  M  W  R
A  M  D  L  G  P  T  V  F  K  B  P
U  O  A  I  N  M  O  S  N  I  O  E
S  V  E  G  O  G  F  S  N  S  X  D
E  H  H  G  C  M  U  Y  V  M  U  K
A  L  L  E  R  G  I  E  S  O  Q  H
```

Answers:

ACUPUNCTURE

DIRECTIONS: Complete the crossword puzzle related to acupuncture.

Across

5. Number of organ meridians in each half of the body.
6. Neurotransmitter that changes brain biochemistry.
8. Chinese name for patterns of energy flow through the body.
9. Acupuncture originated in this country.
10. Results that occur when Qi is disrupted or imbalanced.
13. Body part stimulated in auriculotherapy.
14. May be used in conjunction with acupuncture.

Down

1. Complication resulting when chest needles are inserted too deeply.
2. Key component of Qi described as warm, dry, moving laterally.
3. Nonpainful sensation elicited by acupuncture.
4. Pathways occurring symmetrically on each side of the body.
7. Item that is inserted into the body over strategic points.
11. _____ is applied to the acupuncture sites in moxibustion.
12. Key component of Qi that is described as passive, dark, cold, moist.

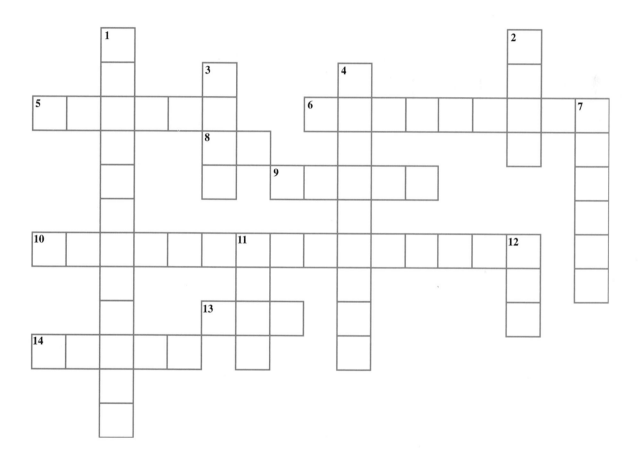

AROMATHERAPY

DIRECTIONS: Find and circle the following terms related to aromatherapy.

Anxiety
Arthritis
Asthma
Colds
Depression

GI distress
Hypertension
Insomnia
Migraines
Muscle pain

Nausea
PMS
Stress relief
Wound healing

H	M	W	H	Y	P	E	R	T	E	N	S	I	O	N
Z	Y	O	L	L	Y	F	T	G	X	T	S	N	F	P
I	F	U	Q	R	O	O	O	H	R	N	V	M	N	C
N	K	N	Y	R	K	Y	T	E	I	X	N	A	K	X
S	X	D	Z	N	A	U	S	E	A	H	G	S	U	F
O	N	H	N	I	S	S	E	R	T	S	I	D	I	G
M	O	E	O	L	R	Z	P	O	U	A	M	L	L	J
N	I	A	P	E	L	C	S	U	M	T	G	O	S	H
I	S	L	L	H	I	E	C	V	S	O	F	C	R	Q
A	S	I	T	I	R	H	T	R	A	M	O	K	Q	G
S	E	N	I	A	R	G	I	M	G	P	I	E	C	L
F	R	G	O	W	H	C	H	Z	W	H	L	I	P	L
O	P	I	D	B	Y	T	A	P	F	Q	G	H	Z	E
M	E	I	D	D	S	M	P	C	W	Q	N	K	A	K
V	D	U	V	A	N	N	H	O	Q	G	G	A	K	L

Answers:

COLOR THERAPY

DIRECTIONS: **Match the phrases in Column A to the appropriate color in Column B.**

Column A

1. _____ Assists in balancing, calming, stability, security.
2. _____ Aids in bleeding, abscesses, congestion, conditions of the ears, nose, eyes, sinuses.
3. _____ Increases red blood cell production, analgesia, and wound healing.
4. _____ Enhances lymphatic system; serves as a sensory stimulant.
5. _____ Soothes the nervous system and relaxes muscles.
6. _____ Increases sexual function, pleasure, and enthusiasm.
7. _____ Enhances communication and used in the treatment of fever, bleeding, and jaundice.

Column B

a. Red
b. Orange
c. Yellow
d. Green
e. Blue
f. Indigo
g. Violet

Answers: 1. d; 2. f; 3. a; 4. c; 5. g; 6. b; 7. e.

FENG SHUI

DIRECTIONS: **Complete the following statements.**

1. Feng shui is translated into English as _____ and _____.
2. Our vitality is dependent on _____ air and _____ water.
3. The objective of feng shui is to improve lives by _____ _____ _____.
4. Yang is the _____ side and symbolizes all things _____, _____, _____, _____, and _____.
5. Yin is the _____ side and symbolizes all things _____, _____, _____, _____, and _____.

Answers: 1. wind, water; 2. fresh, pure; 3. improving the environment; 4. white, masculine, expansive, exterior, hot, heavenly; 5. black, feminine, contracted, interior, cool, earthy.

DIRECTIONS: **Find and circle the following terms related to feng shui.**

Bones	Environment	Jen	Life force	Thunder
Breath	Fame	Kan	Metal	Unity
Building	Feng	Ken	Red	Wind
Chyan	Harmony	Kun	Shui	Wood
Dui	India	Landscape	Shun	Yang
Earth	Japan	Li	Sky	Yin

```
B Q L W Y H A R M O N Y E L U N I T Y
K U R A I T R E D B Y U E I N I O P A
A F I S N D S K Y R N F C G E D O O W
N A N L H D J K L E A Z R X K C T V I
B M D N D M S Q W A P E O S R T H B N
K E I Y U I U C Y T A J F H N H U O D
I U A O I P N A A H J I E U A T N N S
F E N G D F G G N P H U F N Y R D E J
L A T E M K L Z G X E H I C H A E S V
E N V I R O N M E N T S L B C E R N M
```

HOMEOPATHY

DIRECTIONS: **Complete the following statements.**

1. Homeopathy is based on the following three fundamental principles:

   _____, _____,

   and _____.

2. Inherent to the practice of homeopathy is the taking of a meticulous

   _____ _____ of symptoms, what

   the individual exhibits during the illness, and how factors in the

   physical, emotional, and mental environment affect the illness.

3. Homeopathy should not be used for _____

   or _____ conditions.

4. Individuals who practice homeopathy recognize that the symptoms of

   illness are the body's efforts to deal with _____.

5. The process of demonstrating what a substance in its pure form does

   to a healthy body is known as a "_____."

INTUITIVE SPIRITUAL HEALING

DIRECTIONS: **Identify the following statements as *true* (T) or *false* (F).**

1. _____ The anatomic makeup of the physical body creates an electrical field in and around the body.

2. _____ Disturbances in the energy flow through organs in the body may indicate disease.

3. _____ Direct physical contact on the area in which the patient is complaining of symptoms is required for ISH to be effective.

4. _____ ISH is contraindicated in pediatric patients.

DIRECTIONS: **Place a check next to the BEST answer.**

5. A sensation that a patient may experience during a session of ISH is:

   a. _____ Dizziness

   b. _____ Muscle spasm

   c. _____ Nausea

   d. _____ Tingling

6. An expected outcome of ISH is:

   a. _____ A rapid improvement in a patient's physical condition

   b. _____ A need for ongoing sessions until disease is cured

   c. _____ An improved sense of emotional, spiritual, and physical well being

   d. _____ No need for antianxiety and pain relief medications

MAGNETIC THERAPY

DIRECTIONS: **Complete the crossword puzzle related to the actions, side effects, and uses of magnetic therapy.**

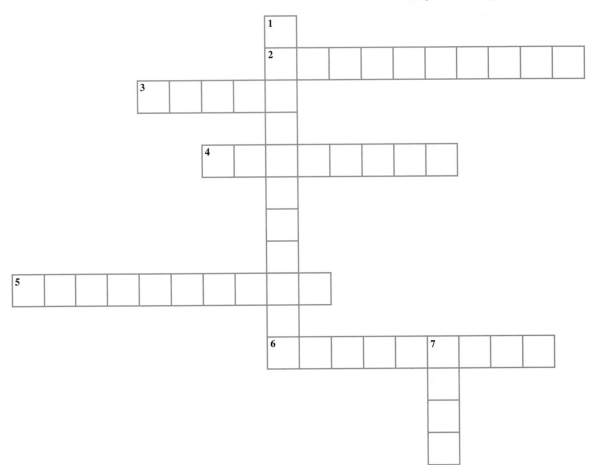

Across

2. Tendon inflammation.

3. Excessive amount of tissue fluid.

4. Seizure disorder.

5. Magnets may interfere with this electrical device in certain cardiac patients.

6. Body's own pain killing substance.

Down

1. Magnetic fields create this on the body.

7. Most common therapeutic use of magnets is to relieve _____.

DIRECTIONS: **Provide the rationale for the following statement.**

8. Magnets may block pain by stimulating nerve endings.

_____

_____

_____

PRAYER

DIRECTIONS: **Complete the crossword puzzle related to prayer. (See the following page for clues.)**

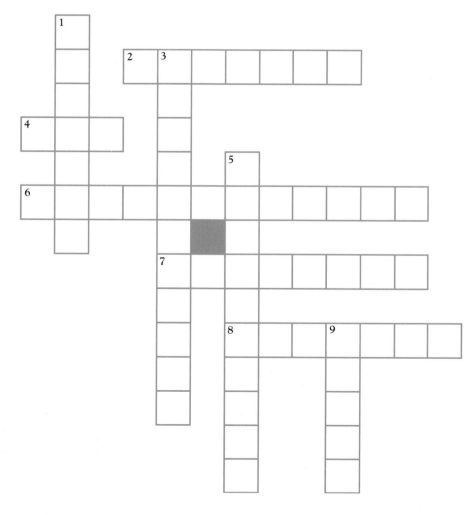

Across

2. Term to describe a type of therapy used in concert with other therapies.
4. Prayer is useful for _____ patient.
6. Prayer is used to seek divine _____ in the healing process.
7. Professional who can provide spiritual and prayer services for patients.
8. Time when prayer can be done.

Down

1. Prayer as a _____ therapy has not been scientifically studied in depth.
3. What occurs during prayer that allows a person to leave behind their immediate problems.
5. Increase in this state of being is a benefit of prayer.
9. Indicator of prayer's success is putting one's _____ in a higher power.

Answers: Across: 2. Adjunct; 4. All; 6. Intervention; 7. Chaplain; 8. Anytime. Down: 1. Healing; 3. Distraction; 5. Relaxation; 9. Trust.

REIKI

DIRECTIONS: **Answer the following questions.**

1. What is centering?

2. Where are the symbols placed during attunement?

3. Where do you place your hands during a session?

4. What is an attunement?

5. For what can Reiki be used?

Answers: 1. Centering is another term for taking a deep breath, exhaling, and entering into a light meditative state in which external events do not intrude; 2. The symbols are placed into certain chakras by the practitioner; 3. The hands are placed in various positions (lightly) on the body of the recipient, usually beginning at the head and working down the front and back of the body; 4. An attunement is when the master-teacher opens certain chakras or energy centers in the recipient's auric field, placing the Reiki symbols into the chakras; 5. Reiki can be used for stress illnesses, emotional or psychological problems, pain reduction, wound healing, and to aid with relaxation.

DIRECTIONS: Find and circle the following terms related to Reiki.

Attuned	Flow	Meditate	Symbols
Aura	Hands	Pain	Therapeutic
Centering	Heal	Rei	Tingling
Chakras	Heat	Reiki	Touch
Chi	IARP	Relaxation	Transfer
Energy	Ki	Stress	Universal life energy
Field	Master teacher		

```
C  E  N  T  E  R  I  N  G  T  Y  U  I  O  P  T  P  O  T
H  X  C  V  H  F  E  H  J  K  N  I  A  P  S  I  Z  N  R
A  M  A  S  T  E  R  T  E  A  C  H  E  R  Y  N  F  V  A
K  T  A  E  H  V  R  A  S  F  L  O  W  O  M  G  I  C  N
R  Q  I  E  R  Q  I  A  R  P  D  F  G  S  B  L  E  S  S
A  T  T  U  N  E  D  U  P  L  C  P  O  T  O  I  L  D  F
S  W  H  E  A  L  T  R  Y  E  U  H  I  R  L  N  D  N  E
E  R  M  E  D  I  T  A  T  E  U  M  I  E  S  G  X  A  R
R  E  I  K  I  A  K  I  Z  X  C  T  V  S  B  N  X  H  B
S  D  R  E  L  A  X  A  T  I  O  N  I  S  T  O  U  C  H
E  N  E  R  G  Y  F  G  H  J  K  L  I  C  Y  Z  W  E  E
U  N  I  V  E  R  S  A  L  L  I  F  E  E  N  E  R  G  Y
```

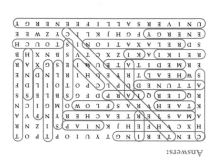

Answers:

THERAPEUTIC TOUCH

DIRECTIONS: In the word puzzle on the following page, find and circle the following uses for therapeutic touch.

Anxiety	Fatigue	Nurse
Bone	Field	Pain
Cancer	Hands	PMS
Centering	Harvest	Pulmonary
Chakra	HIV	Scanning
Diabetes	Infants	Therapeutic touch
Disturbance	Intention	Well being
Energy	Kunz	

```
C P U L M O N A R Y Z X C V B N
M H A G N I E B L L E W S D F H
S C A N N I N G G H J K P L Q A
I G S K I N P R O B L E M S P N
N R H W R E I N F A N T S R T D
T I I Y U A I O R E C N A C P S
E E V O D I S T U R B A N C E P
N F I K U N Z E S R U N X U Y T
T T R R O G E R S E S D I A W S
I Q A E N E R G Y B O N E S D E
O F F I E L D G E U G I T A F V
N H J G S E T E B A I D Y K L R
Z X C E N T E R I N G N I A P A
T H E R A P E U T I C T O U C H
```

Answers:

PART IV

Helpful Cross-References

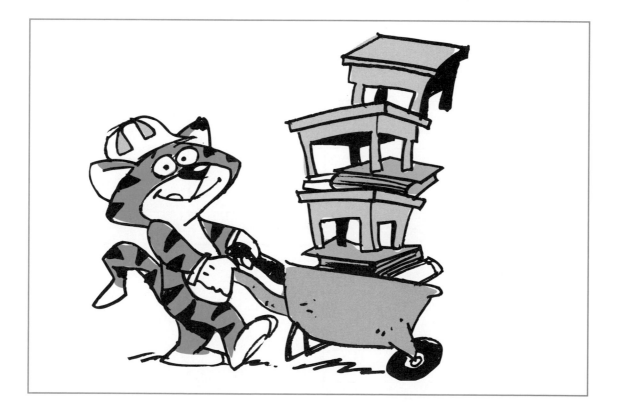

Proposed Pharmacologic Actions of Herbs, Vitamins, and Dietary Supplements

	ANALGESIA	ANTIANXIETY	ANTI-CONVULSANT	ANTI-DEPRESSANT	ANTI-INFLAMMATORY	ANTIOXIDANT	ANTITUMOR	ANTITUSSIVE
HERBS								
Alfalfa								
Aloe vera	■				■			
Astragalus root						■		
Black cohosh								
Capsicum	■							
Chamomile					■			
Cranberry						■	■	
Dandelion					■			
Echinacea								
Ephredra					■			■
Evening primrose								
Feverfew								
Garlic								
Ginger	■				■			
Ginkgo						■		
Ginseng	■					■	■	
Goldenseal								
Hawthorn						■		
Hop	■	■	■	■				
Kava kava	■	■	■					
Licorice					■			■
Passionflower		■						
Red clover					■			■
St. John's wort		■		■				
VITAMINS AND DIETARY SUPPLEMENTS								
Chondroitin					■			
Co-enzyme Q10						■		
Fish oil					■		■	
Glucosamine					■			
Vitamin C						■		
Vitamin E						■	■	

	ANTIVIRAL, ANTIBACTERIAL ANTIFUNGAL	CHOLESTEROL-LOWERING	ENHANCES COGNITION	ESTROGENLIKE	IMMUNE STIMULANT	POSITIVE INOTROPIC	MINERAL-CORTICOID	SYMPATHO-MIMETIC
HERBS								
Alfalfa	■	■		■				
Aloe vera	■				■			
Astragalus root	■				■	■		
Black cohosh				■				
Capsicum								
Chamomile	■							
Cranberry								
Dandelion								
Echinacea					■		■	
Ephredra	■					■		■
Evening primrose	■							
Feverfew								
Garlic	■	■			■			
Ginger						■		
Ginkgo			■					
Ginseng					■			
Goldenseal					■			
Hawthorn						■		
Hop				■				
Kava kava								
Licorice	■						■	
Passionflower	■							
Red clover				■				
St. John's wort								
VITAMINS AND DIETARY SUPPLEMENTS								
Chondroitin								
Co-enzyme Q10					■	■		
Fish oil		■	■					
Glucosamine								
Vitamin C								
Vitamin E			■					

Common Side Effects of Herbs, Vitamins, and Dietary Supplements

	ALLERGEN POTENTIAL	ANTI-COAGULATION	DIURESIS	DIARRHEA	DECREASED FERTILITY	FLUID LOSS	HYPO-GLYCEMIC	INCREASED HEART RATE
HERBS								
Alfalfa	X		X	X			X	
Aloe vera				X		X		
Astragalus root		X	X			X		
Black cohosh								
Capsicum	X	X						
Chamomile	X							
Cranberry								
Dandelion			X			X	X	
Echinacea	X							
Ephredra								X
Evening primrose		X		X				
Feverfew		X						
Garlic		X					X	
Ginger		X						
Ginkgo		X			X			
Ginseng							X	X
Goldenseal								
Hawthorn	X							
Hop	X				X			
Kava kava	X							
Licorice		X			X			
Passionflower		X						
Red clover		X						
St. John's wort	X				X			
VITAMINS AND DIETARY SUPPLEMENTS								
Chondroitin		X						
Co-enzyme Q10				X				
Fish oil		X						
Glucosamine				X				
Vitamin C				X				
Vitamin E		X						

	PROMOTES UTERINE CONTRACTIONS	AFFECTED LIVER ENZYMES/DRUG METABOLISM	SEDATION	INCREASED BLOOD PRESSURE	DECREASED BLOOD PRESSURE
HERBS					
Alfalfa		●			
Aloe vera	●				
Astragalus root					●
Black cohosh	●		●		●
Capsicum					
Chamomile			●		
Cranberry					
Dandelion					
Echinacea		●			
Ephredra				●	
Evening primrose					●
Feverfew	●				
Garlic		●			●
Ginger					
Ginkgo					
Ginseng				●	
Goldenseal	●	●			●
Hawthorn	●		●		●
Hop			●		
Kava kava			●		
Licorice	●	●		●	
Passionflower			●		
Red clover		●			
St. John's wort	●	●	●	●	●
VITAMINS AND DIETARY SUPPLEMENTS					
Chondroitin					
Co-enzyme Q10					●
Fish oil					●
Glucosamine					
Vitamin C					
Vitamin E					

Index of Conditions Treated with Nonpharmacologic Therapies

References

Part I: Pharmacologic Therapies
Section 1: Herbs

Alfalfa

Brinker F: *Herb contraindications and drug interactions*, ed 3, Sandy, Ore, 2001, Eclectic Medical Publications.

Bruneton J: *Pharmacognosy, phytochemistry, medicinal plants*, ed 2, London, 1999, Lavoisier.

Chambers HF: Chloramphenicol, tetracyclines, macrolides, clindamycin, and stretogramins. In Katzumg BG, editor: *Basic and clinical pharmacology*, ed 7, New York, 1998, McGraw-Hill.

Jellin JM et al: *Pharmacist's letter/prescriber's letter natural medicines comprehensive database*, ed 3, Stockton, Calif, 2000, Therapeutic Research Faculty.

Newall C, Anderson L, Phillipson JD: *Herbal medicines: a guide for healthcare professionals*, London, 1996, Pharmaceutical Press.

Physicians' desk reference for herbal medicines, Montvale, N.J., 1999, Medical Economics.

Roland M, Tozer TN: *Absorption. Clinical pharmacokinetics: concepts and applications*, ed 3, Philadelphia, 1995, Lippincott–Williams & Wilkins.

Aloe Vera

Brinker F: *Herb contraindications and drug interactions*, ed 3, Sandy, Ore, 2001, Eclectic Medical Publications.

Bruneton J: *Pharmacognosy, phytochemistry, medicinal plants*, ed 2, London, 1999, Lavoisier.

Jellin JM et al: *Pharmacist's letter/prescriber's letter natural medicines comprehensive database*, ed 3, Stockton, Calif, 2000, Therapeutic Research Faculty.

Mills S, Bone K: *Principles and practice of phytotherapy*, Edinburgh, 2000, Churchill-Livingstone.

Newall C, Anderson L, Phillipson JD: *Herbal medicines: a guide for healthcare professionals*, London, 1996, Pharmaceutical Press.

Astragalus Root

Bratman S, Kroll D: *Natural health bible*, New York, 1999, Prima.

Hoult JRS, Paya M: Pharmacological and biochemical actions of simple coumarins: natural products with therapeutic potential, *Gen Pharmac* 27(4):713, 1996.

Jellin JM et al: *Pharmacist's letter/prescriber's letter natural medicines comprehensive database*, ed 3, Stockton, Calif, 2000, Therapeutic Research Faculty.

Mills S, Bone K: *Principles and practice of phytotherapy*, Edinburgh, 2000, Churchill-Livingstone.

Norred CL, Brinker F: Potential coagulation effects of preoperative complementary and alternative medicines, *Altern Ther Health Med* 7(6):58, 2000.

Pizzorno JE, Murray MT: *Textbook of natural medicine*, vols 1 and 2, Edinburgh, 1999, Churchill-Livingstone.

Wang S, Zi-quiang G, Jia-zhen L: Experimental study on effects of 18 kinds of Chinese herbal medicine for synthesis of TXA2 and PGI2, *Chung Kuo Chung His I Chieh Ho Tsa Chih* 13(3):167, 1993.

Black Cohosh

Blumenthal M, Goldman A, Brinckman J: *Herbal medicine: expanded German E, commission monographs*, Austin, 2000, American Botanical Council.

Brinker F: *Herb contraindications and drug interactions*, ed 3, Sandy, Ore, 2001, Eclectic Medical Publications.

Bruneton J: *Pharmacognosy, phytochemistry, medicinal plants*, London, 1999, Lavoisier.

Grauds C: Black cohosh, *Pharm Times* September:52, 1998.

Jellin JM et al: *Pharmacist's letter/prescriber's letter natural medicines comprehensive database*, ed 3, Stockton, Calif, 2000, Therapeutic Research Faculty.

Mills S, Bone K: *Principles and practice of phytotherapy*, Edinburgh, 2000, Churchill-Livingstone.

Pepping J: Alternative therapies. Black cohosh: cimicifuga racemosa, *Am J Health-Syst Pharm* 56:1400, 1999.

Physicians' desk reference for herbal medicines, Montvale, N.J., 1999, Medical Economics.

Smolinske SC: Dietary supplement adverse reactions and interactions, *Pharm Pract News*, Dec, 20, 1998.

Smolinske SC: Dietary supplement adverse reactions and interactions: 2000 update, *Anesthesiology News* 26(6):24, 2000.

Capsicum

Anonymous: Capsicum, MICROMEDEX, 2002, Greenwood Village, Colo. Available at: www.cooperfitness.com/content/support/pharmaceutical/altmed/detail.asp?DocID=1106. Accessed Jan. 17, 2002.

Brown L, Takeuchi D, Challoner K: Corneal abrasions associated with pepper spray exposure, *Am J Emerg Med* 18:271, 2000.

Caterina MJ et al: The capsaicin receptor: a heat-activated ion channel in the pain pathway, *Nature* 389:816, 1997.

Hautkappe M et al: Review of the effectiveness of capsaicin for painful cutaneous disorders and neural dysfunction, *Clin J Pain* 14:97, 1998.

Norton SA: Useful plants of dermatology: V. capsicum and capsaicin, *J Am Acad Dermatol* 39:626, 1998.

Reilly CA, Crouch DJ, Yost GS: Quantitative analysis of capsaicinoids in fresh peppers, oleoresin capsicum and pepper spray products, *J Forensic Sci* 46(3):502, 2001.

Robbins W: Clinical applications of capsaicinoids, *Clin J Pain* 16:S86, 2000.

Smith CG, Stopford W: Health hazards of pepper spray, *N C Med J* 60(5):268, 1999.

Wachtel RE: Capsaicin, *Reg Anesth Pain Med* 24:361, 1999.

Williams SR, Clark RF, Dunford JV: Contact dermatitis associated with capsaicin: hunan hand syndrome, *Ann Emerg Med* 25:713, 1995.

Zollman TM, Bragg RM, Harrison DA: Clinical effects of oleoresin capsicum (pepper spray) on the human cornea and conjunctiva, *Ophthalmology* 107:2186, 2000.

Chamomile

Benner M, Lee H: Anaphylactic reaction to chamomile tea, *J Allergy Clin Immunol* 52:307, 1973.

Mann C, Staba EJ: *Herbs, spices, and medicinal plants: recent advances in botany, horticulture, and pharmacology*, Phoenix, 1986, Oryx Press.

Savage FG: *The flora and folklore of Shakespeare*, Stratford-on-Avon, England, 1923, Shakespeare Press.

Cranberry

Bruneton J: *Pharmacognosy, phytochemistry, medicinal plants*, London, 1999, Lavoisier.

DeSmet P: The role of plant-derived drugs and herbal medicines in healthcare, *Drugs* 54(6):801, 1997.

Fugh-Berman A: Clinical trials of herbs, *Prim Care* 24(4):889, 1997.

Jellin JM et al: *Pharmacist's letter/prescriber's letter natural medicines comprehensive database*, ed 3, Stockton, Calif, 2000, Therapeutic Research Faculty.

Pizzorno JE, Murray MT: *Textbook of natural medicine*, vols 1 and 2, Edinburgh, 1999, Churchill-Livingstone.

Rand V: Cranberry juice for the prevention of urinary tract infection, *Altern Med Alert* Oct:116, 1999.

Saltzman JR et al: Effect of hypochlorhydria due to omeprazole treatment or atrophic gastritis on protein-bound vitamin B12 absorption, *J Am Coll Nutr* 13:584, 1994.

Dandelion

Blumenthal M, Goldman A, Brinckman J: *Herbal medicine: expanded German E, commission monographs*, Austin, 2000, American Botanical Council.

Brinker F: *Herb contraindications and drug interactions*, ed 2, Sandy, Ore, 1998, Eclectic Medical Publications.

Fetrow CW, Avila JR: *The complete guide to herbal medicines*, Springhouse, Pa, Springhouse.

Jellin JM et al: *Pharmacist's letter/prescriber's letter natural medicines comprehensive database*, ed 3, Stockton, Calif, 2000, Therapeutic Research Faculty.

Kuhn MA, Winston D: *Herbal therapy and supplements: a scientific and traditional approach*, Philadelphia, 2000, Lippincott.

Newall C, Anderson L, Phillipson JD: *Herbal medicines: a guide for healthcare professionals*, London, 1996, Pharmaceutical Press.

Neef H et al: Platelet anti-aggregating activity of Taraxacum officinale Webber, *Phytother Res* 10:S138, 1996.

Echinacea

Brinker F: *Herb contraindications and drug interactions*, ed 3, Sandy, Ore, 2001, Eclectic Medical Publications.

Bone K: Echinacea: what makes it work? *Altern Med Rev* 2(2):87, 1997.

Blumenthal M, Goldman A, Brinckman J: *Herbal medicine: expanded German E, commission monographs*, Austin, 2000, American Botanical Council.

Bruneton J: *Pharmacognosy, phytochemistry, medicinal plants*, London, 1999, Lavoisier.

Budzinski JW et al: An in vitro evaluation of human cytochrome P450 3A4 inhibition by selected herbal extracts and tinctures, *Phytomedicine* 7(4):273, 2000.

Chavez ML, Chavez PI: Monographs on alternative therapies: echinacea, *Hosp Pharm* 33(2):180, 1998.

Combest WL, Nemecz G: Echinacea, *US Pharm* October:127, 1997.

Fugh-Berman A: Clinical trials of herbs, *Prim Care* 24(4):889, 1997.

Kaye AD et al: Nutraceuticals—current concepts and the role of the anesthesiologist, part 1: echinacea, garlic, ginger, ginkgo, and St. John's wort, *Am J Anesthesiol* 27(7):405, 2000.

Kuhn MA, Winston D: *Herbal therapy and supplements: a scientific and traditional approach*, Philadelphia, 2000, Lippincott.

Jellin JM et al: *Pharmacist's letter/prescriber's letter natural medicines comprehensive database*, ed 3, Stockton, Calif, 2000, Therapeutic Research Faculty.

Mills S, Bone K: *Principles and practice of phytotherapy*, Edinburgh, 2000, Churchill-Livingstone.

Newall C, Anderson L, Phillipson JD: *Herbal medicines: a guide for healthcare professionals*, London, 1996, Pharmaceutical Press.

Norred CL: Echinacea. In Roisen MF, Fleischer LA, editors: *Essence of anesthesia practice*, ed 2, Philadephia, 2001, WB Saunders.

Shaw K: Treating cough and colds with OTC alternatives, *Pharm Times* October:62, 1998.

Tracy JW, Webster LT: Drugs used in the chemotherapy of protozoal infections (cont). In Hardman JG, Limbird LE, editors: *Goodman and Gilman's, the pharmacological basis of therapeutics*, Chicago, 2001, McGraw-Hill Medical Publishing Division.

Weiss RF, Fintelmann V: Colds and influenza, *Herbal Med* 2:213, 2000.

Zink T, Chaffin J: Herbal "health" products: what family physicians need to know, *Am Fam Physician* 58(5):1113, 1998.

Ephedra

Adverse events associated with ephedrine containing products—Texas, December 1993-September 1995, *MMWR* 45:689, 1996.

Arch JRS, Ainsworth AR, Cawthorne MA: Thermogenic and anorectic effects of ephedrine and congeners in mice and rats, *Life Sci* 30:1817, 1982.

Astrup A et al: Enhanced thermogenic responsiveness during chronic ephedrine treatment in man, *Am J Clin Nutr* 42:83, 1985.

Astrup A et al: Thermogenic synergism between ephedrine and caffeine in healthy volunteers, *Metabolism* 40(3):323, 1991.

Barrette EP: Metabolife 356 for weight loss, *Altern Med Alert* 3(1):1, 2000.

Blumenthal M, King P: Ma huang: ancient herb, modern medicine, regulatory dilemma, *Herbal Gram* 34:22, 43, 56, 1995.

Brinker F: *Herb contraindications and drug interactions*, ed 2, Sandy, Ore, 1998, Eclectic Medical Publications.

Brinker F: *Herb contraindications and drug interactions*, ed 3, Sandy, Ore, 2001, Eclectic Medical Publications.

Bruneton J: *Pharmacognosy, phytochemistry, medicinal plants*, London, 1999, Lavoisier.

Centers for Disease Control and Prevention: Adverse events associated with ephedrine-containing products, Texas, December 1993-September 1995, *JAMA* 276:1711, 1996.

Dawson JK, Earnshaw SM, Garaham CS: Dangerous monoamine oxidase inhibitor interactions are still occurring in the 1990s, *J Accident Emerg Med* 42:95, 1995.

DeWitt BJ: Ephedra. In Roisen MF, Fleischer LA, editors: *Essence of anesthesia practice*, ed 2, Philadelphia, 2001, WB Saunders.

Dullo AG, Miller DS: The thermogenic properties of ephedrine methylxanthine mixtures: human studies, *Int J Obes Relat Metabl Disord* 10:467, 1986.

Dullo AG: Ephedrine, xanthene and prostaglandin inhibitors: actions and interactions in the stimulation of thermogenesis, *Intern J of Obesity* 17(suppl 10):S35, 1993.

Grauds C: Herbal ephedra and the pharmacist, *Pharm Times* March:60, 1998.

Gurley BJ et al: Ephedrine pharmacokinetics after the ingestion of nutritional supplements containing Ephedra sinica (Ma-huang), *Ther Drug Monit* 20:439, 1998.

Gurley BJ, Wang P, Gardner SF: Ephedrine-type alkaloid content of nutritional supplements containing Ephedra sinica (Ma-huang) as determined by high performance liquid chromatography, *J Pharm Sci* 87(12):1547, 1998.

Haller CA, Benowitz NL: Adverse cardiovascular and central nervous system events associated with dietary supplements containing ephedra alkaloids, *New Eng J Med* 343(25):1833, 2000.

Lefebvre H et al: Pseudo-phaeochormocytoma after multiple drug interactions involving the selective monoamine oxidase inhibitor selegiline, *Clin Endocrin* 42:95, 1995.

Ling M, Piddlesden SJ, Morgan SB: A component of the medicinal herb ephedra blocks activation in the classical and alternative pathway of complement, *Clin Exp Immunmol* 102:582, 1995.

Malchow-Moller A et al: Ephedrine as an anorectic: the story of the Ellsinore pill, *Intern J Obesity* 5:183, 1981.

McGuffin M et al: *Botanical safety handbook*, Boca Raton, Fla, 1997, CRC Press.

McPhee M: *Supplement maker indicted: formula one contained ephedrine instead of labeled herbs*, Denver Post 5B, Oct 21, 1999.

Pizzorno JE, Murray MT: *Textbook of natural medicine*, vols 1 and 2, Edinburgh, 1999, Churchill-Livingstone.

Powell T et al: Ma-huang strikes again: ephedrine nephrolithiasis, *Am J Kidney Dis* 32(1):153, 1998.

Renfrew C, Dickson R, Schwab C: Severe hypertension following ephedrine administration in a patient receiving entacapone, *Anesthesiology* 93:1562, 2000.

Roisen MF, Fleisher LA, editors: *Essence of anesthesia practice*, ed 2, Philadelphia, 2001, WB Saunders.

White LM et al: Pharmacokinetics and cardiovascular effects of Ma-huang (Ephedra sinica) in normotensive adults, *J Clin Pharmacol* 37:116, 1997.

Evening Primrose

Bruneton, J: *Pharmacognosy, phytochemistry, medicinal plants*, London, 1999, Lavoisier.

DeSmet P: The role of plant-derived drugs and herbal medicines in healthcare, *Drugs* 54(6):801, 1997.

Dipro JT, Staffor CT, Schlesselman LS: Allergic and pseudoallergic drug reactions. In Dipiro JT et al, editors: *Pharmacotherapy. A pathophysiologic approach*, ed 4, New York, 2000, McGraw Hill.

Guivernau M et al: Clinical and experimental study on the long-term effect of dietary gamma-linolenic acid on plasma lipids, platelet aggregation, thromboxane formation, and prostacyclin production, *Prostaglandins Leukot Essent Fatty Acids* 51:311, 1994.

Jellin JM et al: *Pharmacist's letter/prescriber's letter natural medicines comprehensive database*, ed 3, Stockton, Calif, 2000, Therapeutic Research Faculty.

Li Wan A: Evening primrose oil, *Pharm J* July:666, 1991.

Mills S, Bone K: *Principles and practice of phytotherapy*, Edinburgh, 2000, Churchill-Livingstone.

Newall C, Anderson L, Phillipson JD: *Herbal medicines: a guide for healthcare professionals*, London, 1996, Pharmaceutical Press.

Norred CL, Brinker F: Potential coagulation effects of preoperative complementary and alternative medicines, *Altern Ther Health Med* 7(6):58, 2001.

Shaw D et al: Traditional remedies and food supplements: a 5-year toxicological study (1991-1995), *Drug Safety* 17(5):342, 1997.

Feverfew

Biggs MJ et al: Platelet aggregation in patients using feverfew for migraine, *Lancet* 2:776, 1982.

Brinker F: *Herb contraindications and drug interactions*, ed 3, Sandy, Ore, 2001, Eclectic Medical Publications.

Bruneton J: *Pharmacognosy, phytochemistry, medicinal plants*, London, 1999, Lavoisier.

Collier HOJ et al: Extract of feverfew inhibits prostaglandin biosynthesis, *Lancet* 2:922, 1980.

DeSmet P: The role of plant-derived drugs and herbal medicines in healthcare, *Drugs* 54(6):801, 1997.

Fugh-Berman A: Clinical trials of herbs, *Complement Altern Ther Prim Care* 24(4):889, 1997.

Gianni L, Dreitlein W: Some popular OTC herbals can interact with anticoagulant therapy, *US Pharm* May, 23:83, 84, 86, 1998.

Groenewegen WA, Heptinstall S: A comparison of the effects of an extract of feverfew and parthenolide, a component of feverfew, on human platelet activity in vitro, *J Pharm Pharmacol* 42:553, 1990.

Jellin JM et al: *Pharmacist's letter/prescriber's letter natural medicines comprehensive database*, ed 3, Stockton, Calif, 2000, Therapeutic Research Faculty.

Lösche W et al: An extract of feverfew inhibits interaction of human platelets with collagen substrates, *Thromb Res* 48(5):511, 1987.

Makheja AM, Bailey JM: The active principle in feverfew, *Lancet* 2:1054, 1981.

Miller L: Herbal medicinals, *Arch Intern Med* 158(9):2200, 1998.

Mills S, Bone K: *Principles and practice of phytotherapy*, Edinburgh, 2000, Churchill-Livingstone.

Murphy J: Preoperative considerations with herbal medicines, *AORN J* 69(1):173, 1999.

Newall C, Anderson L, Phillipson JD: *Herbal medicines: a guide for healthcare professionals*, London, 1996, Pharmaceutical Press.

Norred CL, Brinker F: Potential coagulation effects of preoperative complementary and alternative medicines, *Altern Ther Health Med* 7(6):58, 2001.

Pizzorno JE, Murray MT: *Textbook of natural medicine*, ed 2, Edinburgh, 1999, Churchill-Livingstone.

Tyler V: What pharmacists should know about herbal remedies, *J Am Pharm Assoc* NS36(1):29, 1996.

Voyno-Yasenetskaya TA et al: Effects of an extract of feverfew on endothelial cell integrity and on cAMP in rabbit perfused aorta, *J Pharm Pharmacol* 40:501, 1988.

Garlic

Apitz-Castro R et al: Effects of garlic extract and three pure components isolated from it on human platelet aggregation, arachidonate metabolism, release reaction and platelet ultrastructure, *Thromb Res* 32:155, 1983.

Blumenthal M et al, editors: *The complete German commission E monographs: therapeutic guide to herbal medicines*, Boston, Mass, 1998, American Botanical Council.

Bordia AK et al: Effect of essential oil of garlic on serum fibrinolytic activity in patients with coronary artery disease, *Atherosclerosis* 28:155, 1977.

Bordia A: Effect of garlic on human platelet aggregation in vitro, *Atherosclerosis* 30:355, 1978.

Bordia A, Verma SK, Srivastava KC: Effect of garlic (*Allium sativum*) on blood lipids, blood sugar, fibrinogen and fibrinolytic activity in patients with coronary artery disease, *Prostaglandins Leukot Essent Fatty Acids* 58(4):257, 1998.

Brinker F: *Herb contraindications and drug interactions*, ed 3, Sandy, Ore, 2001, Eclectic Medical Publications.

Burhnam BE: Garlic as a possible risk for postoperative bleeding, *Plast Reconstruc Surg* 95:213, 1995.

Ernst E: Cardiovascular effects of garlic: a review, *Pharmatherapeutica* 5:83, 1987.

German K, Kumar U, Blackford HN: Garlic and the risk of TURP bleeding, *Br J Urol* 76:518, 1995.

Gurley BJ, Gardner SF, Hubbard MA: *Clinical assessment of potential cytochrome P450-mediated herb-drug interactions*, AAPS Ann Mtg and Expo, Indianapolis, Ind, 2000, October 29-November 2, presentation #3460.

Jung EM et al: Influence of garlic powder on cutaneus microcirculation: a randomized placebo controlled double blind cross over study in apparently healthy subjects, *Arzenimittelforschung* 41(6):626, 1991.

Kleinjnen J, Knipschild P, Ter Reit G: Garlic, onion and cardiovascular risk factors: a review of the evidence form human experiments with emphasis on commercially available preparations, *Br J Clin Pharmacol* 28:535, 1989.

Lawson LD, Ransom DK, Hughes BG: Inhibition of whole blood platelet-aggregation by compounds in garlic clove extracts and commercial garlic products, *Thromb Res* 65(2):141, 1992.

Legnani C et al: Effects of a dried garlic preparation on fibrinolysis and platelet aggregation in healthy subjects, *Arzneimittelforschung* 43:119, 1993.

Makheja AN, Bailey JM: Antiplatelet constituents of garlic and onion, *Agents Actions* 29(3/4):360, 1990.

Makheja AN, Vanderhoek JY, Bailey JM: Inhibition of platelet aggregation and thromboxane synthesis by onion and garlic, *Lancet* 7:781, 1979.

Mashour, NH: Herbal medicines for the treatment of cardiovascular disease, *Arch Int Med* 158:2225, 1998.

Mohammad SF, Woodward SC: Characterization of a potent inhibitor of platelet aggregation and release reaction isolated from Allium sativum (garlic), *Thromb Res* 44:793, 1986.

Norred CL, Brinker F: Potential coagulation effects of preoperative complementary and alternative medicines, *Altern Ther Health Med* 7(6):58, 2001.

Oshiba S et al: Inhibitory effect of orally administered inclusion complex of garlic oil on platelet aggregation in man, *Igaku no Ayuma* 155(3):199, 1990.

Pantoja CV, Chiang BC, Concha JB: Diuretic, natriuretic and hypotensive effects produced by *Allium sativum* (garlic) in anaesthetized dogs, *J Ethnopharmacol* 31:325, 1991.

Pedraza-Chaverri J et al: Garlic prevent hypertension induced by chronic inhibition of nitric oxide synthesis, *Life Sci* 62(6):PL71, 1998.

Rietz B et al: The radical scavenging ability of garlic examined in various models, *Boll Chim Farmaceutico Anno* 134(2):69, 1995.

Ronzio RA: Naturally occurring antioxidants. In Pizzorno JE, Murray MT, editors: *Textbook of natural medicine*, ed 2, Edinburgh, 1999, Churchill-Livingstone.

Rose KD et al: Spontaneous spinal epidural hematoma with associated with platelet dysfunction from excessive garlic ingestion: a case report, *Neurosurgery* 26:880, 1990.

Srivastava KC: Aqueous extracts of onion, garlic and ginger inhibit platelet aggregation and alter arachidonic acid metabolism, *Biomed Biochim Acta* 43(S):335, 1984.

Silagy C, Neil A: A meta-analysis of the effect of garlic upon blood pressure, *Hypertens* 12:463, 1994.

Warshafsky S, Kramer RS, Sivak SL: Effect of garlic on total serum cholesterol, *Annal Int Med* 119:599, 1993.

Ginger

Bone ME et al: Ginger root—a new antiemetic: the effect of ginger root on postoperative nausea and vomiting after major gynecological surgery, *Anesthesia* 45:669, 1990.

Brinker F: *Herb contraindications and drug interactions*, ed 3, Sandy, Ore, 2001, Eclectic Medical Publications.

Combest WL: Ginger, *US Pharm* February:74, 1998.

Lumb AB: Effect of dried ginger on human platelet function, *Thromb Haemost* 71(1):110, 1994.

Pancho L et al: Reversed effects between crude and processed ginger extracts on PGF2 alpha-induced contraction in mouse mesenteric veins, *Jpn J Pharmacol* 50:243, 1989.

Phillips S, Ruggier R, Hutchinson SE: Zingiber officinale (Ginger)—an antiemetic for day case surgery, *Anesthesia* 48:715, 1993.

Rivera L et al: Reversal effects between crude and processed ginger extracts on PGF 2 alpha–induced contraction in mouse mesenteric veins, *Jpn J Pharmacol* 50:243, 1989.

Shoji N, Iwasa A: Cardiotonic principle of ginger (Zingiber officinale Roscue), *J Phar Sci* 71(10):1174, 1982.

Suekawa M, Aburada M: Pharmacological studies on ginger. Effect of the spinal destruction on (6)-shoagaol-induced pressor response in rats, *J Pharmacolobio Dyn* 9:853, 1986.

Ginkgo

Cupp MJ: Herbal remedies: adverse effects and drug interactions, *Am Fam Physician* 59:1239, 1999.

Hadley SK, Petry JJ: Medicinal herbs: a primer for primary care, *Hosp Pract* 34:112, 1999.

Knight J: An introduction to common medicinal herbs, *Physician Assist* 12:55, 2000.

Muirhead G: Herbal remedies you can send with confidence, *Patient Care* 33:76, 1999.

Schwetschenau KH, Seaburg D: Update on drug therapies: clinical uses and adverse effects of echinacea, ginkgo biloba, and ginseng, *Hosp Med* 35:49, 1999.

Ginseng

Bratman S, Kroll D: *Natural health bible*, New York, 1999, Prima.

Brinker F: *Herb contraindications and drug interactions*, ed 3, Sandy, Ore, 2001, Eclectic Medical Publications.

Cupp MJ: Herbal remedies: adverse effects and drug interactions, *Am Fam Physician* 59:1239, 1999.

Hadley SK, Petry JJ: Clinical experience: medicinal herbs: a primer for primary care, *Hosp Pract* 34:112, 1999.

Hammond TG, Whitworth JA: Adverse reactions to ginseng, *Med J Austral* 1:492, 1981.

Janetzky K, Morreale AP: Probable interaction between warfarin and ginseng, *Am J Health-Syst Pharm* 54:692, 1997.

Jones BD, Runikis AM: Interaction of ginseng with phenelzine, *J Clin Psychopharmacol* 7:201, 1987.

Jung KY et al: Platelet activating factor antagonist activity of ginsenosides, *Biol Pharm Bull* 21(1):79, 1998.

Knight J: An introduction to common medicinal herbs, *Physician Assist* 12:55, 2000.

Kuo SC et al: Antiplatelet components in Panax ginseng, *Planta Med* 56:164, 1990.

Lei XL et al: Cardiovascular pharmacology of Panax notoginseng (Burk) (F.H. Chren and *Salvia miltiorrhiza*), *Am J Chinese Med* 14:145, 1986.

Li XJ, Zhang BH: Studies on the anti-arrhythmia effects of panaxatriol saponins isolated from Panax notoginseng, *Yao Xue Xue Bao* 23:168, 1988.

Matsuda H et al: Effects of red ginseng on experimental disseminated intravascular coagulation: effects of ginsenosides on blood coagulative and fibrinolytic systems, *Chem Pharm Bull* 34(3):1153, 1986.

Mills S, Bone K: *Principles and practice of phytotherapy*, Edinburgh, 2000, Churchill-Livingstone.

Muirhead G: Herbal remedies you can send with confidence, *Patient Care* 33:76, 1999.

Schwetschenau KH, Seaburg D: Update on drug therapies: clinical uses and adverse effects of echinacea, ginkgo biloba, and ginseng, *Hosp Med* 35:49, 1999.

Siegel RK: Ginseng abuse syndrome, *JAMA* 241:1614, 1979.

Vogler RK, Pittler MH, Ernst E: The efficacy of ginseng: a systematic review of randomized clinical trials, *Eur J Pharmacol* 55:567, 1999.

Wu JX, Chen JX: Negative chronotropic and inotropic effects of Panax saponins, *Acta Pharmacol Sin* 9:409, 1988.

Zhu M et al: Possible influences of ginseng on the pharmacokinetics and pharmacodynamics of warfarin in rats, *J Pharm Pharmacol* 51:175, 1999.

Goldenseal

Bratman S, Kroll D: *Natural health bible*, New York, 1999, Prima.

Budzinski JW et al: An in vitro evaluation of human cytochrome P450 3A4 inhibition by selected herbal extracts and tinctures, *Phytomedicine* 7(4):273, 2000.

Fetrow CW, Avila JR: *The complete guide to herbal medicines*, Springhouse, Pa, 2000, Springhouse.

Jellin JM et al: *Pharmacist's letter/prescriber's letter natural medicines comprehensive database*, ed 3, Stockton, Calif, 2000, Therapeutic Research Faculty.

Newall C, Anderson L, Phillipson JD: *Herbal medicines: a guide for healthcare professionals*, London, 1996, Pharmaceutical Press.

Preininger V: The pharmacology and toxicology of the Papaveraceae alkaloids. In Holmed HL, editor: *Alkaloids* 15:239, 1975.

Hawthorn

Bratman S, Kroll D: *Natural health bible*, New York, 1999, Prima.

Brinker F: Botanical medicine research summaries. In *Eclectic dispensatory of botanical therapeutics*, vol 2, Sandy, Ore, 1995, Eclectic Medical Publications.

Brinker F: *Herb contraindications and drug interactions*, ed 3, Sandy, Ore, 2001, Eclectic Medical Publications.

Gildor A: Crataegus oxyacantha and heart failure, *Circulation* 99(1):2098, 1998.

Gundling K, Ernst E: Complementary and alternative medicine in cardiovascular disease: what is the evidence that it works? *WJM* 1781:191, 1999.

Hahn F, Kinkhammer F, Oberdorf A: Preparation and pharmacological investigation of a new therapeutic agent obtained from Crataegus oxyacnatha, *Arzneim Forsch* 10:825, 1960.

Hobbs C, Foster S: Hawthorn, a literature review, *Herbalgram* 22:19, 1990.

Jellin JM et al: *Pharmacist's letter/prescriber's letter natural medicines comprehensive database*, ed 3, Stockton, Calif, 2000, Therapeutic Research Faculty.

Mashour NH: Herbal medicines for the treatment of cardiovascular disease, *Arch Int Med* 158:2225, 1998.

Mills S, Bone K: *Hawthorn. Principles and practice of phytotherapy: modern herbal medicine*, Edinburgh, 2000, Churchill-Livingstone.

Nasa Y et al: Protective effect of Crataegus extract on the cardiac mechanical dysfunction in isolated perfused working rat heart, *Arzneimittelforschung* 43:945, 1993.

Nemecz G: Hawthorn, *US Pharm* February:52, 1999.

Newall C, Anderson L, Phillipson JD: *Herbal medicines: a guide for healthcare professionals*, London, 1996, Pharmaceutical Press.

Schussler M, Holzl J, Fricke U: Myocardial effects of flavonoids from Crataegus species, *Arzneimittelforschung* 45:842, 1995.

Taskov M: On the coronary and cardiotonic action of Crataegus, *Acta Physiol Pharmacol Bulg* 3:53, 1997.

Trunzler G, Schuler E: Comparative studies on the effects of a Crataegus extract, digitoxin, digoxin and Strophanthin in the isolated heart of homoithermals, *Arzneim-Forsch* 12:198, 1962.

Tyler VE: *Herbs of choice: the therapeutic use of phytomedicinals*, New York, 1994, Pharmaceutical Product Press.

Vibes J et al: Inhibition of thromboxane A2 biosynthesis in vitro by the main components of Crataegus oxyacantha (hawthorn) flower heads, *Prostaglandins Leukot Essent Fatty Acids* 50:173, 1994.

Weikl A et al: Crataegus special extract WS 1442: assessment of objective effectiveness in patients with heart failure (NYHA II), *Fortschr Med* 114:291, 1996.

Zapatero JM: Selection from current literature: effects of hawthorn on the cardiovascular system, *Fam Pract* 16(5):534, 1999.

Hop

Blumenthal M, Goldman A, Brinckman J: *Herbal medicine: expanded German E, commission monographs*, Austin, 2000, American Botanical Council.

Brinker F: *Herb contraindications and drug interactions*, ed 3, Sandy, Ore, 2001, Eclectic Medical Publications.

Bruneton, J: *Pharmacognosy, phytochemistry, medicinal plants*, London, 1999, Lavoisier.

Jellin JM et al: *Pharmacist's letter/prescriber's letter natural medicines comprehensive database*, ed 3, Stockton, Calif, 2000, Therapeutic Research Faculty.

Newall C, Anderson L, Phillipson JD: *Herbal medicines: a guide for healthcare professionals*, London, 1996, Pharmaceutical Press.

Physicians' desk reference for herbal medicines, Montvale, N.J., 1999, Medical Economics.

Weiss RF, Fintelmann V: *Herbal medicine*, ed 2, Stuttgart, 2000, Thieme.

Kava Kava

Attle AS, Xie JT, Yuan CS: Treatment of insomnia: an alternative approach, *Altern Med Rev* 5(3):249, 2000.

Blumenthal M, Goldman A, Brinckman J: *Herbal medicine: expanded German E, commission monographs*, Austin, 2000, American Botanical Council.

Brinker F: *Herb contraindications and drug interactions*, ed 3, Sandy, Ore, 2001, Eclectic Medical Publications.

Brown R: Potential interactions of herbal medicines with antipsychotics, antidepressants and hypnotics, *Eur J Herbal Med* 3(2):25, 1997.

Bruneton J: *Pharmacognosy, phytochemistry, medicinal plants*, London, 1999, Lavoisier.

De Smet P: The role of plant-derived drugs and herbal medicines in healthcare, *Drugs* 54(6):801, 1997.

Fontenot B: *Kava*. Available at: www.findarticles.com/cf_dls/m0GCU/3_16/61500432/print.jhtml. Accessed December 7, 2001.

Gleitz J et al: Antithrombotic action of the kava pyrone (+)-kavain prepared from *Piper methysticum* on human platelets, *Planta Med* 63:27, 1997.

Heiligenstein E, Guenther G: Over-the-counter psychotropics: a review of melatonin, St. John's wort, valerian, and kava-kava, *J Am Coll Health* 46:271, 1998.

Jellin JM et al: *Pharmacist's letter/prescriber's letter natural medicines comprehensive database*, ed 3, Stockton, Calif, 2000, Therapeutic Research Faculty.

Lake, J: Psychotropic medications from natural products: a review of promising research and recommendations, *Altern Ther Health Med* 6(3):36, 2000.

Norred CL, Brinker F: Potential coagulation effects of preoperative complementary and alternative medicines, *Altern Ther Health Med* 7(6):58, 2001.

Piscopo G: Kava kava: gift of the islands, *Altern Med Rev* 2(5):355, 1997.

Pittler MH, Ernst E: Efficacy of kava extract for treating anxiety: a systemic review and meta-analysis, *J Clin Psychopharmacol* 20(1):84, 2000.

Rosenberg RN: Ataxic disorders. In Braunwald E et al, editors: *Harrison's principles of internal medicine*, ed 15, New York, 2001, McGraw-Hill.

Wagner J, Wagner ML, Hening WA: Beyond benzodiazepines: alternative pharmacologic agents for the treatment of insomnia, *Ann Pharmacother* 32:680, 1998.

Licorice

Armanini D et al: Further studies on the mechanism of the mineralocorticoid action of licorice in humans, *J Endocrinol Invest* 19:624, 1996.

Bannister B, Ginsburg R, Shneerswon J: Cardiac arrest due to liquorice-induced hypokalemia, *BMJ* 17:738, 1977.

Bianchi P et al: Comparison of pirenzepine and carbenoxolone in the treatment of chronic gastric ulcers: a double blind endoscopic trail, *Hepatogastroenterology* 32(6):293, 1985.

Brinker F: *Herb contraindications and drug interactions*, ed 3, Sandy, Ore, 2001, Eclectic Medical Publications.

Bruneton J: *Pharmacognosy, phytochemistry, medicinal plants*, London, 1999, Lavoisier.

Budzinski JW et al: An in vitro evaluation of human cytochrome P450 3A4 inhibition by selected herbal extracts and tinctures, *Phytomedicine* 7(4):273, 2000.

Caradonna P et al: Acute myopathy associated with chronic licorice ingestion: reversible loss of myoadenylate deaminase activity, *Ultrastruct Pathol* 16:529, 1999.

Chamberlain JJ, Abolnik, IZ: Pulmonary edema following a licorice binge, *WJM* 167(3):184, 1997.

Chamberlain TJ: Licorice poisoning pseudoaldosteronism and heart failure, *JAMA* 213(8):1343, 1970.

Chen MF et al: Effect of glycyrrhizin on the pharmacokinetics of prednisolone following low dosage of prednisolone hemisuccinate, *Endocrinol Jpn* 37(3):331, 1990.

Combest WL: Licorice, *US Pharm* April:125, 1998.

Famularo G, Corsio, FM, Giacanelli M: Iatrogenic worsening of hypokalemia and neuromuscular paralysis associated with the use of glucose solutions for potassium replacement in a young woman with licorice intoxication and furosemide abuse, *Acad Emerg Med* 6(9):960, 1999.

Ishikawa S et al: Licorice induced hypokalemic myopathy and hypokalemic renal tubular damage in anorexia nervosa, *Int J Eat Disord* 26:111, 1999.

Jellin JM et al: *Pharmacist's letter/prescriber's letter natural medicines comprehensive database*, ed 3, Stockton, Calif, 2000, Therapeutic Research Faculty.

Mashour NH: Herbal medicines for the treatment of cardiovascular disease, *Arch Int Med* 158:2225, 1998.

McGuffin M et al: *Botanical safety handbook*, Boca Raton, Fla, 1977, CRC Press.

Newall C, Anderson L, Phillipson JD: *Herbal medicines: a guide for healthcare professionals*, London, 1996, Pharmaceutical Press.

Norred CL, Brinker F: Potential coagulation effects of preoperative complementary and alternative medicines, *Altern Ther Health Med* 7(6):58, 2001.

Paolini M et al: Effect of licorice and glycyrrhizin on murine liver CYP-dependant monooxygenase, *Life Sci* 62:571, 1998.

Physicians' desk reference for herbal medicines, Montvale, N.J., 1999, Medical Economics.

Saito T et al: An autopsy case of licorice induced hypokalemic rhabdomyolysis associated with acute renal failure: special reference to profound calcium deposition in skeletal and cardiac muscle, *Jpn J Nephrol* 35(11):1308, 1994.

Shintani S et al: Glycyrrhizin (licorice)-induced hypokalemic myopathy, *Eur Neurol* 32:44, 1992.

Passionflower

Blumenthal M, Goldman A, Brinckman J: *Herbal medicine: expanded German E, commission monographs*, Austin, 2000, American Botanical Council.

Brinker F: *Herb contraindications and drug interactions*, ed 3, Sandy, Ore, 2001, Eclectic Medical Publications.

Brown R: Potential interactions of herbal medicines with antipsychotics, antidepressants and hypnotics, *Eur J Herbal Med* 3(2):25, 1997.

Bruneton, J: *Pharmacognosy, phytochemistry, medicinal plants*, London, 1999, Lavoisier.

Fetrow CW, Avila JR: *The complete guide to herbal medicines*, Springhouse, Pa, 1999, Springhouse.

Jellin JM et al: *Pharmacist's letter/prescriber's letter natural medicines comprehensive database*, ed 3, Stockton, Calif, 2000, Therapeutic Research Faculty.

Speroni E, Minghetti A: Neuropharmacological activity of extracts from *Passiflora incarnata*, *Planta Med* 54(6):488, 1988.

Red Clover

Brinker F: *Herb contraindications and drug interactions*, ed 3, Sandy, Ore, 2001, Eclectic Medical Publications.

Budzinski JW et al: An in vitro evaluation of human cytochrome P450 3A4 inhibition by selected herbal extracts and tinctures, *Phytomedicine* 7(4):273, 2000.

Christopher JR: *School of natural healing*, printing 11, Springville, Utah, 1996, Christopher Publications.

Evans AM: Influence of dietary components on the gastrointestinal metabolism and transport of drugs, *Ther Drug Monit* 22(1):131, 2000.

Hoult JRS, Paya M: Pharmacological and biochemical actions of simple coumarins: natural products with therapeutic potential, *Gen Pharmac* 27(4):713, 1996.

Jellin JM et al: *Pharmacist's letter/prescriber's letter natural medicines comprehensive database*, ed 3, Stockton, Calif, 2000, Therapeutic Research Faculty.

Newall C, Anderson L, Phillipson JD: *Herbal medicines: a guide for healthcare professionals*, London, 1996, Pharmaceutical Press.

Norred CL, Brinker F: Potential coagulation effects of preoperative complementary and alternative medicines, *Altern Ther Health Med* 7(6):58, 2001.

Physicians' desk reference for herbal medicines, Montvale, N.J., 1999, Medical Economics.

St. John's Wort

Barone GW et al: Drug interaction between St. John's wort and cyclosporine, *Ann Pharmacother* 34(9):1013, 2000.

Baureithel KH et al: Inhibition of benzodiazepine binding in vitro by amentoflavone, a constituent of various species of *Hypericum*, *Pharm Acta Helv* 72:153, 1997.

Beckman SE, Sommi RW, Switzer J: Consumer use of St. John's wort: a survey on effectiveness, safety and tolerability, *Pharmacotherapy* 20(5):568, 2000.

Bennet DA et al: Neuropharmacology of St. John's wort (hypericum), *Ann Pharmacother* 32:1201, 1998.

Brenner R et al: Comparison of an extract of Hypericum (LI 160) and sertraline in the treatment of depression: a double-blind randomized pilot study, *Clin Ther* 22(4):411, 2000.

Brinker F: *Herb contraindications and drug interactions*, ed 3, Sandy, Ore, 2001, Eclectic Medical Publications.

Brown R: Potential interactions of herbal medicines with antipsychotics, antidepressants and hypnotics, *Eur J Herbal Med* 3(2):25, 1997.

Budzinski JW et al: An in vitro evaluation of human cytochrome P450 3A4 inhibition by selected commercial herbal extracts and tinctures, *Phytomedicine* 7(4):273, 2000.

Calapai G et al: Effects of *Hypericum perforatum* on levels of 5-hydroxytryptamine, noradrenaline and dopamine in the cortex, diencephalons and brainstem of the rat, *J Pharm Pharmacol* 51:723, 1999.

Chatterjee SS et al: Hyperiforin as a possible antidepressant component of Hypericum extracts, *Life Sci* 63(6):499, 1998.

Ciordia R: Beware "St. John's wort," potential herbal danger, *J Clin Monit Comput* 14:215, 1998.

Czekalla J et al: The effect of Hypericum on cardiac conduction as seen in the electrocardiogram compared to that of imipramine, *Pharmacopsychiatry* 30(2):86, 1997.

D'Archy PF: Adverse reactions and interactions with herbal medicines. Part 2—Drug interactions, *Adverse Drug React Toxicol Rev* 12(3):147, 1993.

Gaster B, Holroyd J: St. John's wort for depression: a systematic review, *Arch Int Med* 160:152, 2000.

Gordon JB: SSRIs and St. John's wort: possible toxicity? *Am Fam Physician* 57(5):950, 1998.

Jellin JM et al: *Pharmacist's letter/prescriber's letter natural medicines comprehensive database*, ed 3, Stockton, Calif, 2000, Therapeutic Research Faculty.

Johne A et al: Pharmacokinetic interaction of digoxin with an herbal extract from St. John's wort (*Hypericum perforatum*), *Clin Pharmacol Ther* 66:338, 1999.

Kaehler ST et al: Hyperforin enhances the extracellular concentrations of catecholamines, serotonin and glutamate in the rat locus coeruleus, *Neurosci Lett* 262:199, 1999.

Linde K et al: St. John's wort for depression—an overview and meta-analysis of randomized clinical trials, *BMJ* 313:253, 1996.

Markowitz JS et al: Effect of St. John's Wort (Hypericum perforatum) on cytochrome P-450 2D6 and 3A4A activity in healthy volunteers, *Life Sci* 66(9):133, 2000.

Miller AL: St. John's wort (Hypericum perforatum): clinical effects on depression and other conditions, *Altern Med Rev* 3(1):18, 1998.

Moore LB et al: St. John's wort induces hepatic drug metabolism through activation of the pregnange X receptor, *Proc Natl Acad Sci U S A* 97(13):7500, 2000.

Neary JT, Bu Y: Hypericum LI 160 inhibits uptake of serotonin and norepinephrine in astrocytes, *Brain Res* 816:358, 1999.

Nebel A et al: Potential metabolic interactions between St. John's wort and theophylline, *Ann Pharmacother* 33:502, 1999.

Obach RS: Inhibition of human cytochrome P450 enzymes by constituents of St. John's wort, an herbal preparation used in the treatment of depression, *J Pharmacol Exp Ther* 294(1):88, 2000.

Okpanyi Von SN, Wiescher ML: Experimental animal studies of the psychotropic activity of a Hypericum extract, *Fortschr Arzneimittelforsch* 37:10, 1987.

Phillip M, Kohnene R, Hiller KO: Hypericum extract versus imipramine or placebo in patients with moderate depression: randomized multicenter study of treatment of eight weeks, *BMJ* 319:1534, 1999.

Piscitelli SC et al: Indinavir concentrations and St. John's wort, *Lancet* 355:547, 2000.

Raffa RB: Screen of receptor and uptake-site activity of hypericin component of St. John's wort reveals sigma receptor binding, *Life Sci* 62(16):265, 1998.

Roby CA et al: St. John's wort: effect on CYP3A4 activity, *Clin Pharmacol Ther* 67(5):451, 2000.

Simmen U et al: Extracts and constituents of *Hypericum perforatum* inhibit the binding of various ligands to recombinant receptors expressed with the Semliki Forest virus system, *J Recept Signal Transduct Res* 19(1-4):59, 1999.

Simmen U et al: *Hypericum perforatum* inhibits the binding of α- and β-opioid receptor expressed with the Semliki Forest virus system, *Pharm Acta Helv* 73:53, 1998.

Smolinske SC: Dietary supplement-drug interactions, *J Am Med Womens Assoc* 54:191, 1999.

Snow V, Lascher S, Mottur-Pilson C: Pharmacologic treatment of acute major depression and dysthymia, *Ann Intern Med* 132:738, 2000.

Suzuki O et al: Inhibition of monamine oxidase by hypericin, *Planta Med* 786(3):272, 1984.

Wentworth JM et al: St. John's wort, an herbal antidepressant, activates the steroid X receptor, *J Endocrinol* 166(3):R11, 2000.

Wonnemann M, Singer A, Muller WE: Inhibition of synaptosomal uptake of 3H-L-glutamate and 3H-GABA by hyperforin, a major constituent of St. John's wort: the role of amiloride sensitive sodium conductive pathways, *Neuropsychopharmacology* 23(2):188, 2000.

Section 2: Vitamins and Dietary Supplements

Chondroitin

Bourgeois P et al: Efficacy and tolerability of chondroitin sulfate 1200 mg/day vs chondroitin sulfate 3 x 400 mg/day vs placebo, *Osteoarthritis Cartilage* 6:25, 1998.

Bucsi L, Poor G: Efficacy and tolerability of oral chondroitin sulfate as a symptomatic slow-acting drug for osteoarthritis (SYSADOA) in the treatment of knee osteoarthritis, *Osteoarthritis Cartilage* 6:31, 1998.

Das A Jr, Hammad TA: Efficacy of a combination of fchg49 glucosamine hydrochloride, trh122 low–molecular-weight sodium chondroitin sulfate and manganese ascorbate in the management of knee osteoarthritis, *Osteoarthritis Cartilage* 8:343, 2000.

Deal CL, Moskowitz RW: Nutraceuticals as therapeutic agents in osteoarthritis: the role of glucosamine, chondroitin sulfate, and collagen hydrolysate, *Rheum Dis Clin North Am* 25:379, 1999.

Delafuente JC: Glucosamine in the treatment of osteoarthritis, *Rheum Dis Clin North Am* 26:1, vii, 2000.

Lippiello L et al: In vivo chondroprotection and metabolic synergy of glucosamine and chondroitin sulfate, *Clin Orthop* Dec(381): 229, 2000.

Mazieres B et al: Chondroitin sulfate in osteoarthritis of the knee: a prospective, double-blind, placebo-controlled multicenter clinical study, *J Rheumatol* 28:173, 2001.

McAlindon TE et al: Glucosamine and chondroitin for treatment of osteoarthritis: a systematic quality assessment and meta-analysis, *JAMA* 283:1469, 2000.

O'Rourke M: Determining the efficacy of glucosamine and chondroitin for osteoarthritis, *Nurs Pract* 26:44, 49, 2001.

Verbruggen G, Goemaere S, Veys EM: Chondroitin sulfate: S/DMAOD (structure/disease modifying anti-osteoarthritis drug) in the treatment of finger joint OA, *Osteoarthritis Cartilage* 6:37, 1998.

Coenzyme Q10

Digiesi V et al: Coenzyme Q10 in essential hypertension, *Molec Aspect Med* 15:S257, 1994.

Greenberg S, Frishman WH: Coenzyme Q10: a new drug for cardiovascular disease, *J Clin Pharmacol* 30:596, 1990.

Jellin JM et al: *Pharmacist's letter/prescriber's letter natural medicines comprehensive database*, ed 3, Stockton, Calif, 2000, Therapeutic Research Faculty.

Kuhn MA, Winston D: *Herbal therapy and supplements: a scientific and traditional approach*, Philadelphia, 2000, Lippincott.

Pepping J: Alternative therapies: coenzyme Q10, *Am J Health-Syst Pharm* 56:519, 1999.

Fish Oil

Abeywarden MY, Head RJ: Long-chain n-3 polyunsaturated fatty acids and blood vessel function, *Cardiovasc Res* 52:361, 2001.

Aronson WJ et al: Modulation of omega-3/omega-6 polyunsaturated ratios with dietary fish oils in men with prostate cancer, *Urology* 58:283, 2001.

Barber MD: Cancer cachexia and its treatment with fish-oil-enriched nutritional supplementation, *Nutrition* 17:751, 2001.

Calder PC: Polyunsaturated fatty acids, inflammation, and immunity, *Lipids* 36:1007, 2001.

Hallgren CG et al: Markers of high fish intake are associated with decreased risk of a first myocardial infarction, *Br J Nutr* 86:397, 2001.

Marz RB: *Medical nutrition from Marz*, ed 2, Portland, Ore, 1997, Omni-Press.

Schauss AG: Fish oils. In Pizzorno JE, Murray MT, editors: *Textbook of naturopathic medicine*, ed 2, New York, 2000, Churchill-Livingstone.

Wilson ML, Murphy PA: Herbal and dietary therapies for primary and secondary dysmenorrheal (Cochrane Review), *Cochrane Database Syst Rev* 3:CD002124, 2001.

Glucosamine

Deal CL, Moskowitz RW: Nutraceuticals as therapeutic agents in osteoarthritis: the role of glucosamine, chondroitin sulfate, and collagen hydrolysate, *Rheum Dis Clin North Am* 25:379, 1999.

Delafuente JC: Glucosamine in the treatment of osteoarthritis, *Rheum Dis Clin North Am* 26:1, 2000.

Lippiello L et al: In vivo chondroprotection and metabolic synergy of glucosamine and chondroitin sulfate, *Clin Orthop* Dec(381): 229, 2000.

McAlindon TE et al: Glucosamine and chondroitin for treatment of osteoarthritis: a systematic quality assessment and meta-analysis, *JAMA* 283:1469, 2000.

O'Rourke M: Determining the efficacy of glucosamine and chondroitin for osteoarthritis, *Nurs Pract* 26:44, 49, 2001.

Vitamin C

Brinker F: *Appendix D: drug and mineral interactions with vitamin supplements. Herb contraindications and drug interactions*, ed 3, Sandy, Ore, 2001, Eclectic Medical Publications.

Fetrow CW, Avila JR: *Complete guide to herbal medicines*, Springhouse, Pa, 2000, Springhouse.

Jellin JM et al: *Pharmacist's letter/prescriber's letter natural medicines comprehensive database*, ed 3, Stockton, Calif, 2000, Therapeutic Research Faculty.

Hanrahan C: *Rose hip*. Available at: www.findarticles.com/cf_dls/ g2603/0006/2603000634/print.jhtml. Accessed December 7, 2001.

Ronzio RA: *Textbook of natural medicine*, ed 2, Edinburgh, 1999, Churchill-Livingstone.

Wardlaw GM: *Perspectives in nutrition*, ed 4, Boston, Mass, 1999, McGraw Hill.

Vitamin E

Berdanier CD: *Advanced nutrition*, Boca Raton, Fla, 1999, CRC Press.

Eitenmiller RR, Landen Jr. WO: *Vitamin analysis for the health and food sciences*, Boca Raton, Fla, 1998, CRC Press.

Machlin LJ: *Vitamin E*, New York, 1980, Marcel Dekker.

Meydani M: *Vitamin E*, Lancet 345(8943):170, 1995.

Sauberlich HE: *Assessment of nutritional status*, ed 2, Boca Raton, Fla, 1999, CRC Press.

Part II: Nonpharmacologic Therapies Section 3: Healing with Physical Power

Chiropractic Therapy

Kuhn MA: *Complementary therapies for health care providers*, Philadelphia, 1999, Lippincott–William & Wilkins.

Massage Therapy

Beck MF: *Milady's theory and practice of therapeutic massage*, ed 3, New York, 1999, Milady Publishing.

Billhult A, Dahlberg K: A meaningful relief from suffering: experiences of massage in cancer care, *Cancer Nurs* 24(3):180, 2001.

Birk TJ et al: The effects of massage therapy alone and in combination with other complementary therapies on immune system measures and quality of life in human immunodeficiency virus, *J Altern Complement Med* 6(5):405, 2000.

Contraindications for the use of stroking massage, *WebMD*. Available at: http://my.webmd.com/content/dmk/dmk_article_58933. Accessed November 11, 2001.

Ferrell-Torry A, Glick OJ: The use of therapeutic massage as a nursing intervention to modify anxiety and the perception of cancer pain, *Cancer Nurs* 16(2):93, 1993.

Field T, Scafidi F, Schanberg S: Massage of preterm newborns to improve growth and development, *Pediatr Nurs* 13(6):385, 1987.

Field T: Massage therapy for infants and children, *J Dev Behav Pediatr* 16(2):105, 1995.

Fontaine KL: *Massage in healing practices: alternative therapies for nursing*, Upper Saddle River, N.J., 2000, Prentice Hall.

The history of massage. Available at: http://www.cam.ac.uk/societies/cumass/html/history.htm. Accessed November 11, 2001.

Horrigan B: Maternity massage: another woman's touch eases labor pain, *Choices Health Med* 1(1):10, 2001.

Horrigan C: Massage. In Rankin-Box D, editor: *The nurse's handbook of complementary therapies*, ed 2, Edinburgh, 2001, Bailliere Tindall.

Koehn ML: Alternative and complementary therapies for labor and birth: an application of Kolcaba's theory of holistic comfort, *Holist Nurs Pract* 15(1):66, 2000.

Low Dog T: Conventional and alternative treatments for endometriosis, *Altern Ther Health Med* 7(6):50, 2001.

Massage therapy. Mind, Body, Spirit Clinic at the University of Minnesota. Available at: http://www.fairview.org/mindbodyspirit/massage.html. Accessed November 21, 2001.

Maxwell-Hudson C: *Massage: the ultimate illustrated guide*, New York, 1999, DK Publishing.

Meek SS: Effects of slow stroke back massage on relaxation in hospice clients, *Image J Nurs Sch* 25(1):17, 1993.

Mitzel-Wilkinson A: Massage therapy as a nursing practice, *Holist Nurs Pract* 14(2):48, 2001.

Norred CL: Minimizing preoperative anxiety with alternative caring-healing therapies, *AORN J* 72(5):838, 2000.

Preyde M: Effectiveness of massage therapy for subacute low-back pain: a randomized controlled trial, *Can Med Assoc J* 162(13): 1815, 2000. Also available at: http://www.cma.ca/cmaj/vol-162/ issue-13/1815.htm. Accessed October 29, 2001.

Richards KC: Effect of a back massage and relaxation intervention on sleep in critically ill patients, *Am J Crit Care* 7(4): 288, 1998.

Sansone P, Schmitt L: Providing tender touch massage to elderly nursing home residents: a demonstration project, *Geriatr Nurs* 21(6):303, 2000.

Shealy CN, editor: *The complete illustrated encyclopedia of alternative healing therapies*, New York, 1999, Barnes and Noble.

Smith MC et al: Benefits of massage therapy for hospitalized patients: a descriptive and qualitative evaluation, *Altern Ther Health Med* 5(4):64, 1995.

Snyder M, Cheng WY: Massage. In Snyder M, Lindquist R: *Complementary/alternative therapies in nursing*, ed 3, New York, 1998, Springer Publishing.

Weil A: The healing power of massage, *Self Healing* Aug:2, 1999.

Weil A: A healthier hospital stay, *Self Healing* Aug:2, 2000.

Weil A: Massage soothes back pain, *Self Healing* July:3, 2001.

White JA: Touching with intent: therapeutic massage, *Holist Nurs Pract* 2(3):63, 1988.

Qigong and Tai Chi

Ai AL et al: Designing clinical trials on energy healing: ancient art encounters medical science, *Altern Ther Health Med* 7(4):83, 2001.

Cerrato PL: Tai Chi: a martial art turns therapeutic, *RN* 62(2): 59, 1999.

Chen KM, Snyder M: A research-based use of Tai Chi/movement therapy as a nursing intervention, *J Holistic Nurs* 17(3):267, 1999.

Cohen KS: *The way of Qigong: the art and science of Chinese energy healing*, New York, 1997, Ballantine Books.

Creamer P et al: Sustained improvement produced by nonpharmacologic intervention in fibromyalgia: results of a pilot study, *Arthritis Care Res* 13(4):198, 2000.

Ehling D: Oriental medicine: an introduction, *Altern Ther Health Med* 7(4):71, 2001.

Fontana JA: The energy costs of a modified form of T'ai Chi exercise, *Nurs Res* 49(2):91, 2000.

Fontana JA et al: T'ai Chi chih as an intervention for heart failure, *Nurs Clin North Am* 35(4):1031, 2000.

Hartman CA et al: Effects of T'ai Chi training on function and quality of life indicators in older adults with osteoarthritis, *J Am Geriatr Soc* 48(12):1553, 2000.

Husted C et al: Improving quality of life for people with chronic conditions: the example of T'ai Chi and multiple sclerosis, *Altern Ther Health Med* 5(5):70, 1999.

La Forge R: Mind-body fitness: encouraging prospects for primary and secondary prevention, *J Cardiovasc Nurs* 11(3):53, 1997.

Lai JS et al: Two-year trends in cardiorespiratory function among older T'ai Chi Chuan practitioners and sedentary subjects, *J Am Geriatr Soc* 43(11):1222, 1995.

Mills N, Allen J, Morgan SC: Does Tai Chi/qigong help patients with multiple sclerosis? *J Bodywork Mov Ther* 4(1):39, 2000.

Province MA et al: The effects of exercise on falls in elderly patients: a preplanned meta-analysis of the FICSIT trials, *JAMA* 273(17):1341, 1995.

Sancier KM: Medical applications of qigong, *Altern Ther Health Med* 2(1):40, 1996.

Sherwin DC: Traditional Chinese medicine in rehabilitation nursing practice, *Rehabil Nurs* 17(5):253, 1992.

Simpson W: Qigong, *Pac J Orient Med* 17:5, 2000.

Reflexology

Byers D: *Better health with foot reflexology: the original Ingham method*, St Petersburg, Fla, 2001, Ingham Publishing.

Frankel BSM: The effect of reflexology on baroreceptor reflex sensitivity, blood pressure, and sinus arrhythmia, *Complement Ther Med* 5(2):80, 1997.

Oleson T, Flocco W: Randomized control study of premenstrual symptoms treated with ear, hand, and foot reflexology, *Obstet Gynecol* 2(6):906, 1993.

Stephenson N, Weinrich S, Travakoli A: The effects of foot reflexology on anxiety and pain in patients with breast and lung cancer, *Oncology Nurs Forum* 27(1):67, 2000.

Rolfing

Bruno L: Rolfing. In *Gale encyclopedia of medicine*, 1999, Gale Research. Available at: www.finalarticles.com/cf_d/s/g2601/0012/26001001202/p1/article.jhtml/

Convey A: Rolf therapy, *Muscle Fitness* 4:52, 1993.

Cottingham J, Maitland J: A three-paradigm treatment model using soft tissue mobilization and guided movement awareness techniques for patients with chronic back pain: a case study, *J Orthop Sports Phys Ther* 26(3):155, 1997.

Mixter J: *Rolfing*, Newark, N.J., 1983, Rolf Press.

Pechter K: Hands on health: an illustrated guide to the manipulative arts, *Prevention* 3:50, 1994.

Rolf I: *Rolfing: the integration of human structures*, New York, 1977, Harper and Row.

Yoga

Collins C: Yoga: intuition, preventive medicine and treatment, *JOGNN* 27(5):563, 1998.

Choudhury B: *Bikram's beginning yoga class*, New York, 2000, Penguin Putnam.

Garfinkel M et al: Yoga-based intervention for carpal tunnel syndrome, *JAMA* 280(18):1601, 1998.

Garfinkel M, Schumacher H: Yoga, *Rheum Dis Clin North Am* 26(1):125, 2000.

Iyengar BKS: *Light on yoga*, New York, 1976, Schocken Books.

Iyengar BKS: *Light on the yoga sutras of Patanjali*, London, 1993, Thorsons.

Iyengar BKS: *Yoga: the path to holistic health*, London, 2001, Dorling Kindersley.

Luskin F et al: A review of mind-body therapies in the treatment of cardiovascular disease part one: implications for the elderly, *Altern Ther Health Med* 4(3):46, 1998.

Shaffer H, LaSalvia T, Stein J: Comparing hatha yoga with dynamic group psychotherapy for enhancing methadone maintenance treatment: a randomized clinical trial, *Altern Ther Health Med* 3(4):57, 1997.

Starre B: Yoga: Progressing toward high-level wellness, *Health Values* 13(3):48, 1989.

Section 4: Healing with the Mind

Biofeedback

Andreasi, J: *Psychophysiology: human behavior and physiological response*, ed 3, Hillsdale, N.J., 1995, Lawrence Erlbaum.

Cram J, Kasman G, Holtz J: *Introduction to surface electromyography*, Gaithersburg, Md, 1988, Aspen Publishers.

Green E, Green A: *Beyond biofeedback*, New Castle, Dela, 1977, Knoll Publishing.

Schwartz M: *Biofeedback: a practitioner's guide*, New York, 1995, Guilford Press.

Shellenberger R et al: *Clinical efficacy and cost effectiveness of biofeedback therapy: guidelines for third party reimbursement*, ed 2, Wheatridge, Colo, 1994, Association for Applied Psychophysiology and Biofeedback.

Humor Therapy

Astedt-Kurki P, Liukkonen A: Humor in nursing care, *J Adv Nurs* 20:183, 1994.

Astedt-Kurki P, Isola A: Humor between nurse and patient, among staff: analysis of nurses diaries, *J Adv Nurs* 35(3):452, 2001.

Cousins N: Anatomy of an illness, *N Engl J Med* 295:1463, 1976.

Kennedy K: Have a laugh! Have a healthy laugh! *Nurs Forum* 30:25, 1995.

Pasquali E: Learning to laugh: humor as therapy, *J Psychosoc Nurs Ment Health Serv* 28(3):31, 1990.

Richman J: The lifesaving function of humor with the depressed and suicidal elderly, *Gerontologist* 35:271, 1995.

Sullivan JL, Deane DM: Humor and health, *J Gerontol Nurs* 4:20, 1988.

Williams H: Humor and healing: therapeutic effects in geriatrics, *Gerontion* 1:14, 1986.

Hypnosis

Benham G et al: Self-fulfilling prophecy and hypnotic response are not the same thing, *J Pers Soc Psychol* 75:1604, 1998.

Brown DP, Fromm E: *Hypnotherapy and hypnoanalysis*, Hillsdale, N.J., 1986, Lawrence Erlbaum.

Crawford HJ: Brain dynamics and hypnosis: attentional and disattentional processes, *Int J Clin Exp Hypn* 42:204, 1994.

Crawford HJ, Brown AM, Moon CE: Sustained and attentional and disattentional abilities: differences between low and high hypnotizable persons, *J Abnorm Psychol* 102:534, 1993.

Crawford HJ, Gruzelier JH: A midstream view of the neuropsychophysiology of hypnosis: recent research and future directions. In Fromm E, Nash MR, editors: *Contemporary hypnosis research*, New York, 1992, Guilford Press.

Crawford HJ, Hilgard JR, Macdonald H: Transient experiences following hypnotic testing and special termination procedures, *Int J Clin Exp Hypn* 26:117, 1982.

Crawford HJ et al: Transient positive and negative experiences accompanying stage hypnosis, *J Abnorm Psychol* 101:663, 1992.

Frischholz EJ: Medicare procedure code 9088-(medical hypotherapy): use the code (not the word) [editorial], *Am J Clin Hypn* 40:85, 1997.

Fromm E, Nash MR, editors: *Contemporary hypnosis research*, New York, 1992, Guilford Press.

Hammond CD, editor: *Handbook of hypnotic suggestions and metaphors*, New York, 1990, WW Norton and Company.

Hendler CS, Redd WH: Fear of hypnosis: the role of labeling in patients' acceptance of behavioral interventions, *Behav Ther* 17:2, 1986.

Hilgard ER: *Hypnotic susceptibility*, New York, 1965, Harcourt, Brace, and World.

Hilgard ER: The domain of hypnosis, with some comments on alternative paradigms, *Am Psychol* 28:972, 1973.

Kihlstrom JF: Hypnosis, *Annu Rev Psychol* 36:385, 1985.

Kirsch I, Lynn SJ: The altered state of hypnosis: changes in the theoretical landscape, *Am Psychol* 50:846, 1995.

Kirsch I, Montgomery G, Sapirstein G: Hypnosis as an adjunct to cognitive-behavioral psychotherapy: a meta-analysis, *J Consul Clin Psychol* 63:214, 1995.

Kirsch I et al: The surreptitious observation design: an experimental paradigm for distinguishing artifact from essence in hypnosis, *J Abnorm Psychol* 98:132, 1989.

Lynn SJ et al: Hypnosis as an empirically supported clinical intervention: the state of the evidence and a look to the future, *Int J Clin Exp Hypn* 48:239, 2000.

Lynn SJ, Rhue JW, editors: *Theories of hypnosis: current models and perspectives*, New York, 1991, Guilford Press.

Olness K, Kohen DP: *Hypnosis and hypnotherapy with children*, ed 3, New York, 1996, Guildford Press.

Rainville P et al: Cerebral mechanisms of hypnotic induction and suggestion, *J Cogn Neurosci* 11:110, 1999.

Rhue JW, Lynn SJ, Kirsch I, editors: *Handbook of clinical hypnosis*, Washington, DC, 1993, American Psychological Association.

Spiegel D: *Living beyond limits: new hope and help for facing life-threatening illness*, New York, 1993, Times Books.

Spiegel D, Bierre P, Rootenberg J: Hypnotic alteration of somatosensory perception, *Am J Psychiatry* 146:749, 1989.

Spiegel D et al: Hypnotic hallucination alters evoked potentials, *J Abnorm Psychol* 94:249, 1985.

Weitzenhoffer AM: *The practice of hypnotism: traditional and semi-traditional techniques and phenomenology*, vol 1, New York, 1989, Wiley.

Wickramasekera I: Hypnotherapy. In Jonas WB, Levin JS, editors: *Essentials in complementary and alternative medicine*, New York, 1999, Lippincott–Williams & Wilkins.

Wickramasekera I: *Clinical behavioral medicine: some concepts and procedures*, New York, 1988, Plenum.

Yapko MD: *Essentials of hypnosis*, New York, 1995, Brunner.

Meditation

Anselmo J, Kolkmeier LG: Relaxation: the first step to restore, renew and self-heal. In Dossey BM, Keegan L, Guzzetta C, editors: *Holistic nursing: a handbook for practice*, ed 3, Gaithersburg, Md, 2000, Aspen Publishers.

Benson H et al: Decreased premature ventricular contraction through the use of the relaxation response in patients with stable ischemic heart disease, *Lancet* 7931(2):380, 1975.

Benson H: *Beyond the relaxation response*, New York, 1984, Times Books.

Easwaran E: *Meditation: an eight-point program*, Petaluma, Calif, 1991, Nilgiri Press.

Kabat-Zinn J: *Full catastrophe living: using the wisdom of your body and min to face stress, pain, and illness*, New York, 1990, Bantam/Doubleday/Dell.

Ornish D et al: Can lifestyle changes reverse coronary artery disease? *Lancet* 336:129, 1990.

Watson J: *Postmodern nursing and beyond*, Edinburgh/New York, 1999, Churchill-Livingstone/Harcourt-Brace.

Zaleski P, Kaufman P: *Gifts of the spirit: living the wisdom of great religious traditions*, the Nathan Cummings foundation, New York, 1997, The Fetzer Institute, HarperCollins.

Music Therapy

Allen K, Blascovich J: Effects of music on cardiovascular reactivity among surgeons, *JAMA* 272(11):882, 1994.

Guzzetta CE: Music therapy: hearing the melody of the soul. In Dossey B, Keegan L, Guzetta CE, editors: *Holistic nursing: a handbook for practice*, ed 3, Gaithersburg, Md, 2000, Aspen Publishers.

Heiser RM et al: The use of music during the immediate post-operative recovery period, *AORN J* 65(4):777, 1997.

Hoffman J: Tuning into the power of music, *RN* 52, 1997.

Kaempf G, Amodei ME: The effect of music on anxiety: a research study, *AORN J* 50(1):112, 1989.

Koch ME et al: The sedative and analgesic sparing effect of music, *Anesthesiology* 89:300, 1998.

Lenton SR, Martin PR: Case histories and shorter communications: the contribution of music vs. instructions in the musical mood induction procedure, *Behav Res Ther* 29(6):623, 1991.

Liu EHC, Tan SM: Patient's perception of sound levels in the surgical suite, *J Clin Anesth* 12:298, 2000.

Locsin RG: The effect of music on the pain of selected postoperative patients, *J Adv Nurs* 6:19, 1981.

McCraty R et al: Music enhances the effect of positive emotional states on salivary IgA, *Stress Med* 12:167, 1996.

Moss VA: The effect of music on anxiety in the surgical patient, *Perioper Nurs Q* 3(1):9, 1987.

Nilsson U et al: Improved recovery after music and therapeutic suggestions during general anesthesia: a double-blind randomized controlled trial, *Acta Anaesthesiol Scand* 45:812, 2001.

Palakanis K et al: Effect of music therapy on state anxiety in patients undergoing flexible sigmoidoscopy, *Dis Colon Rectum* 37(5):478, 1994.

Reilly M: An overview of music intervention as an adjunct to pharmacologic pain management, *Anesthesia Today* 10(3):11, 2001.

Rider MS, Achterberg J: Effect of music-assisted imagery on neutrophils and lymphocytes, *Biofeedback Self Regul* 14(3):247, 1989.

Updike P: Music therapy results for ICU patients, *Dimens Crit Care Nurs* 9(1):39, 1990.

Updike PA, Charles DM: Music Rx: physiological and emotional responses to taped music programs of preoperative patients awaiting plastic surgery, *Ann Plast Surg* 19(1):29, 1987.

Whipple B, Glynn NJ: Quantification of the effects of listening to music as a noninvasive method of pain control, *Sch Inq Nurs Pract* 6(1):43, 1992.

Pet Therapy

All AC, Loving GL, Crane LL: Animals, horseback riding, and implications for rehabilitation therapy, *J Rehabil* 65(3):49, 1999.

Allen K: *Coping with life changes and transitions: the role of pets,* 2001. Available at: http://www.deltasociety.org. Accessed Dec, 2001.

Bardhill N, Hutchinson S: Animal assisted therapy with hospitalized adolescents, *J Child Adolesc Psychiatr Nurs* 10(1):17, 1997.

Barker SB, Dawson KS: The effects of animal-assisted therapy on anxiety ratings of hospitalized psychiatric patients, *Psychiatr Serv* 49(6):797, 1998.

Cole KM, Gawlinski A: Animal assisted therapy; the human-animal bond, *AACN Clinic Issues* 11(1):139, 2000.

Connor K, Miller J: Animal-assisted therapy: an in-depth look, *Dimens Crit Care Nurs* 19(3):20, 2000.

Conner K, Miller J: Critical care edition: help from our animal friends, *Nurs Manage* 31(7, part 1):42, 44, 2000.

Davis JH: Animal-facilitated therapy in stress mediation, *Holistic Nursing* 2(3):75, 1988.

Guay DR: Pet-assisted therapy in the nursing home setting: potential for zoonosis, *Am J Infect Control* 29(3):178, 2001.

Hall PL, Malpus Z: Pets as therapy: effects on social interaction in long-stay psychiatry, *Br J Nurs* 9(21):2220, 2000.

Jacobson G, Sata A, Gilmore B: Fish aquarium, animal assisted therapy, and its influence on clients with multiple sclerosis, *Res Theory Nurs Pract* 2:8, 2000.

James K: Animals in health care. In Snyder M, Lindquist R: *Complementary/alternative therapies in nursing,* ed 3, New York, 1998, Springer Publishing.

Johnson RA, Meadows RL: Promoting wellness through nurse-veterinary collaboration, *J Nurs Res* 22(7):773, 2000.

Lynch JJ: *Developing a physiology of inclusion: recognizing the health benefits of animal companions,* 2001. Available at: http://www.deltasociety.org. Accessed Dec, 2001.

Miller J, Connor K: Going to the dogs...for help, *Nursing* 30(11):65, 2000.

Miller J, Ingram L: Perioperative nursing and animal-assisted therapy, *AORN J* 72(3):477, 2000.

Modlin SJ: Service dogs as interventions: state of the science, *Rehabil Nurs* 25(6):212, 2000.

Murrell A: Why a little animal magic brings benefits for patients, *Nurs Times* 97(11):15, 2001.

Owen OG: Paws for thought...pet therapy, *Nurs Times* 97(9):28, 2001.

Ptak AL: *Studies of loneliness: recent research into the effects of companion animals on lonely people.* Available at: http://www.deltasociety.org. Accessed Dec, 2001.

Wallace S: RxRN: making therapeutic strides on four paws, *Altern Complementary Ther* 6(3):166, 2000.

Woods A: Web monitor: sites about animal therapy, cardiac monitoring, and more, *Dimens Crit Care Nurs* 19(3):35, 2000.

Relaxation

Benson H: *The relaxation response,* New York, 1975, William Morrow and Company.

Bourne EJ: *The anxiety and phobia workbook,* ed 2, Oakland, Calif, 1995, New Harbinger Publications.

Carlson CR, Hoyle RH: Efficacy of abbreviated progressive muscle relaxation training: a quantitative review of behavioral medicine research, *J Consul Clin Psychol* 61:1059, 1993.

Carroll D, Seers K: Relaxation for the relief of chronic pain: a systematic review, *J Adv Nurs* 27:476, 1998.

Davis M, Eshelman ER, McKay M: *The relaxation and stress reduction workbook,* ed 4, Oakland, Calif, 1995, New Harbinger Publications.

Forbes EJ, Pekala RJ: Psychophysiological effects of several stress management techniques, *Psychol Rep* 72:19, 1993.

Freeman LW: Relaxation therapy. In Freeman LW, Lawlis GF, editors: *Mosby's complementary and alternative medicine: a research-based approach,* St Louis, 2001, Mosby.

Huntley A, White AR, Ernst E: Relaxation therapies for asthma: a systematic review, *Thorax* 57:127, 2002.

Hyman RB et al: The effects of relaxation training on clinical symptoms: a meta-analysis, *Nurs Res* 38:216, 1989.

Jacobson E: *Progressive relaxation,* Chicago, 1929, University of Chicago Press.

Lehrer PM: Varieties of relaxation methods and their unique effects, *Int J Stress Manage* 3:1, 1996.

Lehrer PM, Woolfolk RL: *Principles and practice of stress management,* ed 2, New York, 1993, Guilford Press.

Matsumoto M, Smith JC: Progressive muscle relaxation, breathing exercises, and ABC relaxation theory, *J Clin Psychol* 57:1551, 2001.

NIH Technology Assessment Panel: Integration of behavioral and relaxation approaches into the treatment of chronic pain and insomnia, *JAMA* 276:313, 1996.

Redd WH, Montgomery GH, DuHamel KN: Behavioral interventions for cancer treatment side effects, *J Natl Cancer Inst* 93:810, 2001.

Sakakibara M, Takeuchi S, Hayano J: Effect of relaxation training on cardiac parasympathetic tone, *Psychophysiology* 31:223, 1994.

Taylor AG et al: Complementary/alternative therapies in the treatment of pain. In Spencer JW, Jacobs JJ, editors: *Complementary/alternative medicine: an evidence-based approach,* ed 2, St Louis, 2003, Mosby.

Storytelling

Aiex NK: Bibliotherapy, *Eric Digest,* June 1993. Available at: http://www.indiana.edu/~eric_rec/ieo/digests/d82.html. Accessed November 21, 2001.

Anderson G: Storytelling: a holistic foundation for genetic nursing, *Holist Nurs Pract* 12(3):64, 1988.

Chelf J et al: Storytelling: a strategy for living and coping with cancer, *Cancer Nurs* 23(1):1, 2000.

Dicke P: Storytelling. In Snyder M, Lindquist R, editors: *Complementary and alternative therapies in nursing*, ed 3, New York, 1998, Springer Publishing.

Fazio LS: Tell me a story: the therapeutic metaphor in the practice of pediatric occupational therapy, *Am J Occup Ther* 46(2):112, 1992.

Kunzman LA: A case for story-telling: honoring the final journey, *Clin Nurse Spec* 14(5):209, 2000.

Larkin DM: Therapeutic storytelling and metaphors, *Holist Nurs Pract* 2(3):45, 1988.

Mayers K: Storytelling: a method to increase discussion, facilitate rapport with residents and share knowledge among long-term care staff, *J Contin Educ Nurs* 26(6):280, 1995.

Mitchell A: Researching healing: a psychologist's perspective, *J Altern Complement Med* 6(2):181, 2000.

Niska KJ: Therapeutic use of parental stories to enhance Mexican-American family socialization: family transition to the community school system, *Public Health Nurs* 18(3):149, 2001.

Nwoga I: African American mothers use stories for family sexuality education, *Am J Mat Child Nurs* 25(1):31, 2000.

Origins of storytelling. Available at: http://falcon.mju.edu/!ramseyil/storyorigins.htm. Accessed June 13, 2001.

Rizza M: *A parent's guide to helping children: using bibliotherapy at home*, National Research Center on the Gifted and Talented, 1997 Winter Newsletter. Available at: http://sp.uconn.edu/~nrcgt/news/winter97/wintr972.html. Accessed November 21, 2001.

Siauliene A: *Bibliotherapy: theory and finding possibilities to develop it in a children's library*. Available at: http://www.goethe.de/ne/rig/siauli2.htm. Accessed June 13, 2001.

Synovitz LB: Using puppetry in a coordinated school health program, *J Sch Health* 69(4):145, 1999.

Ward EM: *Art of storytelling*, Prescott, Ariz, 1990, Educational Ministries.

Ward SL: Caring and healing in the 21st century, *Am J Mat Child Nurs* 23(4):210, 1998.

Weber M: *Bibliotherapy*. Available at: http://maxweber.hunter.cuNew York.edu/pub/eres/EDSPC715_MCINTYRE/Biblio.html. Accessed November 21, 2001.

Wenckus EM: Storytelling: using an ancient art to work with groups, *J Psychosoc Nurs Ment Health Serv* 32(7):30, 1994.

Why storytelling? Available at: http://www.storyarts.org/classroom/index.html. Accessed June 13, 2001.

Section 5: Healing with Subtle Energy

Acupressure

Beal MW: Acupuncture and acupressure, application to women's reproductive health care, *J Nurse Midwifery* 44(3):217, 1999.

Birch S, Kaptchuk T: History, nature and current practice of acupuncture: an East Asian perspective. In Ernst E, White A, editors: *Acupuncture: a scientific appraisal*, Oxford, 1999, Butterworth Heinemann.

Dibble SL et al: Acupressure for nausea: results of a pilot study, *Oncol Nurs Forum* 27(1):41, 2000.

Dundee JW et al: Effect of stimulation of the P6 antiemetic point on postoperative nausea and vomiting, *Br J Anesth* 63:612, 1989.

Harris PE: Acupressure: a review of the literature, *Complement Ther Med* 5(3):156, 1997.

Hyde E: Acupressure therapy for morning sickness, *J Nurse Midwifery* 34(4):171, 1989.

Kroll D: Acupressure therapy for tension headaches, *Altern Complementary Ther* 1(6):357, 1995.

Lee A, Done ML: The use of nonpharmacologic techniques to prevent postoperative nausea and vomiting: a meta-analysis, *Anesth Analg* 88:1362, 1999.

Lewis IH et al: Effect of P6 acupressure on postoperative vomiting in children undergoing outpatient strabismus correction, *Br J Anesth* 61:73, 1991.

Pan CX et al: Complementary and alternative medicine in the management of pain, dyspnea, and nausea and vomiting near the end of life: a systematic review, *J Pain Symptom Manage* 20(5):374, 2000.

Reed Gach M: *Acupressure's potent points*, New York, 1990, Bantam.

Stein DJ et al: Acupressure versus intravenous metoclopramide to prevent nausea and vomiting during spinal anesthesia for cesarean section, *Anesth Analg* 84:342, 1997.

White PF: Are nonpharmacologic techniques useful alternative to antiemetic drugs for the prevention of nausea and vomiting? *Anesth Analg* 84:712, 1997.

Acupuncture

Birch S, Kaptchuk T: History, nature and current practice of acupuncture: an East Asian perspective. In Ernst E, White A, editors: *Acupuncture: a scientific appraisal*, Oxford, 1999, Butterworth Heinemann.

Cohen MR: *The Chinese way to healing: many paths to wholeness*, New York, 1996, Berkeley Publishing Group.

Filshie J, Cummings M: Western medical acupuncture. In Ernst E, White A, editors: *Acupuncture: a scientific appraisal*, Oxford, 1999, Butterworth Heinemann.

Lee A, Done ML: The use of nonpharmacologic techniques to prevent postoperative nausea and vomiting: a meta-analysis, *Anesth Analg* 88:1362, 1999.

Liao SJ, Lee M, Ng LKY: *Principles and practice of contemporary acupuncture*, New York, 1994, Marcel Dekker.

NIH Consensus Conference: Acupuncture: NIH consensus development panel on acupuncture, *JAMA* 280(17):1518, 1998.

Aromatherapy

Baker S: Formation and development of the Aromatherapy Organizations Council, *Complement Ther Nurs Midwifery* 3:77, 1997.

DeSmet P: The role of plant-derived drugs and herbal medicines in healthcare, *Drugs* 54(6):801, 1997.

Price S, Price L: *Aromatherapy for health professionals*, Edinburgh, 1995, Churchill-Livingstone.

Tate S: Peppermint oil: a treatment for postoperative nausea, *J Adv Nurs* 26:543, 1997.

Lis-Balchin M, Hart S: Studies on the mode of action of the essential oil of lavender (*Lavandula angustifolia* P. Miller), *Phytother Res* 13:540, 1999.

Lehrner J et al: Ambient odor of orange in a dental office reduces anxiety and improves mood in female patients, *Physiol Behav* 71:83, 2000.

Schaller M, Korting HC: Allergic airborne contact dermatitis from essential oils used in aromatherapy, *Clin Exp Dermatol* 20:143, 1995.

Stevensen CJ: The psychophysiological effects of aromatherapy massage following cardiac surgery, *Complement Ther Med* 27, 1999.

Color Therapy

Chiazzari S: *The complete book of colour*, Rockport, Mass, Element Books.

Ford-Martin P: Color therapy, *Gale encyclopedia of alternative medicine*. Available at: http://findarticles.com/cf_dls/g2603/0002/2603000292/print.jhtml. Accessed November 12, 2001.

Klotsche C: *Color medicine: the secrets of color/vibrational healing*, Sedona, Ariz, 1993, Light Technology Publishing.

Lad V: *The complete book of Ayurvedic home remedies*, New York, 1998, Three Rivers Press.

Feng Shui

Kennedy DD, Lin Yun: *Feng Shui for dummies*, New York, 2001, Hungry Minds.

Post S: *The modern book of Feng Shui: vitality and harmony for the home and office*, New York, 1999, Dell Publishing.

Rossbach S, Lin Yun: *Feng Shui design: the art of creating harmony for interiors, landscape and architecture*, New York, 1999, Viking Press.

Homeopathy

Anonymous. *An introduction to homeopathy for the practicing pharmacist*, 1994, Boiron Institute.

Barrett S, Tyler VE: Why pharmacists should not sell homeopathic remedies, *Am J Health-Syst Pharm* 52:1004, 1995.

Bidwell GI: *How to use the reperatory with a practical analysis of 40 homeopathic remedies*, New Delhi, India, 1994, B Jain Publishers.

Chavez ML, Chapman RL: Homeopathy. Monographs on alternative therapies, *Hosp Pharm* 33(1):41, 1998.

Jacobs J et al: Treatment of acute childhood diarrhea with homeopathic medicine: a randomized clinical trial in Nicaragua, *Pediatrics* 93(5):719, 1994.

Kleijnen J, Knipschild P, ter Riet G: Clinical trials of homeopathy, *BMJ* 302:316, 1991.

Lange A: Homeopathy. In Pizzorno JE, Murray MT: *Textbook of natural medicine*, ed 2, Edinburgh, 1999, Churchill Livingstone.

Linde K et al: Are the clinical effects of homeopathy placebo effects? A meta-analysis of placebo-controlled trials, *Lancet* 350:834, 1997.

Linde K et al: Critical review and meta-analysis of serial agitated dilutions in experimental toxicology, *Hum Exp Toxicol* 13:481, 1994.

Mayux MJ et al: Controlled clinical trial of homeopathy in postoperative illieus, *Lancet* 5:528, 1988.

Mock D: What's going on here, anyway? A review of Boyd's Biochemical and biological evidence of the activity of high potencies, *J Am Inst Homeopathy*, p 197.

Pray WS: The challenge to professionalism presented by homeopathy, *Am J Pharm Educ* 60:198, 1996.

Reilly D et al: Is evidence for homeopathy reproducible? *Lancet* 344:1601, 1994.

Reilly DT et al: Is homeopathy a placebo response? Controlled trial of homeopathic potency, with pollen in hayfever as a model, *Lancet* 2(8512):881, 1986.

Shipley M: Controlled trial of homeopathic treatment of osteoarthritis, *Lancet* January 15:97, 1983.

Intuitive Spiritual Healing

Benor D: *Healing research: holistic energy medicine and spirituality*, Munich, 1992, Helix Editions.

Brennan B: *Hands of light*, New York, 1987, Bantam Books.

Brennan B: *Light emerging*, New York, 1987, Bantam Books.

Gerber R: *Vibrational medicine: new choices for healing ourselves*, Santa Fe, 1996, Bear & Company.

Myss C: *Anatomy of the spirit*, New York, 1996, Harmony Books.

Naparstek B: *Your sixth sense: activating your psychic potential*, San Francisco, 1997, Harper.

Zukav G: *The seat of the soul*, New York, 1989, A Fireside Book.

Magnetic Therapy

Alfano A et al: Static magnetic fields for treatment of fibromyalgia: a double blind randomized controlled trial, *J Altern Complement Med* 7(1):53, 2001.

Caselli MA et al: Evaluation of magnetic foil and PPT Insoles in the treatment of heel pain, *J Am Podiatr Med Assoc* 87:11, 1997.

Collacott EA et al: Bipolar permanent magnets for the treatment of chronic low back pain: a pilot study, *JAMA* 283:1322, 2000.

Finegold L: Magnet therapy, *Sci Rev Altern Med* 3(1):26, 1999.

Guyton AC, Hall JE: *Textbook of medical physiology*, ed 10, Philadelphia, 2000, WB Saunders.

Jacobson JI et al: Low-amplitude, extremely low-frequency magnetic fields for the treatment of osteoarthritic knees: a double-blind clinical study, *Altern Ther Health Med* 7(5):54, 2001.

Ramey DW: Magnetic and electromagnetic therapy, *Sci Rev Altern Med* 2(1):13, 1998.

Roizen MF: Anesthetic implications of concurrent diseases. In Miller RD et al, editors: *Anesthesia*, ed 5, Philadelphia, 2000, Churchill-Livingstone.

Rosch PJ: Therapeutic use of magnets, *Integr Med Consult* 162, 1999.

Vallbona C, Hazelwood CF, Jurida G: Response of pain to static magnetic fields in postpolio patients: a double blind pilot study, *Arch Phys Rehabil Med* 78:1200, 1997.

Prayer

Byrd R: Positive therapeutic effects of intercessory prayer in a coronary care unit population, *South Med J* (81):826, 1998.

Davidson T: Christian science healing. In *Gale encyclopedia of medicine*, 2001, Gale Research. Available at: www.findarticles.com/cf_0/g2603/0002/2603000280/p1/article.jhtml?term-Christian+Science+Healing. Accessed Jan, 2002.

Koenig HG et al: The relationship between religious activities and blood pressure in older adults, *Int J Psychiatry Med* 28(2):189, 1998.

Koenig HG, George LK, Peterson BL: Religiosity and remission of depression in medically ill older patients, *Am J Psychiatry* 155(4):536, 1998.

Koenig HG, Larson DB: Use of hospital services, religious attendance, and religious affiliation, *South Med J* 91(10):925, 1998.

Matthews D, Marlowe SM, MacNutt FS: Beneficial effects of intercessory prayer ministry in patients with rheumatoid arthritis, *J Gen Intern Med* 13(4):1, 1998.

Meyers D: Is prayer clinically effective? *Reformed Rev* 53(2):95, 2000.

Rauch C: *Probing the power of prayer.* Available at: www.cnn./2000/Health/alternative/01/18/prayer.power/wmd/. Accessed January, 2002.

White EG: *Ministry of healing*, Mountain View, Calif, 1905, Pacific Press.

White EG: *The desire of ages*, Mountain View, Calif, 1898, Pacific Press.

Reiki

Rand WL: *Reiki, the healing touch: first and second degree manual*, Southfield, Mich, 1998, Vision Publications.

Dziemidko HE: *The complete book of energy medicines: choosing your path to health*, Rochester, Vt, 1999, Healing Arts Press.

Weitzel WS: Reiki healing: a physiologic perspective, *J Holistic Healing* 7(1):47, 1989.

Therapeutic Touch

Benor DJ: *Spiritual healing: scientific validation of a healing revolution*, vol 1, Southfield, Mich, 2001, Vision Publications.

Brennan B: High auditory perception and communication with spiritual teachers. In Brennan BA, Smith JA, editors: *Hands of light: a guide to healing through the human energy field*, Toronto, 1987, Bantam.

Bollough VL: Should nurses practice therapeutic touch? Should nursing schools teach therapeutic touch? *J Prof Nurs* 14(4):254, 1998.

Gagne D, Toye RC: The effect of therapeutic touch and relaxation therapy in reducing anxiety, *Arch Psychiatr Nurs* 8(3):184, 1994.

Griffin RL: An overview of therapeutic touch and its application to patients with Alzheimer's disease, *Am J Alzheimer's Dis* 13(4):211, 1998.

Heidt P: Effect of therapeutic touch on anxiety level of hospitalized patients, *Nurs Res* 30(1):32, 1980.

Keller E, Bzek VM: Effects of therapeutic touch on tension headache pain, *Nurs Res* 35(2):101, 1986.

Kreiger D: Healing by the "laying-on" of hands as a facilitator of bioenergetic change: the response of in-vivo human hemoglobin, *Psychoenergetic Syst* 1:121, 1978.

Krieger D: Therapeutic touch: the imprimatur of nursing, *Am J Nurs* 75(5):784, 1975.

Smith MC et al: Outcomes of touch therapies during bone marrow transplant. *Altern Ther Health Med.* In press.

Malinski VM: Therapeutic touch: the view from Rogerian nursing science, *Visions: J Rogerian Nurs Sci* 1(1):45, 1993.

Meehan TC: Therapeutic touch and postoperative pain: a Rogerian research study, *Nurs Sci Q* 6(2):69, 1993.

Meehan TC: Therapeutic touch as a nursing intervention, *J Adv Nurs* 28(1):117, 1998.

Quinn JF: Therapeutic touch as an energy exchange: replication and extension, *Nurs Sci Q* 79, 1988.

Quinn JF, Strelkauskas AJ: Psychoimmunologic effects of therapeutic touch on practitioners and recently bereaved recipients: a pilot study, *Adv Nurs Sci* 15(4):13, 1993.

Ranbarube-Singh S: The surgical significance of therapeutic touch, *AORN J* 69(2):358, 360, 1999.

Reeder F: The science of unitary human beings and interpretive human science, *Nurs Sci Q* 6:1, 13, 1991.

Rosa L, Rosa E, Barrett S: A close look at therapeutic touch, *JAMA* 279(13):1005, 1998.

Shames KH, Keegan L: Touch: connecting with the healing power. In Dossey BM, Keegan L, Guzzetta CE, editors: *Holistic nursing: a handbook for practice*, Gaithersburg, Md, 2000, Aspen Publishers.

Smith M, Reeder R: Outcomes of touch therapies during bone marrow transplant, *Altern Ther Med Health.* In press.

Wirth DP: The effect of non-contact therapeutic touch on the healing rate of full thickness dermal wounds, *Subtle Energies* 1(1):1, 1990.

Wirth DP et al: Full thickness dermal wounds treated with non-contact therapeutic touch: a replication and extension, *Complement Ther Med* 1:127, 1993.

Index